About Island Press

Ecological Integrity

Ecological Integrity

Integrating Environment, Conservation, and Health

Edited by
David Pimentel
Laura Westra
Reed F. Noss

ISLAND PRESS

Washington, D.C. • Covelo, California

Copyright © 2000 Island Press

All rights reserved under International and Pan-American Copyright Conventions. No part
of this book may be reproduced in any form or by any means without permission in writing
from the publisher: Island Press, 1718 Connecticut Avenue NW, Suite 300, Washington
DC 20009.

Library of Congress Cataloging-in-Publication Data

Ecological integrity : integrating environment, conservation,
and health / edited by David Pimentel, Laura Westra, Reed F. Noss.
     p. cm.
Includes bibliographical references and index.
   ISBN 1-55963-807-9 (cloth : acid-free paper) — ISBN
1-55963-808-7 (paper : acid-free paper)
   1. Ecological integrity. I. Pimentel, David, 1925– II.
Westra, Laura. III. Noss, Reed F.
   QH541.15.E245 E36 2000
   304.2—dc21
                                        00-008255

To future generations on the planet

Contents

➤ PART ONE ◄

Introduction and Outline of the Integrity Concept

1 Introduction
   Peter Miller and William E. Rees   3

2 Ecological Integrity and the Aims of the Global Integrity Project
   Laura Westra, Peter Miller, James R. Karr, William E. Rees, and Robert E. Ulanowicz   19

➤ PART TWO ◄

Historical and Philosophical Foundations

3 Ecological Integrity and the Darwinian Paradigm
   Alan Holland   45

4 Ecosystem Design in Historical and Philosophical Context
   Mark Sagoff   61

5 Reconstructing Ecology
   Ernest Partridge   79

6 Toward the Measurement of Ecological Integrity
   Robert E. Ulanowicz   99

➤ PART THREE ◄

The Sustainability and Integrity of Natural Resource Systems

7 Environmental Sustainability and Integrity in the Agriculture Sector
   Robert Goodland and David Pimentel   121

8 Patch Disturbance, Ecofootprints, and Biological Integrity:
    Revisiting the Limits to Growth (or Why Industrial Society
    Is Inherently Unsustainable)
    William E. Rees   139

 9 Can Canadian Approaches to Sustainable Forest Management
    Maintain Ecological Integrity?
    Peter Miller and James W. Ehnes   157

10 Pattern of Forest Integrity in the Eastern United States and Canada:
    Measuring Loss and Recovery
    Orie L. Loucks   177

11 Maintaining the Ecological Integrity of Landscapes and Ecoregions
    Reed Noss   191

12 Health, Integrity, and Biological Assessment: The Importance of
    Measuring Whole Things
    James R. Karr   209

13 Global Change, Fisheries, and the Integrity of Marine Ecosystems:
    The Future Has Already Begun
    Daniel Pauly   227

―――――――――▶ PART FOUR ◀―――――――――

Human and Societal Health

14 Global Environmental Change in the Coming Century:
    How Sustainable Are Recent Health Gains?
    A. J. McMichael   245

15 Epidemiologic Methods for Assessing the Health Impact of
    Diminishing Ecological Integrity
    Colin L. Soskolne, Lee E. Sieswerda, and H. Morgan Scott   261

16 Institutionalized Environmental Violence and Human Rights
    Laura Westra   279

―――――――――▶ PART FIVE ◀―――――――――

The Economics and Ethics of Achieving Global Integrity

17 The Cost of the Wild: International Equity and the Losses
    from Environmental Conservation
    Ted Schrecker   301

18 A Complex Systems Approach to Urban Ecosystem Integrity:
    The Benefit Side
    Philippe Crabbé   317

19 A Biocentric Defense of Environmental Integrity
    James P. Sterba   335

20 Commodity Potential: An Approach to Understanding the Ecological
    Consequences of Markets
    Jack P. Manno   351

21 The State of the Planet at the Five-Year Review of Rio and the
    Prospects for Protecting Worldwide Ecological Integrity
    Donald A. Brown   369

PART SIX

Synthesis

22 Implementing Global Ecological Integrity: A Synthesis
    *Donald A. Brown, Jack P. Manno, Laura Westra, David Pimentel,
    and Philippe Crabbé*   385

    About the Contributors   407

    Index   415

Ecological Integrity

PART I

Introduction and Outline of the Integrity Concept

Introduction

Peter Miller and William E. Rees

> The Easter Islanders, aware that they were almost completely isolated from the rest of the world, must surely have realized that their very existence depended on the limited resources of a small island. After all, it was small enough for them to walk round the entire island in a day or so and see for themselves what was happening to the forests. Yet they were unable to devise a system that allowed them to find the right balance with their environment.   *Clive Ponting, A Green History of the World*

Is humankind fatally flawed, doomed—even in full knowledge—to repeat history on ever greater spatial scales until the brilliant light of civilization is forever snuffed out in one great final crash? After all, the human story is replete with bright beginnings, glorious middles, and tragic ends. In recent millennia advanced civilizations on virtually every continent have collapsed as a result of the destructive overexploitation of their supportive ecosystems. In many cases the descent was marked by famine, disease, and the decline of civil society, ultimately leading to war, social chaos, and cannibalism (e.g., the Maoris in New Zealand and Easter Islanders).

All this we know—and yet industrial civilization willfully imposes a greater burden on the environment than any previous culture. The degradation of natural systems appears in the loss of biodiversity and functionality in aquatic and terrestrial ecosystems; the decline of significant biological populations, including most of the world's wild fisheries; new disease vectors; ozone depletion; global warming; soil loss, salinization, and desertification; and freshwater and groundwater depletion and pollution. Economies that have supported precarious progress for some are unsustainable because aggregate demand exceeds the capacities of natural systems for productivity and waste absorption (Goodland 1992; Karr and Chu 1995; Wackernagel and Rees 1996; following chapters in the present volume). To paraphrase

Ponting (1991, p. 7), we are aware that Earth is completely isolated from the rest of the universe and we realize that our very existence depends on the limited resources of this one small planet. After all, it is small enough for us to fly around in a day or so and see for ourselves what is happening to the forests (and plains and waters). Yet we seem unable to devise a system that allows us to find the right balance with the ecosphere.

Ironically, the very things that define our industrial culture dull the average citizen's sense of vulnerability even as they sweep humanity ever closer to the edge of danger. People are temporarily shielded from the destruction of local ecosystems that have long sustained them. Newfoundland fishers survive the collapse of the cod stocks on transfer payments from the rest of Canada (and we can always import fish from elsewhere); famine in the Sahel is suspended by international relief organizations; and people everywhere are spared the consequences of deteriorating soils by artificial fertilizers that help maintain food production.

A central premise of this book is that such contemporary social and technological buffers merely delay and deepen the ultimate collapse of industrial society. True, trade and technology create the illusion of increasing local carrying capacity. But the reality is that, by enabling continued population and material growth and by dispersing the ecological impacts, the trappings of modernity actually increase the total human load on the ecosphere while simultaneously reducing global carrying capacity (Rees 1996). This ensures that the entire human enterprise will reach critical limits of biophysical integrity at the same time. (Concern over ozone depletion and climate change are thus but early ripples in the sea of contemporary complacency.)

To some readers, this apocalyptic vision will seem excessively pessimistic. Looking back on the past century (and millennium), we who live in North America, Europe, and other high-income countries see our history as a story of progress. In terms of material well-being—the endless parade of globally sourced goods that stock our markets and plentiful supplies of cheap energy—and in terms of the trappings of civilized existence—access to culture, entertainment, travel, education, health care, information, and comfortable homes with clean running water and piped sewage—the material comfort and health of ordinary citizens of the high-income countries today vastly exceeds that of even royalty in previous ages. We are, on average, simply better off by any economic measure than our predecessors. Little wonder our culture has until recently brimmed with confidence in our individual and collective capacity to continue to improve our lot. The late professor Julian Simon perhaps best personified this optimistic spirit. His career was a celebration of human inventiveness and ingenuity, which he deemed "the ultimate resource" (Simon 1981). Simon decried environmental concerns as wastefully groundless, arguing recently that "technology exists now to produce in virtually inexhaustible quantities just about all the products made by nature" (Simon 1995).

Despite such technological hubris, there is justification for the growing unease that much of the progress we have made is precarious and that our present development path is unsustainable. A moment's reflection reminds us that our economic gains, particularly on the global scale, have been mixed, ill-distributed, and costly. While some are as wealthy as Croesus, far more live out their lives in extreme poverty, suffering from malnourishment and disease. Indeed, according to the World Health Organization, we now have the largest number and proportion of malnourished ever in history— 3 billion persons (WHO 1996). How are we to provide for these billions (and the billions more to come) while maintaining ecological integrity if enriching the presently well-off has all but cost the Earth?

The problem is both exacerbated and simplified by a singular global ecological phenomenon—the world is in the midst of the greatest human migration of all time (Rees and Wackernagel 1996). Tens of millions of people are leaving (or being driven from) the countryside every year to eke out a better living in hundreds of ill-prepared, already crowded, smog-bound cities throughout the developing world. The world's urban population is expected to grow by about 50 percent in the 1990s to almost 3 billion. It will increase by another 70 percent to about 5.1 billion people by 2025 (UN 1994). This means that by 2025, the urban population alone is expected to grow by the equivalent of the entire human population in 1930. As early as 2015, there will be 27 mega-cities of 10 million people, 23 of them in less developed countries.

The bad news is that, expectations notwithstanding, life will remain wretched for many of these new urbanites. Millions will be un- or under employed and will suffer from chronic ill-health and malnutrition. Most will lack basic amenities that we in the so-called First World take for granted. Already, 600 million urban dwellers lack adequate sanitation, 450 million have no safe drinking water, and deaths from infectious diseases are rising (NRTEE 1998; Pimentel et al. 1998). The good news is that the concentration of population and consumption in cities creates economies of scale and agglomeration economies that in the best of scenarios could result in considerable energy and material savings in the quest for sustainability (Mitlin and Satterthwaite 1994; Rees and Wackernagel 1996).

In any event, the human animal is psychosocially ill-equipped for a life of crowded deprivation, whether in a disease-ridden city or in the emerging global village. Even without the unprecedented population and environmental pressures to come, political tensions in the twentieth century spawned two world wars, and we seem congenitally condemned to carry on genocidal regional conflicts all over the planet. What is the prognosis for civil society and global peace if material growth falters from resource scarcity or accelerating global ecological change?

On first reading, one might simply say that progress in improving human welfare globally is incomplete; we have a moral duty to extend the benefits of liberal-democratic, free-market, knowledge-based societies to impoverished people everywhere. Indeed, we are morally compelled to do so. But this mainstream interpretation, however compelling in its humanitarian urgency, is itself incomplete. It ignores the crumbling biophysical stage upon which the human drama is being played out. Certainly concerns for human well-being, justice, and equity remain, but these are too often abstracted from the deteriorating state of the planet. Rather late in the play, we are beginning to recognize that a necessary prerequisite for both economic security and social justice is ecological stability. We have no choice but to ensure that economic growth does not further imperil the structural integrity and functional health of the ecosphere.

Herein lies the fundamental challenge to postindustrial civilization. How can progress be decoupled from planetary destruction? Do we have sufficient ingenuity (and generosity) to ensure that Earth's remaining resources and waste assimilation capacity are adequate to sustain the anticipated increase in human numbers—to say nothing of rising material expectations—into the twenty-first century while simultaneously maintaining the basic life support functions of the ecosphere? Can the objectives of enlightened humanism be achieved while preserving the exuberant diversity of nature's garden? Or will the product of 4 billion years of evolution be sacrificed to the brief flowering of humanity?

Perceptual Impediments

Ironically, two of the disciplines that should be well positioned to address this challenge are both seriously misaligned. Economics studies those activities and relationships by which human beings acquire, process, and distribute the material necessities and wants of life, including the energy and material resources needed to power the industrial machine. It therefore subsumes that subset of activities by which humankind interacts with the rest of the ecosphere. However, there is a theoretical problem. Most economic analyses are money- and market-based and are thus thoroughly abstracted from nature. Conventional analyses ignore biophysical conditions and the behavioral dynamics of ecosystems. One egregious result in the present context is that economists place virtually zero marginal value on nonmarket species (and hence on maintaining biodiversity). Such analytic blindness creates a false sense of well-being even as economic growth threatens disastrous ecological consequences.

Ecology does little better. Ecologists do measure and analyze the flows of energy, material, and information between organisms and their ecosystems, and some try to understand ecosystems dynamics. However, ecologists focus almost exclusively on other species, expending little effort on humans as ecological entities in their own right. Even environmental science programs (themselves a response to ecological crises) focus mainly on environmental indicators and human impacts, not so much on humans as components of affected ecosystems.

In short, both economics and ecology are conceptually undermined by the Cartesian dualism that so cleanly severs humans from the rest of nature (and underpins our entire technical–scientific culture). In effect, economists do human ecology with empty theory that ignores natural processes; ecologists have promising theory but ignore the human species. With neither discipline properly focused, it is little wonder that we still have such a poor understanding of so many dimensions of sustainability and the integrity problem.

Our perceptual difficulties do not end there. The foundations for the neoclassical economics that dominates the world today were laid in the nineteenth century on principles borrowed explicitly from Newtonian analytic mechanics. This is the physics (and economics) of reductionist logic, linear cause and effect, simple deterministic law, and complete reversibility. Newton's triumph had been partially to realize Descartes's vision of a universe governed by knowable laws, describable in purely mathematical terms and thus, in theory, completely predictable and open to human manipulation and control.

The unprecedented success of the Newtonian paradigm in describing the simple mechanical world made it a model for others to follow. As noted, economists had already turned their discipline into "the mechanics of utility and self-interest" in the middle of the nineteenth century (W.S. Jevons, in Schenk 1998). Ecology, on the other hand, was just then emerging and initially carried a broader, more holistic perspective. But after a century of failed attempts to discover the kind of simple universal laws that would confer upon their discipline the respectability of Newtonian mechanism, ecologists began to abandon their classical roots. Like economics before it, ecology succumbed to "physics envy" in a mass capitulation to the norms of reductionist science. Holism and integration gave way to atomism and accident, balance and equilibrium to what some see as a "pointless hodge-podge" of fluctuation and change. Even the central concept of the ecosystem has come into question.

Ironically, the real problem here is not a problem with classical ecology but rather with classical physics. For all its inordinate success, analytic mechanics applies to a rather restricted range of simple, well, "mechanical," phenomena. Trying to force the rest of reality to fit this model is simply bad science. Better to reform and extend our models than ignore what reality is telling us, and reality on the macro level seems to talk anything but mechanics.

Indeed, systems ecologists and other systems analysts now recognize that the behavior of most of the natural world is nonlinear, discontinuous, irreversible, and characterized by lags and thresholds. It therefore confounds the assumptions of "normal" predictive science. This does not mean that nature does not behave according to natural laws—it invariably does. However, in the past few decades our artificially stunted linear–mechanical paradigm has given way to a view of nature that, while still fundamentally deterministic, is "relentlessly nonlinear" at higher levels of organization (Stewart 1989). Such terms as "complex systems," "deterministic chaos," "nonlinear dynamics," "autopoiesis," and "Prigoginian self-organization" capture the flavor of the paradigm shift fairly well.

The interaction of the simple laws of physics and chemistry can produce systems behavior of extraordinary complexity and richness (Cohen and Stewart 1994). Perhaps most important, in the present context, is recognition that the interplay of even strictly deterministic rules can quickly generate patterns of systems behavior that are inherently unpredictable even with near-perfect knowledge of the initial state of the system. The internal dynamics of the model system are such that small errors of measurement are folded back and amplified with each iteration. Given sufficient time, any inaccuracy will derail the model. Better measurement doesn't help, at least not for long. The tiniest, unavoidable measurement error can render even the best of models useless as a predictive tool.

The general problem is called "sensitive dependence on initial conditions," and the behavior it produces in both mathematical models and real systems—even simple ones—is called chaos. Such deterministic chaos has always existed, but was generally overlooked in society's pursuit of normal predictive science. Sometimes it was ignored because the mathematics was too difficult. Now that computers are up to the task, "the dreadful truth has become inescapable: chaos is everywhere. It is just as common as the nice simple behavior so valued by traditional physics" (Cohen and Stewart 1994, p. 190). To the extent that such counterintuitive behavior is characteristic of real-world ecosystems, economic systems, and social systems, it requires a serious reevaluation of prevailing analytic models.

Where does this take us in our brief assessment of economics and ecology? It seems that both the economy and the ecosphere are complex, self-organizing systems whose behavior is governed not only by simple Newtonian mechanics but also by evolutionary forces, nonlinear dynamics, and thermodynamic laws. Indeed, the second law of thermodynamics as applied to open, far-from-equilibrium systems provides an important theoretical and heuristic foundation upon which to rebuild our understanding of economy–environment interaction. In this light, ecology's "failure" to deliver simple universal laws and predictive models was really a failure of starting assumptions and cultural expectations. The data were telling it like it is; holistic ecology was on the right track—over broad domains of real time and space, nature is inherently unpredictable. This and not false prediction is the real knowledge. Conversely, economists' simple market models have little basis in empirical reality. They therefore sadly misrepresent both society and nature (Rees 1999).

Contrary to some postmodern philosophers, the failure of positive predictive science in coping with complexity is not a call to deny physical reality and abandon science altogether. Rather, it indicates that the domain of legitimate science must be extended. The mechanical paradigm provided an adequate first approximation of reality for simple systems in simpler times. But new science is needed to interpret reality as humans force nature into domains of unfamiliar and unpredictable behavior. For sustainability, society will have to live with, and adapt to, the increasing uncertainty that this implies. Perhaps the most important adjustment will be the replacement of arrogant certainty with precautionary restraint in our relationship with nature.

In sum, the undisputed success of the old physics in launching industrial society has led us to expect science to produce immediate and dependable solutions to the problems at hand. But the new science suggests that simple answers to the complex issues emerging today will almost certainly be misleading if they are not absolutely wrong. In an era when the sheer scale of the human enterprise rivals that of nature in many dimensions, we can ill afford to blunder ahead in the real world assuming we know enough to be certain of the outcome.

Ironically then, just as our technological wizardry (mechanism again) lends credence to the claim that the knowledge-based society is at hand, society is being forced to acknowledge the inherent ambivalence of knowledge itself. Only a few short years ago, the human story was a matter-of-fact account of the mastery of nature; today, global ecological change has reduced this particular autobiography to cultural myth. The important question is, will heightened awareness of our continuing vulnerability help us find a way out of the Easter Island trap? Will our collective coming to consciousness enable us to devise a socioeconomic system that can achieve balance with the ecosphere?

The Integrity Response to Global Ecological Degradation

The Global Integrity Project is a multipronged response to the combined problems of (a) mixed and threatened human well-being, (b) degradation of the ecosphere, and (c) unsustainable economies. There is a growing body of policy, legislation, regulation, and international agreement that, in response to these problems, establishes local, national, and international mandates to protect and restore ecological integrity and health and create sustainable economies. Our purpose is to clarify and draw the implications of these mandates by giving better definition and operational substance to the notion of ecological integrity and related concepts and to the prescriptions to which they give rise. Our response can be summarized in terms of several interlinked key elements:

1. *Understanding.* Understand the global ecosphere in evolutionary context as a complex system of systems. Human economies are dependent subsystems of the ecosphere that increasingly degrade the whole.

2. *Values.* Adopt an ecological ethic that values natural systems and the multiple forms of life and gives more weight to global and intergenerational equity in humanistic ethics.

3. *Measurement.* Develop indicators of human and ecological well-being consistent with the understanding and values in 1 and 2 and employ them in systems of measurement and reporting.

4. *Prescriptions.* Develop prescriptions to guide conduct based on 1–3, including ecological principles of land-use zoning and sustainable exploitation of resources.

5. *Social Measures.* Recommend effective social mechanisms and institutions for realizing the prescriptions in 4.

This volume elaborates these responses and applies them to health, forestry, agriculture, fisheries, and human settlements.

Understanding, Valuing, and Measuring Ecological Integrity

Ecological perspectives are holistic; they find it important to understand phenomena in their interrelationships as complex wholes and parts. Generically, integrity connotes a valuable whole, "the state of being whole, entire, or undiminished" or "a sound, unimpaired, or perfect condition" (*Random House Dictionary of the English Language* 1967). This nucleus of associations, with both value-laden and descriptive dimensions, has received endless elaboration in many cultural and scientific contexts, as Sagoff points out in chapter 4. Indeed, the multitude of associations signals a powerful and long-standing propensity to see things whole and poses a challenge to separate scientific wheat from mystical, speculative, or romantic chaff. This task is complicated by divergent conceptions of science in general and ecological science in particular, as already noted. Holland (chapter 3) and Partridge (chapter 5) address the question of legitimating ecological theory in response to critics. For Holland, compatibility with Darwinian natural selection is a crucial touchstone. On some interpretations (which Holland rejects), this means that evolutionary history is essentially a string of contingencies that preclude a science of ecosystems, per se. One can only "study the minute particulars that make every place at every time unique" (chapter 4). However, argues Partridge, it is also important and urgent, for both scientific and practical reasons, to see particulars within larger complex wholes, which it is the task of ecology to understand; fortunately we have a body of systematic ecological knowledge that is quite fruitful.

In chapter 2, Westra, Miller, Rees, and Ulanowicz set out approaches to integrity that have guided this project. Ecological integrity is a broad umbrella that covers a variety of themes cutting across scientific and popular thought. In particular, integrity is associated with wild, untrammeled nature and the self-creative capacities of life to organize, regenerate, reproduce, sustain, adapt, develop, and evolve itself. These capacities are displayed spatially in a hierarchy of natural systems and temporally as the legacy of eons of evolutionary and biogeophysical processes with their potential to continue into the future. Finally, "integrity" signifies that the combined functions and components of whole natural systems are valuable for their own sake; their life support functions; their psychospiritual, scientific, and cultural significance; and the goods and services they provide. This multidimensional valuing of the integrity of ecosystems, which is threatened by expanding aggregate human space and resource demands and pollution loads, has led to popular, legislated, and policy insistence on its protection and restoration. In fact, argues Sterba (chapter 19), we would have a moral obligation to protect ecological integrity for the good of other forms of life even if it were of no benefit to us.

A proper diagnosis of and response to deteriorating biological conditions requires a broad scientific base analogous to that in the health sciences. Health, like ecological integrity, is a culturally embedded cluster of concepts that are both descriptive of real conditions and value-laden. Health is of concern to all, whether or not we have any scientific understanding of or solutions to health problems. Note too that there is not a single health science but a multiplicity. Virtually any science, from climatology (see McMichael [chapter 14]) to molecular genetics, becomes a health science if accompanied by a plausible account of its relevance to understanding health, disease, and dysfunction (a fact not lost on researchers seeking grants). Thus, at one level, the health sciences are but a way of organizing many independent scientific endeavors in terms of their contribution to understanding health and its absence. But once brought under a common rubric with common goals, the health sciences promote an interdisciplinary integration of approaches. Analogously, the contents of this volume represent a partially integrated variety of disciplinary approaches to understanding ecological integrity, including epidemiology, forest ecology, marine and river ecology, urban economics (and ecology), thermodynamics, philosophical ethics, political science, and cultural history.

Are integrity and its loss empirically measurable biological conditions? We believe so, and present two basic approaches deriving, on the one hand, from comparisons with a baseline condition in "wild" nature (i.e., places relatively free from human impacts) and, on the other, from complex systems theory.

Karr (chapter 12) pioneered the creation of multimetric indices of biological condition (primarily in streams and rivers) that measure the severity of biological degradation by deviations from a baseline condition of ecological integrity found in wild nature. Loucks (chapter 10) adapted this approach to measure pollution impacts on forest functions in the eastern United States and Canada with his index of mean functional integrity. Miller and Ehnes (chapter 9) also use Karr's index of biological integrity as a point of departure for guiding and assessing the introduction of ecosystems-based Sustainable Forest Management to the midboreal forests of Canada.

Ulanowicz (chapters 2 and 6) has devised a different approach to defining and measuring ecological integrity in terms of several general characteristics of ecosystems. For Ulanowicz, integrity is composed of a system's vigor, organization, and resilience, which can be measured to produce a composite index of integrity. An area with integrity has properties that can be present regardless of whether it is wild or not, although Ulanowicz believes that in most cases high systemic integrity will correspond with high integrity on an index calibrated to a wild benchmark. As in medical diagnosis, multiple convergent indicators of biological condition are an asset.

Conserving Integrity and Living Sustainably

The broad prescriptions that emerge from considering integrity are as simple to state as they are difficult to realize: Conserve integrity and live sustainably. One reason for the difficulty is the perceptual problem mentioned earlier, the separation of humans and nature, economics and ecology. Rees (chapter 8) puts the pieces back together by integrating modern thermodynamics, human ecology, and economics to reveal that the stark global outlook with which we began is a consequence of a materially expanding

economy whose ecological footprint already exceeds the long-range carrying capacity of the planet. Unfortunately, other chapters that follow cor-
roborate that dismal picture. Goodland and Pimentel (chapter 7) point out
the tremendous cost in soil, water, energy and pollution loadings from unsustainable agricultural practices. Loucks (chapter 10) reports an 80 percent
average loss in function for "protected" forest preserves downwind from
midwestern pollution sources. And Pauly (chapter 13) traces the progressive
collapse of global fisheries.

In response, integrity conservation should include, but not be limited to,
a system of buffered protected areas of wild nature of a size and configuration to optimize the conservation of native biodiversity and ecological
processes within their range of natural variation. A protection strategy for
representative wild ecosystems is required because humans, as large social
animals with high material/energy demands, are inherently destructive; like
elephants, we trash the locales we exploit to live (Rees, chapter 8). We are
not alone in this (indeed, all organisms exploit and alter their habitats), but
our destructive impact is so amplified by our numbers, industries, and level
of consumption that only by pulling back can we hope to retain, to some
degree, our life-sustaining natural inheritance. However, measures to conserve integrity cannot stop with protected areas, but must address the exploited landscape matrix between them. Otherwise even protected areas
will fail from impinging pollution loads (Loucks, chapter 10) or loss of connectivity essential for species migration and dispersal. Thus Westra proposes
that in a sense buffers for protected areas must extend everywhere; we
should live as in a buffer (Westra 1998, p. 234). Westra, Miller Rees, and
Ulanowicz (chapter 2) and Noss (chapter 11) elaborate guidelines and a rationale for a protected areas strategy.

Given our requirements, our demands, and our numbers, humans cannot
avoid significant impacts on intensively exploited portions of the globe. The
benchmark condition of integrity in remnant wild ecosystems cannot obtain
everywhere. But we can invoke standards of sustainability and ecological
health as appropriate to exploited and lived-in landscapes. Goodland and
Pimentel (chapter 7) define "environmental sustainability" as "maintenance
of natural capital." This entails that harvest rates of renewable resources must
lie within the system's regenerative capacities and that nonrenewables shall
be depleted at a rate below the rate of their replacement by renewable substitutes. On the output side, waste emissions must lie within the assimilative
capacity of the local environment. Exploited natural systems that can be
maintained in use under such conditions for the long run without degradation to themselves or to other places may be healthy, even if they lack full
integrity (Westra et al., chapter 2). We have already noted that, by these
criteria, many segments of our economy are currently unsustainable.

Undoubtedly the most extensive impacts on natural systems derive from agriculture to feed the world. Goodland and Pimentel (chapter 7), besides cataloging the destructiveness and waste in current agricultural practices, offer numerous suggestions for moving toward sustainability, including incentives to eat lower on the food chain. Even with such measures, however, we are likely to fall short of true sustainability on agricultural lands at current and projected population levels, and trade-offs are inevitable until population size and food consumption are brought under control.

Miller and Ehnes (chapter 9) examine a very different model of resource exploitation than intensive agriculture, namely ecosystems-based sustainable forest management, designed for Canadian midboreal forests and elsewhere. Canadian forest policy is committed to maintaining a condition of forest health approaching integrity even in exploited forests. How close can they come? Both harvest practices to achieve this goal and metrics to measure it are under development. At the same time, Canadian governments have undertaken to complete a network of representative protected areas. These policy directions are congruent with the integrity prescriptions, but it remains to be seen how they will fare in the face of entrenched practices, competing commitments, and limited knowledge.

Inside the Economy: Benefits, Harms, Economic Drivers, and Equity

Our economy is like a giant happiness machine. Dredgelike, it sucks in resources at the front end and spews out wastes at the back, all the while leaking emissions into air, water, and soil. Natural resource industries and agriculture lie at the front end and waste disposal at the back. An outside view of the economy looks at these operations and their leakage and concludes that the economic dredge is a generator of harmful global changes, unsustainable in its operations and progressively destructive of ecological integrity (Miller 1998, p. 139). From these conclusions arises the counsel: Conserve integrity and live sustainably by constraining and redesigning methods, patterns, and rates of resource extraction, processing, consumption, and waste disposal.

Suppose, now, we look inside at the inner workings and the benefits and harms that accrue. In the aggregate, our happiness machine has had some success in improving the lot of humankind. Most obviously, it has generated immense material wealth for many, but wealth isn't happiness, and there is some evidence that, beyond a threshold, increments in wealth are not matched by increments in subjective happiness or other measures of well-being (Durning 1992). Looking at specific measures, it is a triumph of our economy and public health initiatives that there have been "considerable and widespread gains in health and longevity over the past century" (McMichael, chapter 14). Wealth is so highly correlated with health that it overwhelms other effects and thus, to date, diminishing integrity (e.g., deforestation and land conversion) has been positively, if weakly, correlated with favorable health outcomes (Soskolne, Sieswerda, and Scott, chapter 15). The economic machine has succeeded in exploiting nature to net human benefit. Much of this achievement is due to industrialization, which is concentrated in cities. But cities not only concentrate wealth-generating industries, they also enable the flowering of human cultural and intellectual pursuits from the synergies and surplus wealth they create (Crabbé, chapter 18). No wonder, with benefits like these, our society is slow to brake the operations of the happiness machine.

Why, then, be concerned about integrity? From a biocentric ethical standpoint, we ought to be concerned about the impacts our economic choices make on other living things (Sterba, chapter 19). Indeed, major conservation organizations like the World Wildlife Fund are dedicated to acting on this concern by protecting wild spaces around the globe from human encroachment. Schrecker (chapter 17) explores the ethics and politics of such campaigns when they inflict costs inequitably on local economies or individuals deprived of livelihoods by removing a resource from exploitation. Moreover, there are limits to the political will to initiate measures that constrain our economies.

Are there, then, anthropocentric reasons to be concerned about planetary degradation? Indeed there are. Although life expectancy statistics for people generally and infants in particular have shown marked improvement over the last century, Westra (chapter 16) identifies 14 kinds of environmentally mediated hazards that have increased from the operations of our economy, ranging from ultraviolet exposures to toxic hazards to new disease vectors and antibiotic-resistant pathogens. Moreover, many of these hazards are deeply entrenched in current industrial practices and are legally permitted. In that case, argues Westra, they are institutionalized forms of ecoviolence, a kind of assault, which violate fundamental rights of their victims and ought to be outlawed. For epidemiologists, many of these hazards, arising from unsustainable economies causing large-scale global change, present a difficult new challenge for risk assessment and pose the threat that recent health gains might soon be lost (McMichael, chapter 14).

Thus, although an ethical regard for other forms of life may be a factor, it is direct threats to human life, health, and well-being that finally serve to galvanize action. Yet even though many of these threats are widely known, effective action has been very difficult to achieve. We know that we must redesign the happiness machine to decouple human happiness from increased material and energy throughput, but there is a momentum in the other direction. Why? Manno (chapter 20) proposes part of the answer in his account of the commoditization of human welfare. Our market economy systematically privileges market goods and services over nonmarket means to well-being, creating a selective pressure for their increase at the expense of public and nonmarket goods. Commodities attract money, investments, research and development, and overall improvements that make them more attractive vis-à-vis their nonmarket counterparts. Unfortunately for the integrity of the ecosphere, many of these gains are achieved through increased material and energy consumption. It is necessary, then, to use what social and economic levers we can muster to redirect this dynamic.

Conclusion

In the broadest terms, the nations of the world have known since the 1992 Earth Summit at Rio the direction we must turn. How have we fared since then, and what additional measures do we need to take? Brown (chapter 21) examines the recent five-year review of Rio and concludes pessimistically that, despite some positive economic and social trends (though sub-Saharan Africa has fared worse), the ecological indicators have trended downward, leaving us in a worse predicament than in 1992. Northern countries have failed to live up to key provisions of the Agenda 21 agreement struck at Rio. In particular, they have fallen far short of the 0.7 percent of GDP contribution target to assist poor countries to meet the provisions of Agenda 21, and their resource consumption and pollution loads have increased rather than decreased. Until Northern countries take responsibility for their consumption patterns and their obligations to assist the poorer nations financially and technically, the prospects for progress along the path to sustainability are grim.

We began this introduction by asking whether, following the Easter Islanders, "humankind [is] fatally flawed, doomed—even in full knowledge—to repeat history on ever greater spatial scales until the brilliant light of civilization is forever snuffed out in one great final crash?" Although pessimism about the human prospect is not irrational, a widely adopted fatalism would be a self-fulfilling prophecy of doom. We must not let that happen. Our fate, and the planet's, depends in part upon individual and collective actions responding to our planetary condition and its prospects. Our project has been to describe that condition in relation to norms of ecological integrity, sustainability, human welfare, and justice, while addressing more technical problems of theoretical understanding, methodologies, and measurement. On the basis of those values and understandings, we have also recommended many steps to reverse ecological degradation while promoting justice and welfare. In the final chapter (22), Brown, Manno, Westra, Pimentel, and Crabbé summarize our findings, principles, and prescriptions. Our profound hope is that our message of urgency coupled with scientific, moral, and social understanding will lead, not to a paralysis of resignation, but to a creativity of responsible action.

REFERENCES

Cohen, J. and I. Stewart. 1994. *The Collapse of Chaos*. New York: Penguin Books.

Durning, A. 1992. *How Much Is Enough? The Consumer Society and the Future of the Earth*. New York: W.W. Norton.

Goodland, R. 1992. The case that the world has reached limits. In R. Goodland, H.E. Daly, S. El Serafy, eds. *Population Technology and Lifestyle: The Transition to Sustainability*. Washington, DC: Island Press.

Karr, J.R. and E.W. Chu. 1995. Ecological integrity: Reclaiming lost connections. In L. Westra and J. Lemons, eds. *Perspectives on Ecological Integrity*. Dordrecht Kluwer Academic, 34–48.

Miller, P. 1998. Canada's model forest program: The Manitoba experience. In J. Lemons, L. Westra, R. Goodland, eds. *Ecological Sustainability and Integrity: Concepts and Approaches*. Dordrecht: Kluwer Academic, 135–152.

Mitlin, D. and D. Satterthwaite. 1994. *Global Forum 94 Background Document: Cities and Sustainable Development*. London: International Institute for Environment and Development.

NRTEE. 1998. Canada offers sustainable cities solutions for the world. Workshop Discussion Paper. Ottawa: National Round Table on the Environment and the Economy.

Pimentel, D. et al. 1998. Ecology of increasing disease: Population growth and environmental degradation. *BioScience* 48(10):817–826.

Ponting, C. 1991. *A Green History of the World*. London: Sinclair-Stevenson.

Rees, W.E. 1996. Revisiting carrying capacity: Area-based indicators of sustainability. *Population and Environment* 17:195–215.

———. 1999. Consuming the earth: The biophysics of sustainability. *Ecological Economics* 29(1):23–27.

Rees, W.E. and M. Wackernagel. 1996. Urban ecological footprints: Why cities cannot be sustainable (and why they are a key to sustainability). *EIA Review* 16:223–248.

Schenk, R. 1998. Definitions of economics. http://131.93.13.212/econ/ Introduction/Defintns.html.

Simon, J. 1981. *The Ultimate Resource*. Princeton: Princeton University Press.

Simon, J. 1995. *The State of Humanity: Steadily Improving*. Cato Policy Report 17:5. Washington, DC: The Cato Institute.

Stewart, I. 1989. *Does God Play Dice?* Cambridge, MA: Blackwell.

UN. 1994. *World Urbanization Prospects: The 1994 Revision.* New York: United Nations.

Wackernagel, M. and W. Rees. 1996. *Our Ecological Footprint: Reducing Human Impact on the Earth.* Gabriola Island, BC: New Society.

Westra, L. 1998. *Living in Integrity: A Global Ethic to Restore a Fragmented Earth.* Lanham, MD: Rowman & Littlefield.

WHO. 1996. *Micronutrient malnutrition—Half of the world's population affected.* Report from the World Health Organization, 78(13 Nov):1–4.

Ecological Integrity and the Aims of the Global Integrity Project

*Laura Westra, Peter Miller, James R. Karr,
William E. Rees, and Robert E. Ulanowicz*

Despite the bad press that generally follows an El Niño episode, on November 2, 1997 the Italian News Channel (RAI) and the U.S. *Sunday Report* showed a marvel engendered by El Niño: the flowering of the Chilean desert. This phenomenon shows clearly why the insistence on largely unmanipulated (if not "intact," "pristine," or "virgin") systems is so vital to the understanding of integrity and to life on Earth. A desert area in Chile that, to the casual observer in recent times, was seemingly barren changed dramatically after El Niño. Because both the latent biological processes of deserts in general and the specific biota characteristic of the Chilean desert were present, the unusual rains brought in by El Niño produced a wonderland of flowers and grasses, with all the accompanying complement of insects, such as bees, ants, butterflies, and other species.

This burst of life occurred because anthropogenic stress was largely absent from the history of the desert; that is, this Chilean landscape had not been subjected to the chemical and biophysical stresses that prevail in exploited ecosystems around the world. In essence, the desert retained its biological potential (Westra 1994) because its vital state had not been reduced by human disturbance. The main point of this example is to emphasize the difference between a landscape that has been heavily utilized and one that has been left (for the most part) in its natural condition, following its own evolutionary trajectory. At one end of the spectrum, the remote desert area retained most of its capacities for development. Largely untouched, the desert flowered. At the other end, the petroleum-laced fields where Royal Dutch/Shell Oil carries on its ecologically destructive enterprise in Ogoniland, Nigeria (Westra 1998), will not burst into flowers under any circumstances. While most people were completely ignorant of the immense potential for diverse life that was present in that "barren" desert in Chile (although desert ecologists may be familiar with such phenomena), its integrity guaranteed that, under changed conditions, one of its possible developmental trajectories might come to be.

In this chapter we consider, in general terms, the meaning, measurement, and policy implications of the familiar, fundamental, but sometimes puzzling concept of ecological integrity. First we offer a qualitative characterization of six themes associated with the concept of integrity. Then we consider two approaches to the measurement of integrity devised by James Karr and Robert Ulanowicz. Next we address a number of theoretical issues, related concepts, and policy implications associated with integrity. Finally we summarize the approach of Reed Noss and Allen Cooperrider (1994) to implementing the policy of conserving global ecological integrity by protecting, in as wild a condition as possible and with buffers and connections across the landscape, viable areas capable of representing the ecological diversity of the world.

Integrity Revisited and Clarified

The generic concept of integrity connotes a valuable whole, "the state of being whole, entire, or undiminished" or "a sound, unimpaired, or perfect condition" (*The Random House Dictionary of the English Language* 1967). We begin with the recognition that integrity, in common usage, is an umbrella concept that encompasses a variety of other concepts (Westra 1994). The example of the blooming desert illustrates a number of the themes associated with ecological integrity:

1. The example is drawn from wild nature, or nature that is virtually unchanged by human presence or activities. Although the concept of integrity may be applied in other contexts, wild nature provides the paradigmatic examples for our reflection and research. Because of the extent of human exploitation of the planet, such examples are most often found in those places that, until recently, have been least hospitable to dense human occupancy and industrial development, such as deserts, the high-Arctic, high-altitude mountain ranges, the ocean deep, and the less accessible reaches of forests. Wild nature is also found in locations whose capacity to evoke human admiration won their protection in natural parks.

2. The rapid bloom of desert organisms illustrates in a dramatic fashion some of the autopoietic (self-creative) capacities of life to organize, regenerate, reproduce, sustain, adapt, develop, and evolve.

3. These self-creative capacities are dynamically temporal. The present display of living forms and processes in the desert gains significance through its past and its future. Nature's rhythms are displayed over time; no momentary snapshot captures all of nature's potential.

   a. Conjoined with its past, the Chilean desert is a part of nature's legacy, the product of natural history. Because of the relative absence of anthropogenic impacts, the desert biota is the creation largely of "evolutionary and biogeographical processes at that place" (Angermeier and Karr 1994). It thus illustrates what nature is and does in the absence of the human design and influence that dominate the built, modified, and altered environments in which we live most of our lives.

   b. The events of its past and present demonstrate the capacity of desert life forms to maintain themselves and their evolutionary lineages across generations, to respond to changing conditions, to evolve. If those capacities are not destroyed, the system retains its maximum potential to evolve alternative future realizations.

   c. Neither the dry dormancy nor the flowering vibrancy by itself captures the desert's potential to move between these states. Emergent properties result from macro-organic interactions among species and local physical conditions. In another example, an intermediate stage in forest succession does not lack integrity simply because it does not have all the features of a climax forest. Thus, in determining the state of a system, persistent trends and capacities that are only occasionally displayed must be taken into account.

4. Desert conditions, relieved by rains at rare intervals, are themselves the products of larger regional and global weather patterns. Indeed both the biological and geoclimatic processes that led to the blooming desert play themselves out on a stage with much larger spatial scope.

   A major issue for conservation biology is the question of what spatial requirements are needed to maintain native ecosystems. What area and configurations are needed for land and marine ecosystems dedicated to the preservation of the native biodiversity and natural processes, whose joint presence constitutes integrity? How do conditions external to the protected area affect it, and what are effective means to buffer an area against adverse external factors? Global and regional atmospheric and climatic conditions—long-range material, chemical, and biological transport; disease vectors; exotics; refugia; migratory patterns; home ranges; natural disturbance regimes; and the like—are spatial phenomena that impinge on or are constitutive of local ecological integrity. Integrity at a local site requires favorable regional and global conditions.

5. Implicit in the above is the fact that biophysical phenomena constitute a system of interacting and interdependent components that can be analyzed as an open hierarchy of systems. Every organism in the desert comprises a system of organic subsystems and interacts with other organisms and abiotic elements to constitute larger ecological systems of progressively wider scope up to the ecosphere.

6. Note, finally, that ecological integrity is valuable and valued. In the case of the Chilean desert, the dramatic transformation of "barren" desert into a vital and diverse biotic community provoked wonder and appreciation. Other ecological communities, such as reefs and rain forests, display their prolific life in a more continuous, less seasonal or episodic fashion. More generally, the biological and physical processes at work in these instances gave rise to the totality of life on Earth, including ourselves, and maintain the conditions for the continuation of life as we know it. Thus natural ecosystems are valuable to themselves for their continuing support of life on Earth, as well as for the aesthetic value and the goods and services they provide to humankind. Indeed, ecological integrity is essential to the maintenance of ecological sustainability as a foundation for a sustainable society. For these reasons, there is a growing body of policy and law that mandates the protection and restoration of ecological integrity.

As a valuable and valued condition of biological systems, ecological integrity bridges the concerns of science and public policy. For both, we must be able to go beyond general qualitative descriptions to specify empirical and operational standards. Are integrity and its loss empirically measurable biological conditions? We believe so and present two basic approaches derived, on the one hand, from comparisons with a baseline condition in "wild" nature (i.e., places virtually free from human impacts) and, on the other, from complex systems theory. James Karr pioneered the creation of multimetric indices of biological condition (initially in streams and rivers) that measure the severity of biological degradation by deviations from a baseline condition of ecological integrity found in wild nature (Karr et al. 1986; Karr 1991, 1998; Karr and Chu 1999; chapter 12 this volume). Others have adapted this approach to forest (Loucks, chapter 10 this volume; Miller and Ehnes, chapter 9 this volume), shrub–steppe (Kimberling et al., in review), and wetland (Burton et al. 1999) ecosystems. Robert Ulanowicz has devised a different approach to defining and measuring ecological integrity in terms of several general characteristics of ecosystems related to their vigor, organization, and resilience, which can be measured to produce another composite index of integrity (see also chapter 6 this volume). As in medical diagnosis, multiple convergent indicators of biological condition are an asset.

Assessing Biological Condition (Divergence from Integrity): Index of Biological Integrity

Water is both a symbol and a major constituent of life. Humans depend on living waters for many essential goods and services, from drink and food to cleansing of wastes to aesthetic and recreational renewal. However, we have not treated this resource well in the settlement of North America. What a biologist sees in our rivers is a history of damaged landscapes and under-valued, polluted waters. In response to the deteriorating condition of our freshwaters, the U.S. Clean Water Act has as its objective: "to restore and maintain the chemical, physical, and biological integrity of the Nation's waters" [Clean Water Act (CWA) s. 101(a)]. Against this backdrop, the multi-metric index of biological integrity (IBI) was developed to give empirical meaning to the goal of the CWA (Karr 1981; Karr et al 1986; Karr and Chu 1999; Karr, chapter 12 this volume).

Karr defines ecological integrity as "the sum of physical, chemical, and biological integrity" (Karr and Dudley 1981; Karr 1996). Biological integrity, in turn, is "the capacity to support and maintain a balanced, integrated, adaptive biological system having the full range of elements (genes, species, and assemblages) and processes (mutation, demography, biotic interactions, nutrient and energy dynamics, and metapopulation processes) expected in the natural habitat of a region" (Karr and Chu 1995). We can measure the extent to which a biota deviates from integrity by employing an IBI that is calibrated from a baseline condition found "at a site with a biota that is the product of evolutionary and biogeographic processes in the relative absence of the effects of modern human activity" (Karr 1996)—in other words, wild nature. Degradation or loss of integrity is thus any human-induced positive or negative divergence from this baseline for a variety of biological attributes.

Just as the index of leading economic indicators combines many financial measures to assess the state of the national economy, the IBI is holistic in that it integrates measurements of many biological attributes (metrics) to assess the condition of places. Metrics are chosen on the basis of whether they reflect specific and predictable responses of organisms to human activities. Ideal metrics should be relatively easy to measure and interpret. They should increase or decrease as identifiable human influences increase or decrease. They should be sensitive to a range of biological stresses, not narrowly indicative of commodity production or threatened or endangered status. Most important, biological attributes chosen as metrics must be able to discriminate human-caused changes from the background "noise" of natural variability. Human impact is the focus of biological monitoring and assessment (Karr and Chu 1999).

Despite major variations in the structure and function of ecosystems throughout the world, a narrow range of IBI metrics has proven useful in evaluating the condition of places. IBI metrics evaluate species richness; indicator taxa (stress intolerant and tolerant); relative abundance of trophic guilds and other ecological groups; presence of alien species; or the incidence of hybridization, disease, and anomalies such as lesions, tumors, or fin erosion (fish) and head capsule abnormality (in stream insects) (Karr 1996). Note that, unlike the procedures for standard water quality testing, physical and chemical parameters are not measured for the IBI. If such physical attributes are biologically relevant, their impacts will be detected in the biological measures.

Regional calibration of IBI is appropriate because of natural differences between landscapes, just as different body temperatures are normal or healthy for different species of birds or mammals. As human actions touch almost all the different places on Earth, we have no choice but to attempt to understand the specific effects of these actions in each region. This requirement is no more stringent than the requirements of medicine, for instance. The appropriate diagnosis and treatment of a disease may differ among infants, adults, and senior citizens or among species treated with veterinary medicine.

Although rivers and streams represent only a small portion of a landscape, their state is indicative of the condition of the whole watershed. "Rivers, like blood samples from a human, are indicative of the health of the landscape" (Karr 1998). Moreover, although the IBI was developed initially to measure the conditions of streams and rivers, the same principles for the construction of a multimetric index can be applied to terrestrial ecosystems. Karr and colleagues have developed a terrestrial IBI for the shrub–steppe ecosystem at the Hanford Nuclear Reservation in eastern Washington State (Kimberling et al., in review). Orie Loucks (chapter 10) and Peter Miller and James Ehnes (chapter 9) in this volume discuss extensions of the methodology to temperate and boreal forests. Loucks introduces the concept of mean functional integrity (MFI), which is based on several metrics for functions, such as net primary production, hydrologic pumping/evapotranspiration, biomass decomposition, and nutrient/mineral cycling. Miller and Ehnes discuss a framework for linking the IBI concept to current Canadian initiatives to develop criteria and indicators for sustainable forest management. The latter approach includes a benchmark condition that encompasses a range of natural variability derived from sampling multiple sites within a landscape.

For nearly two decades now, university scientists, water resource managers, and citizen volunteers have used the multimetric IBI to evaluate the biological condition of streams and rivers throughout the world. Site-specific assessments of biological condition are used to document the mean condition across a sampling of sites (even statistically representative of a population of places if the site selection is done properly) or the variability in condition of sites within a region. With geographic information systems (GIS) and other technologies one can couple knowledge of biological condition to spatial context, even associating the causes of degradation with specific human activities.

Once a relevant standard and index of integrity have been established, various sites or areas can then be ranked by the extent of their deviation from the integrity standard or benchmark. IBI is a measure designed to document biological condition, the position of a site or landscape on a continuum (see Figure 12.1 this volume) from undisturbed (having biological integrity) to severely degraded. (See chapter 12, this volume, for use of concepts such as benchmark, guide, and goal in biological monitoring and assessment.) A heavily polluted or paved-over area where there is nothing alive has a biological condition marking an extreme of disintegrity, whereas the conditions of agricultural lands and commercial forest plantations lie near the middle of the spectrum. Only pristine or minimally influenced wild lands meet the integrity standard or benchmark. In effect, there are no significant degrees of integrity; it is a standard existing only at the top of the scale of the IBI. Although there is considerable pressure to invoke lower standards of evaluation, that integrity benchmark defined by wild nature should be retained so that citizens, politicians, and policymakers know the level of degradation at sites subjected to the influence of human actions. Having a standard of biological integrity confers the ability to measure the full extent of our impacts on nature in exploited areas, as well as our success in protecting nature's legacy in wild areas. This is essential if we are to make informed social choices about land use.

Human survival depends on many of nature's "goods and services" that are invisible to markets and the economy; some are no doubt invisible to scientists. To know ourselves, we need to understand not only the processes and products of human history, culture, and technology, but also the processes and products of planetary evolution. We cannot hope to understand the effects of human actions on those products and processes without a systematic effort to evaluate trends in the condition of Earth's living systems. Neither can we restore structure and function, the parts and processes of living systems, to previously modified areas if we do not fully understand their role in wild nature. Because IBI is an accurate, empirically derived, and widely tested quantitative method, it is a valuable addition to the toolbox of twenty-first century science. IBI is also valuable because it provides ordinary citizens with locally meaningful indicators that can stimulate a local constituency to understand the condition of its bioregion. It is a practical index that can help make an explicit connection between ecological health and human-population health. In short, IBI provides the kind of information that will ground decisions in a broad understanding of the consequences of human actions, especially the loss of living systems, the basis for our own existence.

Assessing Biological Condition (Ecological Performance): Ascendency and Resilience

The global success and widespread use of IBI have encouraged others who are concerned about trends in ecological systems, especially living systems, to use widely accepted phenomenological conventions to yield alternate quantitative descriptors of ecosystem integrity or health. Some have sought to formulate a generic approach to the measurement of ecological performance that does not require, as the IBI does, a benchmark condition derived from particular wild ecosystems. Such an approach, if successful, could generate a measure of ecological performance for those portions of Earth that have been so widely modified by humans that wild benchmarks no longer exist. A systems-theoretical approach recognizes that the elements and processes of particular ecosystems also exemplify more general physical, chemical, and ecological functions and processes that can be quantified.

In this context, thermodynamic law and, in particular, the concept of "entropy" deserve some attention in that they might be used to measure how "disordered" a system has become. Svirezhev and Svirejeva-Hopkins (1998), for example, suggested that "excess entropy production" to serve human needs (e.g., the excessive dissipation of biomass and fossil energy as indicated by the disruption of ecosystem structure and function) measures the degree to which an ecosystem has been disturbed from its natural state.

Robert Ulanowicz and Bruce Hannon (1988) suggest another measure of integrity based on thermodynamic law. They argue that the rate of entropy production from the dissipation of solar energy by ecosystems can be accurately measured by comparing the spectra of incoming radiation with that leaving the surface. Because the incoming radiation is relatively constant over wide areas, comparison of entropy production rates should be possible by comparing the outgoing radiation profiles. Ecosystems that are performing close to their natural optima are healthier and should be able to extract more useful work from incoming radiation and re-radiate energy at higher entropy (lower effective temperature) than systems that have been disturbed in some way. Integrity, by this measure, should correlate positively with entropy production. Indeed, preliminary results with remote sensors seem to indicate that more mature, less impacted biomes reflect less radiation and appear to have "cooler" spectra than early successional stages or disturbed sites (J.J. Kay, E.D. Schneider, and J. Luval, personal communication). It may, therefore, prove feasible to make a preliminary assessment of the health of ecosystems using a series of measurements from airplanes or satellites.

Unfortunately, knowledge about entropy production tells us nothing about the configuration of ecosystem processes. Ecology is, after all, the study of the relationships among the members of a biotic community and among the community and its physical environment. We therefore need to track the essential processes that link the ecosystem elements. One way to quantify ecological performance more fully, therefore, would be to measure the amounts of material or energy that are actually exchanged among the various parts of the ecosystem. The assumption here is that the magnitude and configuration of trophic interactions in an ecosystem can be quantified and used in assessing the system's relative integrity/health if we know the topology of the system interactions.

All these indicators suggest that a "healthy" system is one that is capable of performing well in multiple ways. In Robert Costanza's (1992) terminology, adequate performance entails both vigor and organization (neither of which should be used in isolation from the other as a criterion of ecological performance). Having decided to emphasize trophic exchanges, the component of vigor inherent in these flows can most readily be quantified as the simple sum of the magnitudes of all the trophic exchanges involved. The corresponding aggregate in the human economy has been called (in ecological economic theory) "total system throughput" (Finn 1976.) It is important to recognize, however, that total system throughput, by itself, does not measure ecosystems integrity. For example, a eutrophic lake, polluted by domestic sewage or agricultural run-off, would be much more productive than the pristine oligotrophic system it displaced, but would lack the latter's biological integrity.

Remaining with trophic exchanges, we can identify the structure or organization of the energy or material flows as a second measurable component of ecological performance. The organization of these trophic exchanges requires somewhat more effort to quantify than their summation (vigor). Suffice it to note that an organized system is one that is constrained to operate in a certain way. Trophic flows do not occur willy-nilly throughout the ecosystem. One need not require microscopic descriptions of the exact signposts that cause material to flow along specific ecosystem pathways. Rather, it is sufficient to measure the degree to which the observed configuration has been constrained by such mechanisms relative to the disorder or indeterminacy these activities might otherwise exhibit.

The measurement of the "overall indeterminacy" is the crux of information theory and may be quantified using the familiar, though not universally accepted, Shannon (1948) index of diversity applied to the types of flows (Ulanowicz and Norden 1990). The formula reveals that when the different types of individual transfers are both many (richness), and more or less of the same magnitude (evenness), then the opportunities (overall indeterminacy) to develop either complex, well-defined, structured flows or confused, arbitrary transfers are high. Thus, overall indeterminacy is a measure of an ecosystem's ultimate developmental capacity. At any point in its developmental history, a system's overall indeterminacy will be partitioned between existing ordered structured flows and a "residual indeterminacy" that represents remaining options for additional order.

To assess the degree to which the ecosystem flows are organized (i.e., well-defined and structured) requires that one calculate an index known as the "average mutual information" of the flow structure. When flows are linked up in a rather arbitrary fashion, the mutual information about where a particle will next be transferred is low. The system is not well organized, trophically speaking, and there is high residual indeterminacy. One would expect to find such ecosystems where the natural and anthropogenic disturbances are irregular and intense, such as in polar ecosystems or highly impacted ones. On the other hand, if a system has been allowed sufficient time to develop within its environment without major external disturbance, cybernetic feedback will emphasize those pathways consisting of the more efficient transfers over and above arbitrary connections that are not cybernetically reinforced. Such a system acquires a complex, highly ordered structure: we say its flow structure has high "average mutual information" and the system has low "residual indeterminacy."

The factor of vigor (system-specific total-system throughput) can now be multiplied by the index of organization (the average mutual information just discussed) to yield a single index of system performance called the system ascendency (Ulanowicz 1980, 1986, 1995, 1997; and chapter 6 this volume). Ascendency assesses the ecosystem's performance at processing material and energy and can serve as a surrogate for ecosystem health.

In addition to ascendency, a further attribute often associated with integrity is the ability to withstand stress. Presumably, the responses to naturally occurring stresses that are encountered on a continuing basis (e.g., seasonal cycles, fire-climax forests, etc.) are incorporated into the organization of the system and contribute to the ascendency. The ability to withstand novel stresses is, however, another matter. The system responds to new perturbations by accessing its repertoire of residual indeterminacies. That is, when the overall indeterminacy is diminished by the average mutual information, the residual indeterminacy is a direct measure of the freedom the system has to reconfigure itself in response to any new perturbation. It serves as a measure of potential resilience and suggests why a tropical rain forest has low resilience, because of its high-average mutual information that leaves little residual indeterminacy.

The astute reader will have noticed that system performance (ascendency) and resilience are antagonistic, that is, mutually exclusive to a degree. Expressed in the language of information theory, each of the two attributes is quantified by one of two complementary terms (mutual information and residual indeterminacy) that sum to yield the overall indeterminacy of the system. The "overall indeterminacy," then, represents the system's developmental capacity, or "the greatest possible [number of] ongoing developmental options within its time/location" (Westra 1994). It is the closest one can come (under the thermodynamic and information-theoretic assumptions made here) to quantifying the integrity of an ecosystem. Because the overall indeterminacy explicitly gauges the diversity of trophic processes that are occurring in the system, the need to conserve biodiversity becomes an immediate corollary of the need to maintain systems integrity.

In conclusion, integrity is not a unitary attribute of an ecosystem. Its various aspects require more than a single index for their quantitative description. This section has shown that the triad: natural capacity (overall indeterminacy); ascendency (based on mutual information); and residual indeterminacy provides a 3-tuple with which to gauge the multifaceted integrity of a functioning ecosystem. In particular, systems exhibiting the "full integrity" described by Karr above are likely to be characterized by full natural capacity, high ascendency, and low residual indeterminacy.

IBI and Ascendency Compared

The development and advance of integrative approaches to ecological assessment such as IBI and ascendency demonstrate the growing concern among scientists about diverse environmental trends, especially the threat to Earth's living systems. Both approaches recognize that no single measure can adequately reflect the health of those systems, so they have adopted multiple measures of system condition. Both have foundations in ecological theory. Both provide analytical approaches that cut across ecosystem types. Both provide an approach to observation that is systematic and holistic. Both provide important insights about the condition or status of living systems, and thus the supply of goods and services those systems provide to human society.

The two are also fundamentally different in several respects. The triad of measures advanced by Ulanowicz—capacity, ascendency, and residual indeterminacy—emphasizes theoretical foundations in thermodynamic laws and function or process. Ulanowicz develops a logical framework for the development, empirical testing, and application of these measures. To date, empirical tests have been limited; their application in public policy contexts would be premature until more extensive empirical validation is accomplished.

The theoretical foundations of IBI derive from diverse wings of ecological science (demography, trophic dynamics, and competition theory) as well as from the principles of toxicology and the health sciences (dose-response curves). The 10 to 12 metrics (e.g., taxa richness, relative abundance of trophic or other groups, and incidence of disease) commonly incorporated into an IBI reflect this broad range of biological contexts. Incorporation of both structural (parts) and functional (processes) measures, either directly or indirectly, is an explicit goal of multimetric indexes. Although not called an IBI, Theo Colborn (Colborn et al. 1996) uses the condition of birds' eggshells, of fish's health and reproductive capacities, and even of certain human psychological and anatomical considerations to draw inescapable conclusions about the state of the Great Lakes basin ecosystem. Loucks's (Chapter 10) MFI is a multimetric index that emphasizes functional measures to assess both specific functional disorders and the *extent* of the problem. That is, he examines which particular ecological functions are curtailed, and how seriously, and thus where the sub-optimal or dysfunctional system should be placed on a continuum from full integrity to the opposite extreme of dissipative disorder. Karr, Colborn, and Loucks examine the integrity of the biota of a landscape, while fully recognizing the relevance and the role of abiotic elements within the system under consideration.

Furthermore, the general principles for development and use of IBI apply to a wide range of ecosystems and human influences on those systems. Since the original application of multimetric indexes (IBI, Karr 1981) in biological monitoring and assessment, empirical tests have been extensive. They have repeatedly validated the core IBI principles while they improved understanding of how to use multimetric indexes to communicate with diverse constituencies. Perhaps most important, their influence in the public policy arena is widespread and growing. From their incorporation as components of water-quality standards in a number of states in the United States (Davis et al. 1996) to the focus given to biological monitoring and assessment in regions throughout the world (e.g., European Union Water Framework Directive; Moog and Chovanec 2000), multimetric biological indexes influence diverse public policy issues. They have escaped from the halls of science, a critical step if human society is to protect its future by altering current environmental trends.

The Work of the Global Integrity Project: Issues and Prescriptions

The Global Integrity Project has been guided by two complementary policy imperatives: conserve integrity and live sustainably. Living sustainably in turn requires that we halt the spiral of ecological degradation. Other chapters in this volume document the degradation in different sectors and make recommendations for response. But in whatever sphere we act, in order to conserve integrity and live sustainably, we must be guided by an understanding of our dependence on the ecological condition of the planet and knowledge of the consequences of our actions. To know those consequences, we must learn how to measure and evaluate the condition of places and learn how to use that information to make it possible to protect the long-term interest of human society and of living systems indefinitely into the future. Learning how to conserve integrity means we must learn how to define and measure it. Learning how to live sustainably means we have to understand the consequences of human actions and avoid those actions that degrade life.

The preceding sections summarize our current effort to define and operationalize (give empirical significance to) the concept of ecological integrity. They revisit and extend earlier work of Laura Westra (1994) and colleagues, which focused on the capacities of a system to retain its specific functions as well as its components (the parts and processes) as central to the integrity of the system.

It is very important to emphasize that "specific function" here refers to critical natural life-support processes and not to any function dedicated to specific human interests beyond survival needs (Westra 1998, see chapter 8 definition of *sustainability*). Westra has defended and defined the maintenance of primary life-support functions as sustainability 1, or S-1, in contrast to sustainability 2, or S-2. The latter refers to the conditions necessary for the sustainability of human enterprises such as forestry or the fishing industry. This volume, with its emphasis on linking sustainability with integrity rather than with development, focuses principally and primarily on "the elements and processes of living systems to protect biological integrity" (Karr, chapter 12 this volume). In contrast, the "functions" defined narrowly "in a utilitarian context for humans" (Karr 1996; Karr, chapter 12 this volume) may be used to define a system's "health," but not its integrity. Thus, an exclusive policy emphasis on systems' "health" in relation to human–related functions beyond survival is inadequate for the preservation of biological integrity.

Nevertheless, ecological health (linked with Westra's sustainability 2) is a very important complementary concept to integrity, because it articulates a

norm for ecosystems that are exploited or impacted to meet human needs—
the places where we live, grow our food, harvest natural and plantation
products, extract resources, create and use infrastructure, engage in intensive recreation, and dump our wastes and sewage. Although these areas may
have lost the biological integrity of wild areas, our use of them is sustainable
if their exploited condition is adequately productive and stable. Thus, we
adopt Karr's definition of ecological health as a norm that applies to sites
modified by human activity. It incorporates two criteria: "no degradation
of the site that would impair its productive future use" (e.g., no loss of soil
or groundwater) and "no degradation of areas beyond that site" (e.g., no
production of acid rain that adversely affects vegetation and lakes elsewhere)
(Karr 1996, Karr and Chu 1995). When these two conditions are met at a
site, human activity is sustainable at that site. For a society to be ecologically
sustainable, every site on which it depends must be healthy in this sense.

The work of Loucks (1998 and chapter 10 this volume), which focuses
on the impacts of atmospheric pollution transport in "protected" forest
areas in the eastern United States and Canada, is particularly significant in
demonstrating how ecological integrity and health are compromised by off-
site pollution sources. Some of the forests he studied show a shocking 80
percent loss of function. His research also raises questions about the links
between loss of functionality and loss of species, whether there is a time lag
between functional losses and certain species losses, and, if so, which pre-
cedes the other.

Ecological footprint analysis, developed by William Rees and his students, is another important tool for diagnosing unsustainability in relation
to off-site impacts (Wackernagel and Rees 1996; Rees 1995, 1996, 1999;
and Rees, chapter 8 this volume). It is not enough that one's immediate
habitat or environment is stabilized, or even flourishing, in its biological
condition. We need to ensure that the distant terrestrial and aquatic ecosystems we "appropriate" through trade and by exploitation of the global
commons to support ourselves also remain in a productively healthy state.
Ecological footprint analysis shows that our species, using prevailing technologies, has already exceeded global carrying capacity by one-third. This
means that we currently maintain our consumer lifestyles and economies, in
part, by degrading and liquidating natural capital. The empirical evidence is
clear in the form of ozone depletion, greenhouse gas accumulation, soils
degradation, biodiversity loss, and the depletion of various natural capital
stocks, from old-growth forests and wild fish populations to minerals,
ground water, and petroleum, as documented in the other chapters in this
volume.

In short, whether or not we experience such degradation directly, consumer societies inevitably degrade large areas ecologically and appropriate

the biophysical output of a vast hinterland scattered all over the planet. Indeed, the present human population at current average consumption levels is dismantling and dissipating the ecosphere. We are currently losing biomass, species, and ecosystem structure (the very essence of integrity loss) on all scales, from local to global. In this light, without significant reductions in total energy and material demand, any bioreserves (as proposed in the next section and Noss, chapter 11 this volume) will be temporary. Potential human demand is so great that, given present values, consumer behavior, and technology, we will eventually need—and take for ourselves—everything the world has to offer. The United Nations World Commission on Environment and Development anticipates the need for a five-to-ten-fold expansion of industrial activity (WCED 1987). The addition of a quarter million people to Earth each day renders these problems even more acute (Pimentel et al. 1992).

It is precisely this sort of scenario that the ethics and policy directives of integrity are intended to prevent. Humans can be part of natural systems, but with our present beliefs and values, technologically "enhanced" humans, the consumers in so-called advanced affluent societies, are aliens in nature whose expanding ecological footprints threaten the basic life-support needs of all for the sake of satisfying an escalating plethora of wants. We have derailed the natural evolutionary processes in the landscapes we have come to dominate—and we dominate almost everywhere.

How, then, can we conserve integrity and live sustainably? Westra (1998) proposes eight second-order principles (SOPs) to define an ethics of integrity.

SOP 1 In order to protect and defend ecological integrity, we must start by designing policies that embrace complexity.

SOP 2 We should not engage in activities that are potentially harmful to natural systems and to life in general. Judgments about potential harms should be based on the approach of "post-normal" science.

SOP 3 Human activities ought to be limited by the requirements of the precautionary principle.

SOP 4 We must accept an "ecological worldview" and thus reject our present "expansionist worldview" and reduce our ecological footprint.

SOP 5 It is imperative to eliminate many of our present practices and choices as well as the current emphasis on "technical maximality" and on environmentally hazardous or wasteful individual rights.

SOP 6 It is necessary for humanity to learn to live as in a "buffer." Zoning restraints are necessary to impose limits both on the quality of our activities, but also on their quantity. Two corollary principles follow: (a) we must respect and protect "core"/wild areas; (b) we must view all our activities as taking place within a "buffer" zone. *This is the essential meaning of the ethics of integrity.*

SOP 7 We must respect the individual integrity of single organisms (or micro-integrity), in order to be consistent in our respect for integrity and also to respect and protect individual functions and their contribution to the systemic whole.

SOP 8 Given the uncertainties embedded in SOPs 1, 2, and 3, the "Risk Thesis" must be accepted, for uncertainties referring to the near future. We must also accept the "Potency Thesis" for the protection of individuals and wholes in the long term (Westra 1998).

The contrast between the Chilean desert and Ogoniland with which we began reminds us of the importance of maintaining wild core areas of ecological integrity. But Loucks's research on stagnating and dying forests in "protected areas" indicates that even intense human use outside core areas must be modified immediately and drastically if we are to succeed in protecting integrity. The basic effect of the ethics of integrity is that modern humans must live their lives as if "living in a buffer" (Westra 1998).

This requirement demands the elimination of many accepted and institutionalized practices that ultimately rob us and nonhuman life of a normal future (Colborn et al. 1996). A further requirement is a more ecologically sensitive process for designing and implementing public policy, while reducing corporate autonomy that can ignore the public good and the requirements of global integrity and health (Korten 1995).

Note that the effect of the "live as in a buffer" maxim is to stretch the common meaning of *buffer* in natural resource management as a protective barrier lying between incompatible forms of land use. Under Westra's treatment, there is no "other side" of the buffer where we are free to engage in human activities that would be incompatible adjacent to protected wild areas. Noss's tripartite zonation of the landscape into areas of core wild lands, buffers, and a matrix of intensely utilized lands is reduced to a dichotomous core and buffer (Noss 1992). The counsel is that *wherever* we live out our lives and produce the goods we need, we should do so as though our activities were taking place adjacent to wild lands, that is, as in a buffer. Westra's dictum reminds us that, for many of nature's processes, particularly those involving pollution transport in water or air, climate change, and migratory species, we are as good as next door to the most remote of locations. Nursing Inuit mothers in the Canadian arctic feed heavy metals and other compounds originating in the industries of Asia to the infants suckling their breasts.

Are We Saving Nature's Legacy?

Given the present world situation and the environmental problems that afflict us, we must acknowledge that the clean up and restoration job that faces us is daunting. Moreover, because large areas in a condition of ecological and biological integrity are essential to the task, we must acknowledge this as our starting point. We know that the percentage figures referring to "wild" areas provided by the Brundtland Commission and others are arbitrary and grossly insufficient, especially as they stand with little or no effort to curb harmful activities beyond their immediate borders (Westra 1994). Twelve or 15 percent of all global landscapes, including land and water, is not enough. Hence, a major question posed by the Global Integrity Project is, how much is necessary? How much is enough?

The protection of integrity, in both its structural and functional dimensions, recognizes the connection between the presence of biological integrity and the production of "services" by ecosystems or nature (Daily 1997). To this end, the protection and restoration of health to exploited areas is also vital. Again, protecting small organisms in all habitats is critically important to the functioning of natural systems (Pimentel et al. 1997).

In previous sections of this chapter, we have focused on the conceptual, theoretical, and methodological difficulties connected with the notion of integrity and the ecosystem approach that upholds it. The purpose of the Global Integrity Project is to identify appropriate scientific concepts and methods, but also to prescribe moral directives to guide and correct public policy. In this respect, it is an eminently practical project.

Our research was originally inspired by the work of Reed Noss, a conservation biologist intent on preserving biodiversity and one of the cofounders of the Wildlands Project (Noss 1992; Westra 1995). The science and policy underpinning the Wildlands Project are given both scope and precision in *Saving Nature's Legacy* (Noss and Cooperrider 1994). The task they set is to break the chain of causation leading to extinction (Figure 2.1).

Several points raised by Noss and Cooperrider are worthy of emphasis. First, although people too seldom think of themselves as biological entities (Rees, chapter 8 this volume), humans are part of the biota that loses health under these threats and may eventually fatally harm themselves. The problem is that accelerating habitat fragmentation everywhere as a result of population and economic growth and export-led development strategies imposes a heavy burden on the natural systems that provide necessary "services" for all biota, including humans. Although some species may be able to survive in highly fragmented landscapes and smaller protected areas, even small gaps like roads can pose "a severe threat to sensitive wildlife and natural ecosystems" (Noss and Cooperrider 1994).

Second, wilderness areas represent an ethical restraint on the human manipulation of nature. There must be untrammeled spaces for other living

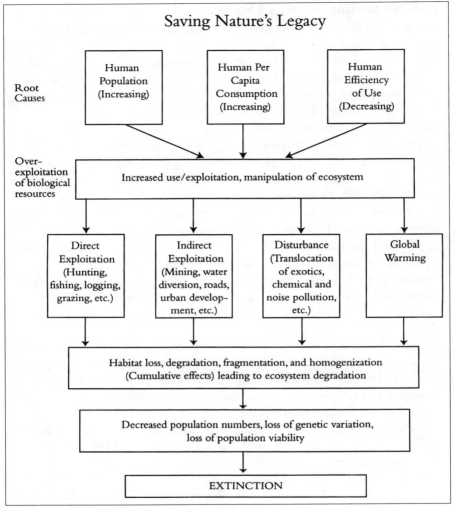

FIGURE 2.1

Relationship between root causes, overexploitation of resources, and loss of biodiversity.
The final result is extinction (Noss and Cooperider 1994, p. 51).

things and ecological processes to flourish, interact, and evolve in their own
way. Ecologically representative protected areas provide the best prospect
for ensuring the survival of the full diversity of the planet's cohabitant
species, populations, and ecological processes. These, and the coincident
benefits to humans of life support, ecological knowledge, and spiritual
value, are compromised or lost if we view the whole of nature as a domain
for our unfettered manipulation and appropriation. There is an absolute im-

perative to protect wild areas if we hope to be able to preserve and restore enough of the planet's ecological integrity to ensure the continuation of critical life-support systems. As previously noted, protecting wild areas requires that we live elsewhere "as if in a buffer."

Noss and Cooperrider (1994) maintain that society's ability to restore large carnivores provides "a critical test of society's commitment to conservation." The sheer amount of land that must be set aside for large animals is daunting. "The required area of 32 million acres for a long-term viable population (of grizzlies) is roughly 60 percent of the U.S. northern Rockies region" (Noss and Cooperrider 1994, p. 163).

Equally worthy of note, Noss speaks of integrity and of biodiversity as desirable states, without offering detailed definitions of either concept. Nevertheless, he is prepared to suggest strategies to "begin turning degenerative trends around" (Noss and Cooperrider 1994).

Noss and Cooperrider suggest four fundamental objectives:

1. Represent, in a system of protected areas all native ecosystem types and seral stages across their natural range of variation.

2. Maintain viable populations of all native species in natural patterns of abundance and distribution.

3. Maintain ecological and evolutionary processes, such as disturbance regimes, hydrological processes, nutrient cycles, and biotic interactions.

4. Manage landscapes and communities to be responsive to short-term and long-term environmental change and to maintain the evolutionary potential of the biota.

Although these goals support "conservation planning" and are conveniently pursued at a "regional scale," the ultimate scope of Noss's strategy is global. "Land-use planning and zoning for biodiversity must be applied to all lands at local, regional, national, and international scales" (Noss and Cooperrider 1994, pp. 89–90).

Thus the task at hand is two-fold: we must select appropriate areas for reserves, "designing for reserve networks," and provide for standard buffers and corridors. We must also decide on the ideal size and shape for each based on the primary biota targeted for protection and restoration. In addition, qualitative and quantitative changes are necessary to our material-intensive activities to restore health to all utilized areas globally.

What about humans? People need both wild land and a healthy modified habitat, but the question of exactly how much, particularly as it regards wild lands, remains unanswered. For many people, particularly in less-developed countries, conditions in their over-crowded, under-serviced cities are already less tolerable than those we would impose on animals living in zoos. Things would be a good deal worse, even terminal, without the life-support services provided by naturally evolving large areas of biological and ecological integrity. Westra (1998) argues that although humanmade environments, in principle, should be as ecologically benign as beaver lodges or beehives, in practice, our "hives" are built and function in conflict with "natural biogeographical evolutionary processes" (Karr 1996).

But when Westra's (1998) ethics of integrity propose principles that lead to the selection of wild areas of similar size to those required for human habitation and use, we have a revolutionary constraint on the expansion of the human enterprise. Grizzlies need large areas of wild lands to survive. This will certainly compromise some human plans and activities (but keep in mind that the large wild areas also provide natural services that support human life). "Protection should not imply a 'lock-up,' as many core reserves and buffer zones can accommodate a variety of human uses, so long as they are compatible with conservation objectives" (Noss and Cooperrider 1994, p. 88).

How much wild land might suffice? While 12 or 15 percent is not enough, and would be hard enough to achieve in most densely populated countries, various authors press for much larger reserves. Deep ecologist Arne Naess, for example, proposes a 30/30/30 percent guideline: 30 percent human activities, 30 percent carefully orchestrated activities compatible with the wild ("buffers," in the language of the ethics of integrity), and 30 percent wild areas of biological integrity. This appears to be an ecologically appropriate goal but would clearly face insurmountable implementation difficulties in most of the human-occupied world.

Clearly, the imperatives to conserve integrity and live sustainably, the prerequisites for the continuation of life as we know it, make radical demands. And while meeting these demands may be essential, it is a paradox that even in matters of life and death, we perversely continue in our ways. Part of the reason, of course, is that many economists, technological optimists, and even world leaders do not acknowledge the existence of a serious crisis. As economist Richard Gordon recently declared: "The tendency to technical progress is viewed as the most critical economic law. . . ." "Human ingenuity has been remarkable at advancing the real standard of living and warding off the pressures of resource depletion. . . . The immediate need, then, for avoiding depletion is nil. . . ." (Gordon 1994). It is also clear that policy choices and preferences, even in democratic nations, are manipulated by economic interests that promote their own goals against the wider public interest. Major corporations may reject independent studies that find against their products and even suppress internal data that threaten corporate interests, particularly the bottom line (Korten 1995; Westra

1998). The harmful deceptions and secret strategies of the tobacco industry over many years to deny the harmful effects of smoking and to actually increase levels of nicotine addiction are a case in point.

We assert that the reasons most often offered in support of the status quo (especially in affluent Northwest countries) do not stand up to scrutiny. First, the damage we wreak is potentially destabilizing to critical biophysical systems in the short term and interferes with slower natural evolutionary processes of change over the long term. Second, even democratic choices, if manipulated and uninformed, do not validate decisions that attack our life-support systems and our lives (Westra 1998).

If humans need the wild for aesthetic and psychological reasons, and the wild is essential to conserve biodiversity and vital life-support functions, then targets—percentages and specified areas—for preservation must be established and implemented globally. As difficult as it will be to implement specific reserve plans as public policy, strict controls on the rest of our activities within the human dominated "buffer" will be even harder to bring into force.

Nevertheless, if we fail in this vision, ultimately no area will be safe for nonhuman life, and we will put our own security at risk. Is it not sufficient warning that in 1988 a record number of natural disasters caused massive property damage and drove more people from the land and their homes than war and civil conflict combined? Singular events such as Hurricane Mitch and the El Niño weather phenomenon, plus declining soil fertility and deforestation, drove a record 25 million people from the countryside into crowded under-serviced shanty towns around the developing world's fast growing cities. This is 58 percent of the world's total refugees (International Red Cross 1999). Experts predict that developing countries in particular will continue to be hit by super disasters driven by human-induced atmospheric and climatic change, ecological degradation, and rising population pressures. The miners' canary has toppled from its perch. It is time to act, if only to save ourselves.

REFERENCES

Angermeier, P. L. and J. R. Karr. 1994. Biological integrity versus biological diversity as policy directives. *BioScience* 44:690−697.

Burton, T. M., D. G. Uzarski, J. P. Gathman, J. A. Genet, B. E. Keas, and C. A. Strikcer. 1999. Development of a preliminary invertebrate index of biotic integrity for Lake Huron coastal wetlands. *Wetlands* 19:869−882.

Colborn, T., D. Dumanoski, and J. P. Myers. 1996. *Our Stolen Future*. Dutton, Penguin, New York.

Costanza, R. 1992. Toward an operational definition of health. In R. Costanza, B. Norton, and B. Haskell (eds.), *Ecosystem Health: New Goals for Environmental Management.* Island Press, Washington DC, pp. 239–256.

Daily, G. (ed.). 1997. Introduction to *Nature's Services.* Island Press, Washington, DC, pp. 3–4.

Davis, W. S., B. D. Snyder, J. B. Stribling, and C. Stoughton. 1996. Summary of state biological assessment programs for streams and rivers. EPA 230-R-96-007. Office of Policy, Planning, and Evaluation, US Environmental Protection Agency, Washington, DC.

Finn, J. T. 1976. Measures of ecosystems structure and function derived from analysis of flows. *Journal of Theoretical Biology* 56:363–380.

Gordon, R.L. 1994. Energy, Exhaustion, Environmentalism, and Etatism. *The Energy Journal* 15:1–16.

International Red Cross. 1999. *1999 World Disasters Report.*

Karr, J. R. 1981. Assessment of biotic integrity using fish communities. *Fisheries* 6(6):21–27.

———. 1991. Biological integrity: A long-neglected aspect of water resource management. *Ecological Applications* 1:66–84.

———. 1996. Ecological integrity and ecological health are not the same. In P. Schulze (ed.), *Engineering within ecological constraints.* National Academy Press, Washington, DC, pp. 97–109.

———. 1998. Rivers as sentinels: Using the biology of rivers to guide landscape management. In R. J. Naiman and R. E. Bilby (eds.), *The Ecology and Management of Streams and Rivers in the Pacific Northwest Coastal Ecoregion.* Springer-Verlag, New York.

Karr, J. R. and E. W. Chu. 1995. Ecological integrity: Reclaiming lost connections. In L. Westra and J. Lemons (eds.), *Perspectives on Ecological Integrity.* Kluwer Academic Publishers, Dordrecht, The Netherlands, pp. 34–48.

———. 1999. *Restoring Life in Running Waters: Better Biological Monitoring.* Island Press, Washington, DC.

Karr, J. R. and D. R. Dudley. 1981. Ecological perspective on water quality goals. *Environmental Management* 5:55–68.

Karr, J. R., K. D. Fausch, P. L. Angermeier, P. R. Yant, and I. J. Schlosser. 1986. Assessment of biological integrity in running waters: A method and its rationale. *Illinois Natural History Survey Special Publication* 5, Champaign, Illinois.

Kimberling, D. N., J. R. Karr, and L. S. Fore. Manuscript. Responses of terrestrial invertebrates to human disturbance in shrub-steppe in eastern Washington. *Ecological Applications,* in review.

Korten, David. 1995. *When Corporations Rule the World.* Kumarian Press, Berret Koehler Publishers, West Hartford, CT

Loucks, O. L. 1998. The epidemiology of forest decline in eastern deciduous forests. *Northeastern Naturalists* 5(2):143–154.

Moog, O. and A. Chovanec. 2000. Assessing the ecological integrity of rivers: Walking the line among ecological, political and administrative interests. *Hydrobiologia* 422/423:99–109.

Noss, R. F. 1992. The Wildlands Project: Land conservation strategy. *Wild Earth* (Special Issue):10–25.

Noss, R. F. and A. Y. Cooperrider. 1994. *Saving Nature's Legacy*. Island Press, Washington, DC.

Pimentel, D., U. Stachow, D. A. Takacs, H.W. Brubaker, A. R. Dumas, J. J. Meaney, J. A. S. O'Neil, D. E. Onsi, and D. B. Corzilius. 1992. Conserving biological diversity in agricultural/forestry systems. *BioScience* 42:354–362.

Pimentel, D., C. Wilson, C. McCullum, R. Huang, P. Dwen, J. Flack, Q. Tran, T. Saltman, and B. Cliff. 1997. Economic and environmental benefits of biodiversity. *BioScience* 47(11):747–757.

Rees, W. E. 1995. Achieving sustainability: Reform or transformation? *Journal of Planning Literature* 9(4):343–361.

———. 1996. Revisiting carrying capacity: Area-based indicators of sustainability. *Population and Environment* 17:195–215.

———. 1999. The built environment and the ecosphere: A global perspective. *Building Research and Information* 27(4/5):206–220.

Shannon, C. E. 1948. A mathematical theory of communication. *Bell System Technical Journal* 27:379–423.

Svirezhev, Y. M. and A. Svirejeva-Hopkins. 1998. Sustainable biosphere: Critical overview of the basic concept of sustainability. *Ecological Modeling* 106:47–61.

Ulanowicz, R. E. 1980. An hypothesis on the development of natural communities. *Journal of Theoretical Biology* 85:223–245.

———. 1986. *Growth and Development: Ecosystems Phenomenology*. Springer-Verlag, NY.

———. 1995. Ecosystem integrity: A causal necessity. In L. Westra and J. Lemons (eds.), *Perspectives on Ecological Integrity*. Kluwer Academic Publishers. Dordrecht, The Netherlands, pp. 77–87.

———. 1997. *Ecology, The Ascendant Perspective*. Columbia University Press, NY.

Ulanowicz, R. E. and B. Hannon. 1988. Life and the production of entropy. *Proceedings of the Royal Society of London* B 232:181–192.

Ulanowicz, R. E. and J. Norden. 1990. Symmetrical overhead in flow networks. *International Journal of Systems Science* 21(2):429–437.

Wackernagel, M. and W. E. Rees. 1996. *Our Ecological Footprint*. New Society Publishers, Gabriola Island, B.C.

World Commission on Environment and Development (WCED). 1987. *Our Common Future*. Oxford University Press, NY.

Westra, L. 1994. *An Environmental Proposal for Ethics: The Principle of Integrity*. Rowman Littlefield, Lanham, MD.

Westra, L. 1995. Ecosystem integrity and sustainability: The foundational value of the wild. In Westra, L. and J. Lemons (eds.), *Perspectives on Ecological Integrity*. Kluwer Academic Publishers, Dordrecht, The Netherlands, pp. 12–33.

Westra, L. 1998. *Living in Integrity: A Global Ethic to Restore a Fragmented Earth*. Rowman Littlefield, Lanham, MD.

PART II

Historical and Philosophical Foundations

The Global Integrity Project brought together scientists and philosophers who were interested in clarifying the concept of ecological integrity. The authors in this part grapple with the historical and philosophical foundations of this concept. This part summarizes the arguments of those who have questioned certain elements of the concept of ecological integrity and offers refutations and clarifications of issues raised by skeptics.

In chapter 3, "Ecological Integrity and the Darwinian Paradigm," Alan Holland examines the idea of ecological integrity through a Darwinian lens. Holland explains why any theory of ecological integrity must be compatible with Darwin's. He is concerned with how one can reconcile the role of contingency central to Darwin's theory of evolution with the idea that ecosystems have structure and pattern. Holland demonstrates that even if one agrees that radically contingent forces affect ecosystems, they still have pattern, structure, and predictability. Therefore, there is no basic conflict between the idea of ecological integrity and an acknowledgment that ecosystems are created in part by random events.

In chapter 4, "Ecosystem Design in Historical and Philosophical Context," Mark Sagoff presents several challenges to the idea of ecological integrity. First he sketches the intellectual history of the idea of ecology and then he argues that holistic mathematical theories of ecology, will never be falsifiable. Next, Sagoff asserts that ecosystems have no essence; they have only a natural history. Because they have no essence, he challenges the very idea of ecological integrity. Yet because ecosystems have natural histories, Sagoff sees value in nature on aesthetic grounds.

In chapter 5, "Reconstructing Ecology," Ernest Partridge analyzes and rebuts many of Sagoff's conclusions, while agreeing with others. In particular, Partridge stresses that ecosystems are systems; that ecology is capable of prediction; that ecosystems exhibit the kind of structure, resilience, and integrity found in organisms; that there are reasons to prefer "natural" ecosystems to those "cultivated" by human societies; and that scientific uncertainty about ecosystems has moral significance.

In chapter 6, "Toward the Measurement of Ecological Integrity," Robert E. Ulanowicz, like Partridge, refutes many of the skeptics' arguments regarding the idea of integrity and describes methods for measuring ecosystem performance and thereby operationalizing the concept of ecological integrity. Ulanowicz develops his theory of ecosystem ascendency as a method for measuring integrity. This theory incorporates elements from information, economics, and network theory to measure a system's performance, reliability, creativity, and options for self-organization. Ulanowicz also suggests how these methods of measuring integrity might be extended to provide greater usefulness.

Ecological Integrity and the Darwinian Paradigm

Alan Holland

We shall assume that any theorizing in the ecological domain, if it is to carry weight, must work within the broad framework of Darwinian theory. In particular, ecological concepts and theories must be compatible with the broad thrust of the theory of natural selection. This "condition of adequacy," therefore, must be shown to be satisfied by the concept of "ecological integrity." Articulating the condition of adequacy, however, is not straightforward, since Darwinian theory itself is not a settled domain, but is characterized by a number of unresolved, and keenly debated, issues. Examples include the conflicting accounts of the conditions required for speciation to occur (Ridley 1985, ch. 8), and the disagreement over whether evolutionary change has been relatively constant, or whether, as the advocates of "punctuated equilibrium" maintain, it has been irregular (Dawkins 1988, ch. 9).

The debate that forms the background to the present discussion has rumbled along more or less since the inception of the theory. It is the issue of whether there is even such a thing as a "principle of natural selection," or whether evolution amounts to nothing more, nor less, than a radically contingent *historical* process—for if the history of living nature (evolution) should turn out to be characterized by radical contingency, the problem arises of how there could be room in the evolutionary process, so conceived, for applying the concept of "ecological integrity." How are integrity and contingency compatible?

The first section will outline the nature of the problem, and the second will flesh out the radically historical interpretation of Darwin. The third section will suggest reasons for thinking the problem less severe than it first appears, and the fourth will identify two approaches to integrity—(a) historical and (b) functional—and indicate how they may jointly serve to determine a usable criterion of integrity even under conditions of radical contingency. Finally, and before drawing some conclusions, we shall consider the question, How much integrity should there be?

Nature of the Problem

One reason that has been given for excluding notions such as "integrity" completely from the realm of scientific ecology is that "integrity" is a normative concept: it carries suggestions about how things should (or should not) be. Science, on the other hand, is said to deal with how things are (or are not). It is for this reason, among others, that Mark Sagoff writes: "[T]he idea that there are such qualities as the 'health' or 'integrity' of ecosystems and that species are their indicators seems less a refutable proposition of empirical science than a first principle of a certain ecological faith" (Sagoff 1997, p. 845). Others have objected to integrity that it is a "mystical" notion. For Sagoff, "outside of medicine, most natural sciences avoid normative terms such as 'health' and 'integrity'" (Sagoff 1997, p. 918). Apparent exceptions—as when nature is said to "abhor" a vacuum—are explained as a *façon de parler*.

This reason for excluding concepts such as integrity from the realm of scientific ecology appeals to a problematic dichotomy of fact and value, and will not be pursued further here. Suffice it to say that it may prove rather more difficult than Sagoff appears to allow, to exclude *façons de parler* from scientific discourse. From the notion of a "pioneering" species or plant "colony," through that of embryo "development," and even "reproduction," right down to that of the "decay" of a radioactive particle, it is a moot point what is, and what is not, a *façon de parler*. The same might be said of much of the discourse surrounding molecular genetics, involving notions such as "instruction," "information," "copy," "blueprint," and the like.

Sagoff's main objection is more challenging. It is that a concept such as integrity, construed as a property of ecosystems, presupposes notions of structure, order, and design that belong to an "old equilibrium ecology, that is now defunct" (Sagoff 1997, p. 893). Now whether the various forms of order that integrity presupposes are shared with an older paradigm is not really the important question, especially since Darwin's concern was not at all to deny order, but to explain it. The important question is the extent to which any conception of the natural world as ordered does or does not belong in the post-Darwinian paradigm. A radically historical understanding of Darwinian theory appears to undermine the view that there are any structures, wholes, or patterns in the natural world such as integrity theory seems to require; it delivers us instead a picture of pure contingency everywhere—of everything just happening to be what it is where it is. "In the final analysis, nothing is guiding the ship," as F. E. Smith observes (quoted in Rolston 1979, p. 8). It appears to follow that there is no place for ecological integrity within the Darwinian paradigm, for as Donald Worster has remarked: "What is there to love or preserve in a universe of chaos?" (1990, p. 16).

"Radically Contingent" Evolution

The full implications of construing Darwinian evolution as radically contingent can be most readily grasped by looking at one of the longest-standing objections to the "theory" of natural selection—the objection that says it is mere tautology. According to Ridley (1985, p. 29), the objection is traceable to the Bishop of Carlisle around the year 1890. Briefly stated, the objection is that according to the theory, an individual is marginally better equipped to reproduce if it has inherited what Darwin calls a "useful variation." However, a useful variation can only be explained as one that makes its owner better equipped to survive and reproduce. Hence, the notion of a useful variation—or, in more popular terms, "fitness"—has no explanatory force whatever.

Many of those who advance this objection, such as T. Bethell (1989), believe that it totally undermines Darwin's theory. They hold that a theory wholly lacking in explanatory force cannot be taken seriously as a theory. Defenders of Darwin (Gould 1980, Ridley 1985, Dawkins 1988) appear to agree with their opponents that the objection would undermine the theory of natural selection if it were sound, but they deny that it is sound. They claim that the notion of a useful variation is indeed explanatory, and that it captures the notion of being "well designed," or "better adapted," for the environment in which it finds itself. Hence there is a "principle" governing natural selection, namely the advancement of the "better designed." Such a principle is not just explanatory, but might even license modest predictions about future events.

It has to be doubted, however, whether this defense is as persuasive as its popularity might lead one to expect. The chief difficulty is whether we are entitled to assume that there is an independently identifiable concept of the "environment," in relation to which an organism can be said to be "adapted" or "well designed," for the suspicion lurks that we know what to count as an organism's environment only when we know what specific features prove in the event to be relevant to its survival. Even in the famous case of the peppered moth, *Biston betularia*, it can be argued that camouflage explains survival only retrospectively, because we need to know which moths survive if we are to know that camouflage is relevant in the first place. Camouflage instantiates fitness (or being "well designed") because it results in differential survival. Fitness is not independently identifiable, and hence not explanatory of survival.

There is, however, a third and rather less familiar interpretation of the "theory" of natural selection, adumbrated, for example, in a paper by A. Manser (1965). Differing slants on the basic idea can be detected in several more recent papers in the journal *Biology and Philosophy*, with titles like "Natural Selection without Survival of the Fittest" (Waters 1986), "The Non-existence of a Principle of Natural Selection" (Shimony 1989), and "What Is This Stuff Called Fitness?" (Ollason 1991). According to this view, the tautology objection is sound, but it does not undermine the principle of natural selection, because there is no principle of natural selection to undermine. Darwin's genius is simply to show how all the facets of life on Earth as we know it can be explained as a result of the accumulation of countless haphazard and humdrum events: a slip here, a chance meeting there, a ray of sun, a drop of rain, and occasionally, it may be, acts of judgment. The theory is precisely that no "theory" is needed. Where we are now is just where this accumulation of events happens to have landed us. Everything is contingent, though nothing is unexplained. And partly *because* it provides the stoniest ground of all (but partly also because I think it correct), it is this interpretation of the Darwinian paradigm that we shall take as the ground upon which to test whether the concept of ecological integrity can take root.

Responses to the Problem

It is important to notice, first, that on this most radical construal of the Darwinian paradigm, contingency goes right down to the level of the species and the organism. Yet despite this contingency, as Sagoff himself must admit, we nevertheless find structure, pattern, and predictability. Thus we find, remarkably, a clustering of organisms around norms, which we call species; we find, as Fisher argued (Dawkins 1988, p. 231), that major variations are likely to prove disadvantageous; and, possibly, that genetic variation is positively correlated with species longevity. Moreover, we already know that some ecosystems at any rate are identifiable: we call them organisms. What we also find are identifiable ecological items, such as species, that do not satisfy the kind of criteria that Sagoff affirms are necessary for the identification and reidentification of ecological items—namely, some account of "which of [an object's] properties are constitutive and which are accidental" (Sagoff 1997, n. 318). For the species concept most readily suited to this radical construal of Darwin is that of the cladists, who deny that species exhibit constitutive characteristics, but claim that they are defined in terms of relational and historical properties—specifically, inter-breeding and lineage (Ridley 1989). There is, it appears, no incompatibility between order and contingency. Either Darwinian happenstance is enough to explain the degree of structure and pattern that we find at the level of species and organism, or it is not. If it is, then contingency is no reason in itself for supposing that we cannot find structure and pattern at the level of patch, habitat, or ecosystem also. If it is not, and we need to suppose other principles operating—say Kauffman's "order for free" (1996, ch. 4)—then we can equally suppose them to be operating at the level of patch, habitat, and ecosystem.

Moreover, Darwin himself both recognizes, and tries to explain, structure and pattern at ecological levels more comprehensive than those of organism and species. His work on the formation of coral reefs is one example. It sets out to explain, most beautifully, why we find just three kinds of coral reef formation: the fringe reef, the barrier reef, and the atoll. His account exhibits the three formations as stages of a continuous process involving both the elevation of the coral and the "prolonged subsidence" of the intervening land (1984, p. 147). On the basis of such an account, it is possible to predict the future state of an "ecosystem" of this kind from its present state, with some moderate degree of confidence.

A key role is played in Darwin's reasoning, and in the phenomenon described, by the fact that "in ordinary cases, reef-building polypifers do not flourish at greater depths than between 20 and 30 fathoms" (1984, p. 86). This signals a third point, which is that all these events involving organisms, species, and ecosystems take place under the constraints of boundary conditions, and of relevant principles or even laws from other fields such as chemistry, physics, geology, and physiology. And while we cannot assume, without a commitment to some form of reductionism, that any of these outlying laws or principles will *determine* ecological phenomena, it should not come as a complete surprise if ecological patterns do emerge. What we have is not contingency merely, but contingency constrained. In the case of organisms and species, one of the more notable constraining factors is the principle of Mendelian inheritance; but similar constraints can be identified at the more comprehensive levels too. For all his endorsement of contingency in *Wonderful Life*, Stephen J. Gould rhetorically asks: "Am I really arguing that nothing about life's history could be predicted, or might follow directly from general laws of nature?" And he answers: "Of course not: the question that we face is one of scale, or level of focus" (1991, p. 289). Observing that obedience to physical principle still obtains, he cites the "laws of surfaces and volumes," which constrain the relations between the size, shape, and surface area of any organism. Another example is the way that food webs (almost) invariably exhibit a pyramidal structure due to the availability of energy as it moves through the food chain.

Of course, it is not only Darwinian contingency that is supposed to undermine attempts to find order and structure in the natural world, but also the more recently developed "chaos theory." As titles such as *Order Out of Chaos* (Prigogine and Stengers 1984) signify, however, what most impresses writers in this field is not chaos as such, but the order that manages to coexist with it. Nor should the chaotic be confused with the random, for it is possible to give an entirely deterministic rendering of chaos theory, with all unpredictability being attributed to sensitivity to initial conditions. Moreover, we think we know of mechanisms that serve to dampen the effects of variation in initial conditions. One such mechanism is redundancy, a phenomenon that has been observed both at the level of genes and at the level of functional descriptions of ecosystems. It also bears mention that some writers in the field find reason to attach special significance to the "edge" of chaos—a region dominated neither by order nor by chaos (Goodwin 1994, pp. 169-70). So the point about ecosystems in the larger picture is not that they are ordered, but that they exhibit just enough disorder to permit the characteristics of organisms and species as we know them to emerge (cf. Rolston 1987).

Two Interpretations of Integrity

Might we be able to avoid the problem of contingency altogether by adopting J. Karr's "historical" characterization of integrity as a "condition of minimum human influence" (Karr 1996)? For it does seem plausible to put some version of this condition at the theoretical heart of the concept of integrity. And some would claim that, besides providing an empirical point of reference for measuring human disturbance, the *normative* burden of the concept of integrity is to place a value upon nature that goes its "own way," regardless of whether that way exhibits order and structure or not. At the same time, as we shall see, this is not to say that the condition of minimum human influence exhausts the meaning of integrity, or that it is even a sufficient condition. Nor is it to say that such an understanding of integrity will everywhere serve as an operational guide. There needs also to be in place what I shall label, crudely, a "functional" understanding of integrity—the idea that natural systems are characterized by a range of conditions—relating to soil composition, species complements, mineral and nutrient cycling, trophic exchange, nature and rates of decomposition, and so forth—which are materially affected by human interventions. Let us consider some of the problems whose resolution points toward these conclusions.

First, some account needs to be given of why integrity matters. This is the problem Worster raises when he asks what there is to love or preserve in a universe of chaos. The trouble with love is that it can be blind, obdurate, and misplaced. We cannot therefore simply invite others to share our love of nature, without also undertaking the hard task of showing that, and why, nature is lovable. Now the objection is that if all that matters is that nature should go its own way, and it doesn't matter whether it goes this way or that, how can it matter whether we make it go the way that some humans want it to go? And even if some (other) humans want it the way it is, this is now simply a disagreement between some humans and others about what they want. In response to this problem, one can offer both moral and instrumental reasons for saving (i.e., loving and preserving) as much nonhuman nature as is possible. And both kinds of consideration carry weight. But the instrumental reason, at any rate, cannot rest merely on the historical notion of integrity. Any such argument must in addition be able to point to causally effective properties of natural systems that anthropogenic systems lack—certain life-support functions perhaps. Otherwise, the most that could be demonstrated would be the desirability, not the necessity, of integrity. In fact, for reasons touched on later, it may turn out to be unwise to rely exclusively on the moral and instrumental case. It may be worth holding out for the point that what is important *is* precisely the fact that nature goes its *own* way—not which way it goes—and that this is important even if, and probably because, it makes things uncomfortable for humans.

A second point to consider is that of human influence as opposed to, or as a part of, biological integrity. In a recent issue of *Environmental Values*, Baird Callicott poses to the integrity theorist this characteristically sharp dilemma concerning how to incorporate indigenous human influence into the definition of biological integrity: "Ignoring a significant influence on nature is bad natural science and regarding any group of people as wildlife is bad social science (as well as questionable ethics)" (1995, p. 357). In fact, the problem is not about indigenous peoples only, but a general problem about how to construe the implications of certain kinds of human impact, whether the humans in question are indigenous peoples or modern "eco-tourists." And this dilemma is itself part of a broader dilemma: whether to discount significant human influence (and be guilty of bad natural or social science), or to acknowledge it and be forced to admit that natural integrity is almost nowhere to be found, since very little of the globe is free from human influence. (The other side of the same problem is how to construe major disruptions occasioned by natural events such as earthquakes or hurricanes. If human influence is the sole source of disintegrity, then we must say that natural disasters leave integrity intact, even if their effects differ in no way from the effects of some human interventions.)

I believe that these critical challenges can be deflected, but not if we understand integrity exclusively in terms of minimum human influence. The following two strategies suggest themselves:

1. It is possible to distinguish between different *kinds* and *degrees* of human impact. Conceptually speaking, at any rate, there seems to be room for refining the notion of human impact by distinguishing different dimensions such as geographical extent, ecological range, depth, character, etc., and distinguishing between minimal and not so minimal impact along each dimension. Thus a distinction one might think important is between the kind of impact that allows the nonhuman world to respond for itself, and the kind of impact where humans themselves have a hand in shaping the response. To illustrate the point at the level of organisms, an urban fox, one might argue, is still nature responding for itself—albeit responding to the human presence; its activities still exhibit integrity. As the phenomenon of the "commuter fox" indicates, it has not lost its wild nature. Not so the labrador, deliberately rendered docile. To acknowledge the presence of integrity in the face of human influence is not, I suggest, a watering down of historical integrity, but a more modulated understanding of it. What does seem clear, however, is that to register differences in kind and degree of human influence, we shall need to appeal to an assortment of *functional* indicators.

2. It is also possible to distinguish between actual and potential integrity. On this view, even natural systems that have actually been modified (by humans) may be thought of as retaining integrity potentially, if the modification is not beyond nature's powers of recuperation. In a connected vein, it is commonly thought that on the historical view, integrity once lost is gone forever. But this judgment is perhaps too hasty, for integrity is not simply a matter of original cause, but also of ongoing process. So it is not clear why an initially significant human impact should not gradually lose its significance over time, in the wake of continuing natural processes. And here again, it is clear that underlying functional criteria must be used to establish when the human influence might have become "minimal" once more. (It should be noticed that neither of these suggested "modulations" involves resorting to a notion of "degrees" of integrity.)

A third difficulty with relying exclusively on the historical notion concerns contexts in which reference needs to be made to integrity hypothetically—when, for example, some project to restore integrity is mooted. The historical reading of integrity must speak, hypothetically, of "what this patch would be like without human influence." At worst, such an expression is incoherent. Since there *were* humans, one has to construct a hypothetical history beginning with some false or invented incident, and it is hard to see how this could count as the onset of a *natural* sequence. At best, this conception faces the problem of sensitivity to initial conditions. For whatever starting point is chosen, the onset of contingencies would quickly generate any number of plausible pathways leading to the present. To deal with hypothetical integrity, it seems that here, too, functional criteria must be used, albeit tentatively and provisionally.

Although it plays an important role in making integrity operational, nevertheless the functional reading should not be thought to provide defining properties or essential characteristics of integrity, nor as being what integrity consists of. The characteristics it identifies should be viewed as marks, signs, or indicators of integrity only. Otherwise, if it were held, with Odum, that the development of a natural ecosystem was "directed toward achieving as large and diverse an organic structure as is possible within the limits set by the available energy input," then all kinds of human intervention might be licensed as compatible with the demands of integrity. The first of two "cautionary tales" from the United Kingdom serves to illustrate the point. It concerns the proposal of Shell (U.K.) to sink the Brent Spar oil platform into the North Sea. A major problem with the proposal was the amount of metals contained in the tanks and ballast. In an article published in *Nature* (1995), Nisbet and Fowler observe that metals abound naturally on the ocean floor, especially around midocean-ridge hydrothermal systems. Accordingly, they argue that the metals of the Brent Spar "would not be out of the ordinary, and indeed might be beneficial as a mimic of vent activity." They claim as a result that "the addition of extra dumped metals would probably act as a nutrient to the local ecosystem." It is clear that the promotion of integrity, so understood, would run counter to the historical notion.

To understand how the historical and functional readings may combine and not conflict, it is important to see that the functional reading is not committed to any kind of "essentialist" view of natural processes. It is not being supposed, and need not be supposed, that what is being studied are inherent properties of natural processes, but rather, particular properties of a particular process, and what we might call its "near neighbors." Thus the functional reading is, I maintain, compatible with a purely *nominalistic* understanding of ecosystems as "sets of neighboring patches" (where "neighboring" refers to some notion of ecological, not geographical, closeness), and conformable therefore to the governing notion of contingency. Comparisons are then made with neighboring patches subject to varying degrees of human impact, and locally generalizable data derived about the effects of such impacts. (Darwin adopts a similar approach to the "monstrosity" of artificially selected types. He treats this not as a property of artificial types as such, but as a property of artificial types in relation to the species in nature "to which they are nearest allied" (1968, p. 74).

But in supposing that natural systems exhibit distinct characteristics in comparison with those of anthropogenic systems "to which they are nearest allied," are we guilty of incorporating a notion of direction in evolution that is not consistent with the presumption of radical contingency? Not if we distinguish between a "direction"—which presupposes a specific end point or destination, and a de facto "trend," which does not. The distinction can be illustrated with reference to the debate over whether evolution has exhibited a "trend" toward complexity (McShea 1991). Colin McGinn, in a review of *Darwin's Dangerous Idea* (by Daniel Dennett), suggests that the trend toward complexity in evolution is problematic since one would expect natural selection to favor simpler organisms (McGinn 1995). In regarding the situation as problematic, it appears that McGinn is construing the trend in question—whether the one that there "ought" to be, toward simplicity, or the one that there is, toward complexity—as having a direction. This is shown by the fact that he thinks the trend as such to require explanation. An alternative reading, however, is to regard the trend as a de facto trend, not requiring any explanation in its own right, but just coming about as the accumulation of individually explicable events. The point is that the detection of trends is sufficient to justify interventions when such trends are perceived to be "disturbed." Although there *might* also be directional processes in nature, we do not need to suppose that there are, in order to take human impact on natural systems with the utmost seriousness.

Functional measures of integrity in terms of structure, pattern, and trend, therefore, should not be taken to be what *constitute* integrity, just in case humans may get clever enough to create anthropogenic systems that simulate whatever "measures" of integrity of this kind ecologists produce. Nor should they be taken as sufficient conditions of integrity, as the cautionary tale of the Brent Spar indicates. They are however, *indispensable* for plotting the presence and extent of human impact and therefore measuring the extent to which we are succeeding in allowing nature to "go its own way." The historically oriented condition of minimal human influence likewise does not fully capture the concept of integrity, nor can it guide us in what to do in situations that lack integrity. Thus both understandings of integrity are necessary, but neither is sufficient by itself for making integrity operational.

How Much Integrity Do We Need?

My contention is that it is unwise to attempt to answer the question, How much integrity do we need? and that we should attempt instead to answer a different question. There are several reasons for refusing to answer the question as given.

First, it would create the entirely misleading impression that it is possible to attain some measure of precision and accuracy about such things. The fact is that we live in a world increasingly characterized by radical uncertainty and indeterminacy, in which (1) the size, gravity, extent, and likelihood of impacts are difficult or impossible to predict or estimate; (2) even innocent and justifiable actions can conspire to produce devastating consequences that are slow to materialize, are cumulative in their effects, and combine in unpredictable ways; and (3) resulting harms become less and less specific, as do assignable agents of harm. Given this account of our current human predicament, the attempt to quantify the amount of integrity required to serve human needs is bound to be virtually meaningless.

The second reason concerns the perils of quantification as such, both for environmentalists and for policymakers more generally. The point can be illustrated by a second "cautionary tale" from the United Kingdom. In its attempt to get reductions in the Thames Water Company's extraction of water from boreholes near the river Kennet, the English Environment Agency produced figures suggesting that the "nonuse value" that would accrue from increasing the river flow might be as high as £13.2 million. The water company contested the figures and there was a public inquiry. The inquiry inspector ruled against the Environment Agency and slashed the crucial figure attached to nonuse value from £13.2 million to a mere £0.3 million (ENDS 1998). In a competition over figures where the rules are unclear, private companies usually have the advantage over public agencies of being able to hire more and better-paid economists. It is not unreasonable to fear that similar disputes will develop over ecologists' figures, especially if the ecologists are asked to make judgments about human needs. And it is hard to believe that this will result in good policy making.

A third and more substantive reason is that the answer to the question, How much integrity do we need? is radically indeterminable, not because integrity is unfathomable, but because needs are. It depends upon who "we" are, and how our needs are specified—in other words, upon conceptions of what makes life worthwhile. Among the less calculable determinants of a worthwhile life, for example, is the question of what risks it is acceptable to ask people to bear. And even an apparently straightforward determinant such as freedom from disease creates insoluble problems, since we do not know what diseases lie around the corner, nor what is needed or what it would cost to eradicate them. Similar reasoning suggests the need for caution before making instrumental claims, on scientific grounds, that ecological integrity is indispensable for the health and well-being of the human race. At any rate, it is hard to see how such claims can be substantiated without some account also being offered of the requirements for a decent human life.

A fourth and final reason is that to ask ecologists to calibrate integrity in relation to needs is to suppose that the demands resulting from and associated with present socioeconomic systems are an acceptable touchstone by which to set levels of integrity. However, it is only because we have reason to believe that present socioeconomic demands are not sustainable (and therefore not acceptable) that we are bothering to ask questions of this kind in the first place. The same reasoning, again, should make us wary of setting too much store by notions of environmental sustainability and ecosystem health. Holmes Rolston remarks with some justice that "what sustainably gets people fed . . . can and probably will sacrifice a great deal of biodiversity" (1998, p. 351). The great risk in espousing environmental sustainability as the touchstone for environmental policy is that it protects the natural world just insofar as, and in the form that, it has the capacity to sustain human economic systems—or more precisely, in whatever form makes the relation between ecological and economic systems sustainable. And without some stand being taken on the character of the economic system in question, this requirement contains no guarantee of the continuance of the wild world. The special virtue of the principle of integrity, for an environmentalist, is that it clearly and unambiguously defends nature in its own right—the idea of nature going its own way.

Accordingly, rather than attempt to answer the question, How much integrity do we need? we should seek instead to answer the question, How much forbearance does the nonhuman world require to retain its integrity? We should seek, in other words, to answer the question in terms of what is required to enable (what remains of) the wild world to go its own way, free from any significant human direction and significant human impact. Thus to ensure the continuation of old-growth forests, Foster et al. observe that "these areas must be maintained within a landscape that is adequate in size to allow for the continuing mosaic of disturbance and for the dispersal of organisms and processes among patches" (1996, pp. 421-22). Specifications of what is required will, of course, have all the provisional and revisable status that is the hallmark of scientific inquiry, and may not be free of cultural judgment, but will at least be free of the need to engage in cultural speculation. The relevant data will specify requirements for maintaining viable populations, representative varieties of community types, and so forth. The specifications will also use data on nutrient loss, changes in energy capture, trophic exchange, and suchlike, gathered from comparative studies of similar areas that have undergone differential human impact—the sort of data supplied elsewhere in this volume.

Conclusion

Environmentalists are right to protest the depiction of our predicament as a matter of choosing between nature and jobs, or nature and health. It is arguable, however, that they give too many hostages to fortune by claiming that a particular amount of natural integrity is a necessary condition for jobs and health. The reason is that the amount of integrity required is radically conditional upon the kind of conception people have of a worthwhile human life. Of course, policymakers would dearly love their decisions to be made for them by scientists. But what makes life worthwhile is an ethical and political question, not a scientific one. A wiser strategy is to engage in the normative debate about what makes human life worthwhile, and insist that, from the standpoint of practical wisdom—a standpoint that strives to look long term and take a full range of factors into account—the named and nonnegotiable presence of the nonhuman is constitutive of a superior ideal of the human good. At the same time one can insist that this is precisely not to abandon the fight against poverty, hunger, and disease, because this fight is not best conducted by appropriating more and more of the natural world, but by dealing with its social, economic, institutional, and political causes. One can certainly add that there are independent moral reasons for protecting nature, but it always seems likely that such reasons will be canceled out by short-term appeals to the human suffering that might be alleviated if we forgo such protection. Moreover, it always seems likely that both kinds of moral appeal will themselves be submerged by broader social goals. One may like to think that moral claims silence (or ought to silence) all other claims. But the truth may be something less: that moral claims cannot be silenced. They can, however, be ignored. The French will continue to line their avenues with poplar trees, even though they know for certain that it costs human lives to do so, when the trees fall into the path of vehicles.

The claim of integrity therefore needs to be placed in a larger sociopolitical context, even though this is a strategy that no doubt has its risks—of distraction, and of misappropriation by other agendas. But my belief is that the case for nature is certain to be lost if any other strategy is adopted. The problem with relying on notions such as "ecosystem health" or "environmental sustainability" to carry the flag for nature is precisely that they leave conceptions of the worthwhile life untouched: the aim of perpetuating an environment that is capable of supporting a tolerable human life indefinitely does not guarantee a place for the natural world—for it is certainly conceivable, and probably true, that many people's notions of a decent human life will find little if any role for the nonhuman world. And as Mark Sagoff has argued, there are those who believe that humans could *only* live tolerable lives in a world that was domesticated through and through. Conversion of the whole planet into the niche of *Homo sapiens* is one of the most depressing prospects it is possible to imagine. But, in a version of Hardin's "tragedy of the commons," it is too easy to imagine the series of entirely plausible, reasonable—and even morally admirable—steps that would bring this about.

REFERENCES

Bethell, T. 1989. "Darwin's Mistake." In *Philosophy of Biology*, edited by M. Ruse, 85–92. London: Macmillan.

Callicott, J. B. 1995. "The Value of Ecosystem Health." *Environmental Values* 4: 345–361.

Darwin, C. 1968 [1859]. *The Origin of Species*. Harmondsworth: Penguin.

———. 1984 [1842]. *The Structure and Distribution of Coral Reefs*. Tucson: University of Arizona Press.

Dawkins, R. 1988. *The Blind Watchmaker*. Harmondsworth: Penguin.

ENDS [Environmental Data Services (UK)]. 1998. "Water Abstraction Decision Deals Savage Blow to Cost-Benefit Analysis." *ENDS Report* 278 (March): 16–18.

Foster, D. R., D. A. Orwig, and J. S. McLachlan. 1996. "Ecological and Conservation Insights from Reconstructive Studies of Temperate Old-Growth Forests." *TREE* 11, no. 10: 419–424.

Goodwin, B. 1994. *How the Leopard Changed Its Spots*. London: Weidenfeld & Nicolson.

Gould, S. J. 1980. "Darwin's Untimely Burial." In *Ever Since Darwin*. Harmondsworth: Penguin.

———. S. J. 1991. *Wonderful Life*. Harmondsworth: Penguin.

Karr, J. R. 1996. "Ecological Integrity and Ecological Health Are Not the Same." In *Engineering within Ecological Constraints*, edited by P. C. Schulze, 97–109. Washington, DC: National Academy Press.

Kauffman, S. 1996. *At Home in the Universe*. Harmondsworth: Penguin.

Manser, A. 1965. "The Concept of Evolution." *Philosophy* 40: 18–34.

McGinn, C. 1995. "Left-Over Life to Live." *Times Literary Supplement* (November 24): 3–4.

McShea, D. W. 1991. "Complexity and Evolution: What Everybody Knows." *Biology and Philosophy* 6: 303–324.

Nisbet, E. G., and C. M. R. Fowler. 1995. "Is Metal Disposal Toxic to Deep Oceans?" *Nature* 375 (June 29): 715.

Ollason, J. G. 1991. "What Is This Stuff Called Fitness?" *Biology and Philosophy* 6: 81–92.

Prigogine, I., and I. Stengers. 1984. *Order out of Chaos*. New York: Bantam.

Ridley, M. 1985. *The Problems of Evolution*. Oxford: Oxford University Press.

———. 1989. "The Cladistic Solution to the Species Problem." *Biology and Philosophy* 4: 1–16.

Rolston, H. 1979. "Can, and Ought We to Follow Nature?" *Environmental Ethics* 1: 7–30.

———. 1987. "Duties to Ecosystems." In *Companion to A Sand County Almanac*, edited by J. B. Callicott, 246–274. Madison: University of Wisconsin Press.

———. 1998. "Saving Nature, Feeding People, and the Foundations of Ethics." *Environmental Values* 7: 349–357.

Sagoff, M. 1997. "Muddle or Muddle Through? Takings Jurisprudence Meets the Endangered Species Act." *William and Mary Law Review* 38, no. 3: 825–993.

Shimony, A. 1989. "The Non-Existence of a Principle of Natural Selection." *Biology and Philosophy* 4: 255–273.

Waters, C. K. 1986. "Natural Selection without Survival of the Fittest." *Biology and Philosophy* 1: 207–225.

Worster, D. 1990. "The Ecology of Order and Chaos." *Environmental History Review* 14: 1–18.

Ecosystem Design in Historical and Philosophical Context

Mark Sagoff

The tombstone of Walter Savage Landor, an English poet and essayist, bears the epitaph, "Nature I loved, and next to Nature, Art."[1] Poets, theologians, and scientists in the eighteenth and nineteenth centuries thought that Nature had much in common with Art—indeed, as God's creation, Nature was a kind of Art. Alexander Pope, in his "Essay on Man," captured as follows the eighteenth-century conception of the hierarchical organization with which the Creator had endowed the natural world:

> Vast chain of being! which from God began,
> Natures aethereal, human, angel, man,
> Beast, bird, fish, insect, what no eye can see . . .
> Where, one step broken, the great scale destroyed
> From Nature's chain whatever link you strike,
> Tenth, or ten thousandth, breaks the chain alike.

According to eighteenth-century sensibilities, God displayed his beneficence to man by designing nature to serve human needs. Accordingly, humanity should respect and protect the self-sustaining plan on which God created the living world or risk Armageddon—the terrible consequences we now associate with ecological collapse.

In this same vein, contemporary biologists, such as Paul Ehrlich, warn us that species work like rivets holding together the ecological airplane that supports all life. The insight that God does nothing in vain—that the living world conforms to a hierarchical, self-regulating, mathematical plan—connects the insights of "Great Chain of Being"[2] cosmology with the findings of biologists, ecologists, and other scientists today.

The Design of Living Systems

This chapter attempts to examine in historical and philosophical perspective two opposed approaches ecologists and others have taken to understand the design of living systems. The first approach, which has roots as far back as Lucretius and more recent antecedents in Charles Darwin and John Stuart Mill, denies that ecological communities or systems exhibit any kind of design at all. To be sure, species are shaped by natural selection. Evolution accounts for their structural and functional properties. No such organizing force or principle, however, applies to the arrangement of plants and animals in communities or ecosystems. From this perspective, nature pursues no purpose, embodies no end, and develops in no direction. Unifying principles and concepts in ecology, such as "autocatalysis," "homeostasis," "exergy," and "integrity," may have theological but not biological significance. Nature has no essence; it has a history.

Ecologists who favor this cautious approach often work as detectives might to trace the causal paths that produce phenomena of interest. They gather specimens, construct experiments, and record observations in order to explain in terms of natural history the biological goings-on at a specific place. The result of this kind of inductive inquiry may be a thick description of a site, an explanation of a puzzling event (the decline of a species of frog, for example), or a rich historical narrative. By appreciating the contingency, indeed, the improbability, of ecological phenomena, these biologists help us appreciate the wonder of nature, and they increase our reverence for life.

The second approach, which takes up themes that stretch from Neoplatonic sources, particularly Plotinus, to poets and theologians of the eighteenth century, seeks reasons beyond the contingency of local affairs to explain the abundance and distribution of plants and animals. To discover the patterns and principles that underlie ecological phenomena, ecologists who take this view elaborate general theoretical models that explain how nature works. As James H. Brown has written, these ecologists believe "there is a common conceptual basis for linking activities of species with biogeochemical processes. It has not yet been well developed, however, because it represents a new kind of integration between the biological and physical sciences."[3]

The problem with unifying mathematical models and concepts in ecology, such as those Brown calls for, however, is that there are so many of them. Theoreticians have proposed a myriad of mathematical approaches to serve as "the common conceptual basis" needed to integrate the ecological and other phenomena. Brown himself has suggested that ecological phenomena are explicable under the laws and principles that govern "complex adaptive systems."[4] In the 1960s E. P. Odum described a universal "strategy of ecosystem development" replete with homeostasis, feedback mechanisms, and equilibria "directed toward achieving as large and diverse an organic structure as possible within the limits set by the available energy input and prevailing physical conditions of existence."[5] Robert Sterner of the University of Minnesota, in contrast, has written that stoichiometry "is a framework that serves to organize a set of otherwise disparate observations about biological systems."[6]

Peter Yodzis of the University of Guelph emphasizes "multiple domains of attraction" and "deterministic dynamics."[7] Robert Ulanowicz at the University of Maryland has proposed a conception of "ascendency" to measure "both the size and the organizational status of the network exchanges that occur in an ecosystem."[8] Sven Jorgensen, a Danish ecologist, offered "the maximum exergy hypothesis" to explain ecosystem reactions as increasing exergy. Michael Conrad of Wayne State described the ecosystem as an "existential computer" concatenating an "elaborate hierarchy of informational processes."[9] In their zeal to create new mathematical "paradigms" and achieve novel conceptual breakthroughs, theoretical ecologists do not pause very often to test any of them or even show how they may be tested.

Models and mathematical theories in ecology might be easier to test if agreed-upon ways existed to define ecosystems and to reidentify them through time and change. It is easy for any theory to be true of the ecosystem it defines—since the definition can always change or adjust to save the phenomena. To say that an ecosystem is "self-organizing," for example, is to presuppose some criterion for determining when that system remains the same thing through change and when it changes so much that it becomes something else. A theory can always prove an ecosystem is "self-organizing," because, if the ecosystem no longer meets the criterion, whatever it may be, the theory can claim that it no longer remains "the same ecosystem."

"Despite the importance of self-identity," Steward Pickett and colleagues have written, "there is no consensus on how to define and measure it." Instead, ecologists assume that ecosystems are "given as such in nature" and "therefore have to be found and identified instead of being defined and delimited."[10] Each theory may define the ecosystem differently, so that the ecological object becomes an artifact of the theory, which is as a result true of it. Ecologists F. Gilbert and J. Owen conclude that relationships in ecological communities that theorists posit are largely imaginary. What structure had been thought to exist is merely "a biological epiphenomenon, a statistical abstraction, a descriptive convention without true emergent properties but only collective ones."[11]

This chapter is organized into the following parts. First, it reviews some of the reasons that Charles Darwin and John Stuart Mill believed that living nature has no design beyond or above the level of the organism. The chapter then considers problems theoreticians encounter in ascribing integrating concepts to ecosystems, for example, the difficulty of defining or delimiting ecosystems in ways that do not reduce these ascriptions to tautologies. The chapter traces to a particular view in the philosophy of science the belief that order or organization underlies the apparent contingency of ecological events. The challenge to theoretical ecology posed by reductionist approaches is next described. The chapter concludes by recalling the historical role of philosophers, poets, and others in reflecting on the findings of the natural sciences.

Darwin and Historical Explanation

In the third chapter of *The Origin of Species*, Darwin describes the "Complex Relations of all Animals and Plants to each other in the Struggle for Existence." He notes that the slightest change—the introduction of a single species, for example—can radically alter the course of natural history. "In Staffordshire," Darwin writes,

> there was a large and extremely barren heath, which had never been touched by the hand of man; but several hundred acres of exactly the same nature had been enclosed twenty-five years previously and planted with Scotch fir. The change in the native vegetation of the planted part of the heath was most remarkable, more than is generally seen in passing from one quite different soil to another: not only the proportional numbers of the heath-plants were wholly changed, but twelve species of plants (not counting grasses and carices) flourished in the plantations, which could not be found on the heath. The effect on the insects must have been still greater, for six insectivorous birds were very common in the plantations, which were not to be seen on the heath. . . . Here we see how potent has been the effect of the introduction of a single tree, nothing whatever else having been done.[12]

In this passage, Darwin observes that the introduction of a single species turned a barren heath into a rich forest community. What principle of ecological organization, succession, development, or integrity might this example illustrate? To answer such a question, we would need to know whether the heath disappeared and was replaced by a forest or whether it simply became a forest while remaining the same ecosystem. If the former, we should say that the heath was an unstable system, possibly because it lacked diversity, since the appearance of a single new species caused its demise. If the latter, the heath might exhibit a great deal of resilience and stability insofar as it increased in richness and diversity in response to the introduction. Does it make a difference that the Scotch fir did not volunteer but was planted? Would the ecosystem have retained its essential design had the fir alighted there naturally rather than by the hand of man?

Darwin never asked these questions or thought them worth asking. He did not see any reason to believe that what we now call ecosystems had a design—or even an identity—to be theorized about. Darwin distinguished between inanimate objects, the behavior of which conforms to mathematical laws of nature, and collections of living organisms, which he thought follow a contingent historical path. Darwin draws this distinction while reflecting on a landscape cleared by AmerIndians.

> Throw up a handful of feathers, and all fall to the ground according to definite laws; but how simple is the problem where each shall fall compared to that of the action and reaction of the innumerable plants and animals which have determined, in the course of centuries, the proportional numbers and kinds of trees now growing on the old Indian ruins![13]

It would be a mistake to infer from this passage that Darwin considered the explanation of the trajectory of the falling feathers to differ only in degree of complexity from the explanation of the numbers and kinds of trees on the Indian burial ground. On the contrary, he thought the two explanations differed not in degree of complexity but in kind. The falling of the feathers instantiates timeless laws of nature; the fate of the forest, Darwin thought, results from the unpredictable vicissitudes of contingent events.

Darwin approached the study of the abundance and distribution of plants and animals as a historical science like geology, paleontology, or anthropology. These historical sciences, as paleontologist Stephen J. Gould has written, avoid mathematical deduction while "treating immensely complex and nonrepeatable events (and therefore eschewing prediction while seeking explanation for what has happened) and using the methods of observation and comparison."[14] Evolutionary biologists such as Gould have proposed that nature works by a sort of make-do, catch-as-catch-can tinkering[15] and, accordingly, that its phenomena may be understood largely in terms of local, ephemeral accidents.[16] Gould advocates thick description, in the sense Clifford Geertz gives to this method, to explain ecological phenomena in terms of the contingencies of time and place.[17]

Darwin's great accomplishment was to show how the forces of random mutation and natural selection could explain the traits of particular plants and animals, for example, the nearly perfect way a finch's beak was formed to fit a particular seed upon which the bird fed. Darwin understood that plants and animals evolve in association with one another. He attributed the course of these dependencies, however, not to higher-level principles but to the contingencies of time and place. Thus Darwin would reject the idea that ecosystems evolve. Natural selection and random mutation, the creative forces of evolution, apply only to objects that breed true, that is, to things that reproduce. Since ecosystems have no genomes, their evolution cannot be explained in terms of random mutation or natural selection but only by appeal to some independent, creative force.

Mill on Nature

In 1850, the year after Landor wrote his "Dying Speech of the Old Philosopher," John Stuart Mill, then 44, started to publish the writings he would later collect under the title *Three Essays on Religion*. In the first of these essays, "On Nature," Mill questioned the Romantic view that nature exhibits an order or plan. He wanted in part to refute the well-known argument from design, which infers the existence of God from the orderliness of the natural world. Biologists in the nineteenth century would have been unable to account for design in nature or elsewhere without presupposing the existence of a designer. After all, if in the forest you come upon a piano or a watch, you would not say it was self-organizing. Similarly, if the forest itself turned out to be intelligibly arranged or designed, this, too, would point to the existence of a beneficent Creator.[18]

Rather than concede this argument for the existence of God, Mill wrote that nature is "too clumsily made and capriciously governed" to justify the attribution of order, purpose, or design to its spontaneous course. "In sober truth," Mill declared, "nearly all the things which men are hanged or imprisoned for doing to one another, are nature's every day performances. Killing, the most criminal act recognized by human laws, Nature does once to every being that lives; and in a large proportion of cases, after protracted tortures such as only the greatest monsters whom we read of ever purposely inflicted on their living fellow-creatures."[19] How could so vicious an arrangement be thought of as the creation of a beneficent deity?

To make his argument, Mill distinguished between two senses of the term "nature." First, the term "nature" may refer to everything in the universe, that is, everything to which the laws of physics apply. In this context, the "natural" constitutes the opposite of the "supernatural." Second, "nature" may refer to the spontaneous arrangement of things, that is, to all that which is independent of or unaffected by human agency. If nature remains unfallen and uncorrupted, human beings, especially in pursuit of profit, may disturb its inherent order, that is, its original integrity. The idea of the "natural," in this context, is defined in terms of its significant opposite, the "artificial" or "cultural."

Mill asks whether nature in either of these senses possesses a design, organization, order, or—as we might say—an "integrity." Does nature, either in the sense of "everything" or in the sense of "untouched by mankind," embody patterns, follow principles, or display uniformities that humanity should reckon with and respect?

The answer is plainly affirmative insofar as we refer to nature in the sense of "everything in the world." The laws of nature—for example, of gravitation and motion—apply to human beings as to all objects. In this context, however, the admonition to "obey nature" or "design with nature," while excellent advice, would be unnecessary, since no one can perform miracles today. By knowing and taking advantage of the laws of physics, humanity can command nature, as it were, only by obeying it. Mill concludes:

> To bid people to conform to the laws of nature when they have no power but what the laws of nature give them—when it is a physical impossibility for them to do the smallest thing otherwise than through some law of nature—is an absurdity. The thing they need to be told is, what particular law of nature they should make use of in a particular case.[20]

Now consider the term "nature" in the sense in which it means not everything that happens, but only that which takes place without human agency. Recently, environmental writer Bill McKibben framed this conception of nature in terms of that which is free of human influence. In his appropriately titled book, *The End of Nature*, McKibben described the view from his window looking out on an Adirondack forest:

> What happens in here I control; what happens out there has always been the work of some independent force. . . . In our modern minds nature and humanity are separate things. It is this separate nature I am talking about when I use the word—nature.[21]

Mill asks if humanity should follow the design of nature in this sense, in other words, to preserve rather than to alter nature's spontaneous course. He answers that the injunction to respect nature in the sense of maintaining its spontaneous course "is not merely, as it is in the other sense, superfluous and unmeaning, but contradictory." Human beings cannot at once live and leave nature alone. Mill explains:

> For while human action cannot help conforming to Nature in the one meaning of the term, the very aim and object of action is to alter and improve Nature in the other meaning. If the natural course of things were perfectly right and satisfactory, to act at all

would be a gratuitous meddling, which as it could not make things better, must make them worse. . . . If the artificial is not better than the natural, to what end are all the arts of life? To dig, to plough, to build, to wear clothes, are direct infringements of the injunction to follow Nature.[22]

To benefit themselves, Mill thought, human beings have to alter nature. For example, plant and animal breeding had greatly transformed virtually every food Mill's contemporaries ate and every flower and shrub they planted in their gardens. (In the United States today, very little remains of the ecosystems that greeted the early settlers, for example, in New England.[23]) Many of the changes human beings make in the natural world—by polluting water, for example—are counterproductive or even destructive. Mill understood this, of course. He denied, however, that the natural is normative—that we do better overall or as a rule to leave nature alone than to alter it for our use.

According to Mill, the distinction between Nature "out there" and nature we control can be a moral or theological but not a biological one. Mill did not argue that the design of what we call ecosystems can somehow be "reduced" to the physical sciences; rather, like Darwin, he denied that they had any particular order, goal, tendency, or purpose on which such a reduction might be attempted. Of course, if God (the independent force McKibben mentions) created ecosystems for some purpose or to some end, one could speak of their function, their structure, their organization, and their integrity. We would look for the key to nature's ecological order, however, in scripture, not in science.

According to religious sentiment, Mill wrote, "whatever man does to improve his condition is . . . a thwarting of the spontaneous order of Nature" and therefore "probably offensive" to the Supreme Being "of whose will the course of nature was supposed to be the expression."[24] Mill would see no reason to distinguish between the Great Chain of Being cosmology of his time and the models of hierarchy, stoichiometry, or ascendency that theoretical ecologists elaborate today. The theological presuppositions of all of these theories of nature's integrity or design would seem to Mill to be about the same.

What Is a Living System?

Theoretical ecologists today seek to define ecosystem-level properties, but they are in no better position than Darwin to identify ecosystems, delimit them, or determine under what conditions they survive change. As Simon

Levin points out, "[E]cosystems are not uniquely identified entities, nor are they defined by sharp boundaries. Instead, they are loosely defined assemblages that exhibit characteristic patterns on a range of scales of time, space, and organization complexity."[25]

The oxymoron "loosely defined" may be taken as a euphemism for undefined or constructed *in silico* (on a computer) to illustrate or vindicate a particular theory. Each theory interprets data to find the "signal" beneath the "noise"; each makes its own decision about which phenomena are incidental and which are essential to the persistence of the ecosystem. Each theory constructs the system in its own way—so that what is "signal" to one theorist may be "noise" to the other.

Consider an example. In one study, Robert Ulanowicz writes: "In the absence of overwhelming external disturbances, living systems exhibit a natural propensity to increase in ascendency."[26] In this hypothesis, what counts as a "living system"? Any organism, for example, any animal or plant, would count as a living system. Organisms show a natural propensity to senescence and death, and this differs from ascendency. In any event, as ecologist Volker Grimm has written, "Organisms and ecological systems do not share the same ontological status." Grimm observes: "Organisms have clearly defined boundaries and can be said to have a clear objective: to produce as many reproducing offspring as possible. By contrast, ecological systems usually have no clear boundaries, and they have no objective or purpose. It is, therefore, generally accepted among ecologists that the analogy of ecological systems to organisms cannot be accepted."[27]

What counts as a "living system" besides organisms such as plants and animals? Perhaps nothing does. Perhaps anything counts as a living system if it contains living things. Perhaps some assemblages constitute living systems while others do not. Consider the following: a toxic waste dump; a rotting garbage pail rampant with rodents; a latrine after months of use in hot weather; a yeast infection; a head full of lice; a school system; a transportation system; a banking system. Which of these are and which are not "living systems" for purposes of testing the hypothesis that living systems possess some property (e.g., dynamic equilibrium) or progress in some direction (e.g., ascendency)? What criterion tells us that one place where life goes on is a "living system," but another place is not?

Theoretical ecology differs from inductive natural history precisely insofar as it posits universal generalizations of the form, "All S is P," where "S" refers to some kind of object (living system) and "is P" refers to some property or predicate ("tends toward ascendency"). The requirement imposed by epistemology is that the subject "S" must be defined independently of the predicate "is P." This is a requirement because the predicate "is P" must designate an empirical, not a logical, property of the system. Otherwise, ecology is not an empirical science. Having met that single epistemological requirement, the scientist tests his or her theory on examples of "S" least likely to have the property "is P"—and this makes references to cesspools, pig farms, and rotting carcasses relevant.

Since ecologists have no agreed-upon method of reidentifying living systems, communities, mosaics, patches, or what-have-you through time and change, they cannot empirically test generalizations about them. Rather, these generalizations—e.g., all living systems exhibit a natural propensity to increase in ascendency—follow logically from the background theory that decides what counts as a living system (e.g., a lake but not a lavatory) and how to reidentify that system through time and change. Absent an independent criterion for identifying and reidentifying an ecosystem, theoretical models cannot be falsified because they entail the qualities they profess to discover. They offer analytic, not empirical truths—that is, tautologies that may satisfy moral or religious predilections but would wither in the glare of skepticism.

Theory in Ecology

Simon Levin, a prominent mathematical ecologist who teaches at Princeton, spoke for many of his mathematically inclined colleagues when he wrote that general theory constitutes the indispensable framework for ecological science. Levin and others argue that mathematical theory in ecology "provides an antidote to the helpless feeling engendered by the view that nature is so complicated, and evolutionary processes so contingent on accident and history, that all we can ever hope to achieve is detailed understanding of specific situations . . . rather than any general rules and patterns."[28]

Now, many field ecologists may not agree that they experience a "helpless feeling" as they try, like detectives, to determine the specific causes of particular ecological phenomena. Indeed, the detailed understanding of specific situations is often exactly what society needs in order to find solutions to particular problems, for example, the decline of some endangered plant or animal. Rather than experiencing the helpless feeling that all they can do is natural history, many empirical ecologists assume that just this kind of patient and careful observation provides the basis for any empirical science.

Natural historians, even if they do not feel helpless, however, may be daunted by the amount of work that is involved in the careful observation of a site over time. After all, field biologists must observe a site long enough and well enough, first, to recognize the details that others do not easily see;

second, to observe details that even they did not initially see; and, third, to infer details that no one can see. This activity often takes years, decades, and longer, as in the exemplary research of Peter and Rosemary Grant, who found that genetic changes in different breeds of finches can be modeled mathematically, although the evolutionary path of these birds cannot be predicted, because it depends on the vagaries of climate, weather, invasions, and other contingent events.[29]

The theoretical ecologist, in contrast, is often able to discover predictive rules and patterns in a matter of moments. A mathematical model of a particular ecosystem, from which to deduce its structural and functional properties, may require little more than the choice of software, while any number of general models of any ecosystem can be generated by applying equations drawn from other sciences—information theory, optimization theory, cybernetics, oscillation theory, or whatever. Not only is theorizing faster, easier, and more convenient than empirical work—for example, one does not have to leave the office to do it—but the rewards are far greater. A. O. Hirschman explains:

> Several factors are responsible for the compulsion to theorize, which is often so strong as to induce mindlessness. In the academy, the prestige of the theorist is towering.[30]

Hirschman points out that policymakers cannot wait for the results of slow, painstaking empirical research; they need immediately to understand in mathematical terms "reality and its 'laws of change.'" As a result of these various factors, the quick theoretical fix has taken its place in our culture alongside the quick technical fix."[31]

The plethora of theory in ecology, however, has drawn two kinds of criticism. First, critics note that theory-building goes on apart from and seems to bear no relationship to empirical work in ecology. For example, in his recent *Primer of Ecological Theory*, Jonathan Roughgarden includes virtually no mention of any particular species or ecological site; he does not encumber his abstract mathematical models with any sense that they are to be tested. "I am not going to discuss much data in this book," writes the author of another typical introduction to theoretical ecology. "I am just going to discuss theory . . . and will leave it to each reader to fill in examples from his or her other studies in biology and ecology, and experience of particular organisms."[32] E. O. Wilson delightfully characterized theoretical speculations of this kind as follows: "One gets the feeling he is receiving secrets of the universe from a space visitor anxious to be on his way."[33]

A second difficulty with theory in ecology is that there is so much of it. Theorists themselves complain, with Simon Levin, of "a glut of mathematical publications, often neither good mathematics nor good biology."[34]

Levin himself noted, "[M]uch of mathematical ecology is simply mathematics dressed up as biology, and is dismissed by field biologists as being of no relevance to their interests."[35] Lev Ginzburg goes further:

> [O]ur journals are full of stability conditions, often expressed in terms of the eigenvalues of unknown matrices, diversity and complexity measures having very little to do with reality and a growing number of "theorems" which, I suspect, appear in publications on theoretical biology because they are too trivial for a mathematical journal.[36]

If ecologists believe their science is already burdened with too much theory, why do they produce more and more of it? The reason, apparently, lies in their philosophy of science. Some ecologists argue that patient, inductive research, even if it results in historical narratives that explain the causes of phenomena, does not count as science, which must promulgate universal mathematical models. Canadian ecologist Robert H. Peters, for one, argues that insofar as ecology is a science, it must discover "a set of theories that make simple, quantitative, and reasonably accurate predictions of biological phenomena."[37] Levin agrees: "To the theoretician, models are a part of the real world. In studying the logical consequences of assumptions, the theoretician is discovering, not inventing."[38]

The purpose of ecological science, according to Jack B. Waide, is to provide "a comprehensive synthetic theory of the ecosystem."[39] A scientist, Peters agrees, "explains an observation by showing that the observation could have been predicted by an existing theory or law." He declares, "Ecology is not to be confused with natural history." It is "a science intent on the development and assessment of objective scientific theory."[40] Peters concludes, "[H]istorical explanations have their legitimate purposes but we gain nothing by confusing these with science."[41]

The faith that the ecological is orderly—that it manifests an intelligible design to be captured by general mathematical models—is consistent with centuries of theological doctrine. Theologians have argued that God does not play dice or, if he did, the dice are loaded in our favor. Those who maintain this faith today, like Peters, insist on general mathematical models as the characteristic of science. Of course, once nature has been corrupted by human activity, it no longer may manifest its original design, and thus the theory may no longer apply. To think otherwise—to suppose that all nature is one—would be to reduce ecology to the study not of natural history but of genetics, chemistry, physics, and so on. The factory farm, the toxic dump, and the sewage treatment plant would then follow the same scientific principles and thus count as ecosystems—with just as much design, order, and integrity as the Edenic communities they pollute and replace.

The Reductionist Challenge to Theoretical Ecology

Biotechnologists—including silviculturalists, aquaculturalists, and agro-ecosystem engineers who work for bioindustrial giants such as Monsanto and Novartis—do not study theoretical or mathematical ecology. They are more likely to master methods of gene transfer, tissue culture, growth hormone morphology, protoplast fusion, somatic embryogenesis, microbial inoculation, photosynthetic efficiency enhancement, monoclonal antibody development, cloning, somaclonal variation, and batch fermentation processing, among many other techniques that teach nature new tricks. Rather than concern themselves with mathematical models describing nature's spontaneous course, biotechnologists fabricate large-scale, computer-managed, vertically integrated, genetically recombined, patented agri-aqua-silvicultural bioindustrial systems. One commentator has said, "The living world can now be viewed as a vast organic Lego kit inviting combination, hybridization, and continual rebuilding. Life is manipulability."[42]

Accordingly, some ecologists have identified biotechnology as the future of their science. Frank Forcella has written in the *Bulletin of the Ecological Society of America*:

> Ecologists are the people most fit to develop the conceptual directions of biotechnology. We are the ones who should have the best ideas as to what successful plants and animals should look like and how they should behave, both individually and collectively. Armed with such expertise, . . . should we take the forefront in biotechnology, and provide the rationale for choosing species, traits, and processes to be engineered? I suspect this latter approach will be more profitable for the world at large as well as for ourselves.[43]

The distinction Mill drew between two conceptions of nature helps us frame the dilemma biotechnology poses to ecological theory. Mill distinguished between two senses of the word "nature"—the first refers to everything under the sun, and the second refers only to that which has been affected by human agency. If ecologists believe their science embraces nature in the first sense, then they would have to endorse the reductionist, mechanistic, or materialistic approach associated with biotechnology and environmental engineering. After all, biotechnologists have shown they can construct biological systems to fit commercial specifications, for example, to increase yields of fish, flesh, and fiber. The rather unsentimental and unmathematical methods of bench biotechnologists can make nature yield virtually anything. The reductionist approach biotechnology takes toward nature gets results, at least if the falling prices of crops suggest anything. To the extent that they get marketable results rewarding investment, biotechnologists succeed where ecological theorists fail in showing us how nature works.

On the other hand, ecologists might endorse the other side of Mill's distinction and argue that their holistic and integrative theories tell us how Nature works insofar as it remains independent of human agency. Ecologists might then have to provide a criterion for determining the degree to which human beings have altered Nature's spontaneous course at any particular site. This might require as a baseline some concept of the original ecosystem. Since ecosystems constantly change—they present a Heraclitean flux in which one cannot step once without altering its course—no plausible way exists to characterize the pristine and original system. As biologist Michael Soulé has written, "[A]ny serious attempt to define the original state of a community or ecosystem leads to a logical or scientific maze."[44]

The idea that Nature possesses intrinsic ordering principles that human beings can disrupt, moreover, deeply divides ecology from other natural sciences. By analogy, imagine that certain Newtonian laws of motion held only to the extent to which a system had not been impacted by human beings. Suppose, for example, that the gravitational constant applied in pristine places but not to sites debauched by multinational corporations. Suppose raindrops obeyed the Poisson distribution when they fell into naturally occurring cisterns but not into humanmade buckets. We might then speak meaningfully of integrative patterns and principles that account for the direction or tendencies of motion, say, in pristine forests but not in factory farms. In effect, this is how theoretical ecology asks us to think about the biological world.

Rather than surrender to reduction on the one hand or to natural history on the other, ecological theory identifies a separate Nature for study. It is a Nature in which ecosystems evolve even though they have no genomes and no mates. It is a Nature in which principles of order, autocatalysis, ascendency, exergy, and stoichiometry are true, even though they do not hold equally of landscapes altered by human beings. (If they did apply, humans would use those rules to control or corrupt nature even more.) It is a Nature that multinational corporations have yet to disturb and desecrate. It is a Nature that provides the services that support all life and that we alter at our peril. It is a Nature that knows her business better than we do because she is unfallen, while humanity has sinned. It is a Nature that corresponds to general mathematical models—nature with an intelligible essence, not just a contingent history. Ecology in large part has become the science of Eden—of Nature "out there" in McKibben's sense. This is the sense in which Nature has ecological integrity and design because it is directed by an independent Force.

Was Lucretius Right?

In a verse about Landor's epitaph, Robert Frost teases a dean of humanities with whom he had discussed the meaning of the term "nature." In his poem "Lucretius versus the Lake Poets," Frost writes:

> For I thought Epicurus and Lucretius
> By Nature meant the Whole Goddam Machinery,
> But you say that in college nomenclature
> The only meaning possible for Nature
> In Landor's quatrain would be pretty scenery,
> Which makes opposing it to Art absurd.[45]

In this light verse, Frost announces that he understands nature as Lucretius did, which is to say, to mean the machinery of matter. By this, Frost refers to the principles and mechanisms that form the subject matter of physics, chemistry, biochemistry, and other reductionist or materialistic sciences. Frost, who described himself in another poem as "a plain New Hampshire farmer," had too much experience culling rocks out of his fields and watching crops die to believe that nature embodied a normative or beneficent design. New Hampshire farmers must fight nature every step of the way, and they depend on advances in biotechnology—rather than theoretical ecology—to force nature's otherwise recalcitrant hand.

It is amusing to consider how the views of poets and those of scientists have changed during the past two centuries. At the time of Pope, Landor, and Wordsworth, poets defended the coherence of Nature; they found in independent Nature an organization that seemed to them divine. Biologists such as Darwin and philosophers such as Mill challenged this view and asserted an empiricist and materialist vision of the contingencies of the natural world. They denied that a Great Chain of Being or any other intelligible or organizing principle characterized the living environment. Today, these positions are reversed. A poet like Frost, perhaps because he was also a farmer, finds nothing in nature but competition and contingency. It is our ecologists and philosophers who now impute overarching order, purpose, or design to the natural world.

ACKNOWLEDGMENTS

The author wishes to thank Robert McIntosh, whose comments greatly improved this chapter. The author gratefully acknowledges support from the National Science Foundation (Grant No. SBR-9422322), but he alone is responsible for the views presented here.

NOTES

1. The line is taken from the "Dying Speech of the Old Philosopher," a poem Landor published in 1849. See http://library.utoronto.ca/utel.rp/poems/landor14.html.
2. The classic history of this image is A.O. Lovejoy, *The Great Chain of Being* (New York: Harper Torchbooks, 1936, pbk. ed. 1960).
3. James H. Brown, "Organisms and Species as Complex Adaptive Systems: Linking the Biology of Populations with the Physics of Ecosystems," in Clive G. Jones and John H. Lawton, eds., *Linking Species and Ecosystems* (New York: Chapman and Hill, 1995), p. 17.
4. Brown, "Organisms and Species as Complex Adaptive Systems," p. 16. In seeking to link species interactions and biogeochemical processes, theoretical ecologists today give a mathematical patina to efforts long underway, for example, those of H. C. Cowles early this century.
5. E.P. Odum, "The Strategy of Ecosystem Development," *Science* 164(18 April 1969), p. 266.
6. Robert W. Sterner, "Elemental Stoichiometry of Species in Ecosystems," in Clive G. Jones and John H. Lawton, eds., *Linking Species and Ecosystems*, p. 252.
7. Peter Yodzis, *Introduction to Theoretical Ecology* (Cambridge: Harper and Row, 1989), pp. 36–49.
8. Robert Ulanowicz, "Life after Newton: An Ecological Metaphysic," unpublished ms. 1998, citing R. Ulanowicz, "An Hypothesis on the Development of Natural Communities," *Journal of Theoretical Biology* 85(1980): 223–245.
9. Michael Conrad, "The Ecosystem as an Existential Computer," in Bernard C. Patten and Sven E. Jorgensen, eds., *Complex Ecology: The Part–Whole Relation in Ecosystems* (Englewood Cliffs, NJ: Prentice Hall, 1995), pp. 609–622; quotation at p. 620.
10. Kurt Jax, Clive G. Jones, and Steward T.A. Pickett, "The Self-Identity of Ecological Units," *Oikos* 82(1998): 253–264; quotation at p. 253.
11. F. Gilbert and J. Owen, "Size, Shape, Competition, and Community Structure in Overfills," *Journal of Animal Ecology* 59(21)(1990): 21–39; quotation at p. 33.
12. Charles Darwin, *The Origin of Species* (New York: New American Library Mentor Book, 6th ed., 1872), p. 80.
13. Darwin, *Origin,* p. 82.
14. Stephen J. Gould, "Balzan Prize to Ernst Mayr," *Science* 223(1984), p. 255.
15. See F. Jacob, "Evolution and Tinkering," *Science* 196(1977): 1161–1166.
16. For discussion, Stephen J. Gould, "Is a New and General Theory of Evolution Emerging?" *Paleobiology* 6(1980): 125.
17. Clifford Geertz, "Thick Description: Toward an Interpretative Theory of Culture," in *The Interpretation of Cultures* (New York: Basic Books, 1973), pp. 3–30.
18. Robert McIntosh, in a comment to the author, points out that the early ecologist Charles Elton took seriously the watch metaphor and argued that the animal gears could move each other—in other words, that ecosystems did function like watches!

19. John Stuart Mill, "Nature," in *Three Essays on Religion* (New York: Greenwood Press, [1969] Reprint of the 1874 ed.), pp. 28–29.
20. Mill, "Nature," p. 16.
21. Bill McKibben, *The End of Nature* (New York: Random House, 1989); quoted in a review of the book by Lynn Margulis and Edwin Dobb, *The Sciences* (Jan.–Feb. 1990): 46.
22. Mill, "Nature," pp. 19–20.
23. For discussion, see William Cronon, *Changes in the Land: Indians, Colonists and the Ecology of New England* (New York: Hill and Wang, 1983), which argues that nothing of the ecosystem that greeted the Puritans remained even by the time of Thoreau.
24. Mill, "Nature," p. 23.
25. G.A. De Leo and S. Levin, "The Multifaceted Aspects of Ecosystem Integrity," *Conservation Ecology* [online] 1(1)(1997): 3. See www.consecol.org/vol1/iss1/art3.
26. Robert Ulanowicz, *Ecology: The Ascendent Perspective* (New York: Columbia University Press, 1997).
27. Grimm observes that the old organismic ecology still haunts the science like a ghost. He writes, "[T]he organismic notion is still deeply and unconsciously ingrained in the minds of most ecologists, as exemplified by the broad, loose usage of ontological terms, such as 'community' and 'ecosystem.'" Volker Grimm, "To Be, or to Be Essentially the Same: The 'Self-Identity' of Ecological Units," *Trends in Ecology and Evolution* 13(1998): 298–299; quotation at 298.
28. Jonathan Roughgarden, Robert M. May, and Simon Levin, "Introduction," pp. 3–10 in *Perspectives in Ecological Theory* (Princeton University Press, 1989); quotation on p. 8, citing Clifford Geertz, *The Interpretations of Cultures* (Basic Books: New York, 1973) as a source of the "thick description" view of explanation that provides an alternative to theory.
29. Jonathan Weiner celebrates this kind of commitment in his Pulitzer Prize–winning book, *The Beak of the Finch: A Story of Evolution in Our Time* (New York: Knopf, 1994).
30. A.O. Hirschman, 1979, "Paradigms as a Hindrance to Understanding," in P. Rabinow and W. Sullivan, eds., *Interpretive Social Science* (Berkeley: University of California Press), pp. 163–179. Quotation at pp. 163–164.
31. Hirschman, "Paradigms as a Hindrance," p. 164.
32. Peter Yodzis, *Introduction to Theoretical Ecology* (New York: Harper and Row, 1989), p. 3.
33. E.O. Wilson, *The New Population Biology* (book review), *Science* 163(March 14, 1969):1184–1185 (reviewing *Population Biology and Evolution,* R. Lewontin, ed., 1968).
34. Simon Levin, "Mathematics, Ecology, and Ornithology," *Auk* 97(1980): 422–423.
35. Levin, "Mathematics, Ecology, and Ornithology," pp. 422–423.
36. Lev Ginzburg, "Ecological Implications of Natural Selection," in Claudio

Barigozzi, ed., *Lecture Notes in Biomathematics* 39 (Springer-Verlag, 1980), p. 171.

37. Robert H. Peters, *A Critique of Geology* (New York: Cambridge University Press, 1991).

38. Simon Levin, "The Role of Theoretical Ecology in the Description and Understanding of Populations in Heterogeneous Environments," *American Zoologist* 21(1981): 865–875; quotation at p. 866.

39. Jack B. Waide, "Ecosystem Stability: Revision of the Resistance-Resilience Model," in Patten and Jorgensen, *Complex Ecology: The Part–Whole Relation in Ecosystems*, pp. 372–396; quotation at p. 378. Waide points out, "Such a theory would provide the basis not only for analyzing ecosystem dynamics and processes regulating them across scales of space and time, but also for viewing ecosystems abstractly as conditionally stable attractors within environmentally defined basins of attraction."

40. Peters, *Critique,* p. 175.

41. Peters, *Critique,* p. 177.

42. Edward Yoxen, *The Gene Business: Who Should Control Biotechnology?* (New York: Harper and Row, 1983), p. 2.

43. Frank Forcella, "Ecological Biotechnology," *Bulletin of the Ecological Society of America* 65(1984): 434.

44. Michael Soulé, "The Social Seige of Nature," in Michael Soulé and Gary Lease, eds., *Reinventing Nature: Responses to Postmodern Deconstruction* (Washington, DC: Island Press, 1995), p. 143. For a similarly jaundiced view of the community concept in ecology, see Margaret B. Davis, "Climatic Instability, Time Lags, and Community Disequilibrium," in J. Diamond and T. J. Case, eds., *Community Ecology* (New York: Harper and Row, 1986).

45. Robert Frost, "Lucretius Versus the Lake Poets," in Edward Connery Lathem, ed., *The Poetry of Robert Frost* (New York: Holt, Rinehart, and Winston, 1969), pp. 393–394.

Reconstructing Ecology

Ernest Partridge

The Challenge of "The New Ecology"

In the canon of environmental ethics, Aldo Leopold wrote the fundamental credo: "A thing is right when it tends to preserve the integrity, stability and beauty of the biotic community; it is wrong when it tends otherwise."[1] However, ecology is a science, and environmental ethics is pursued most scrupulously by philosophers. And to scientists and philosophers, there is no holy text. Thus even Leopold's maxim is fair game for circumspect analysis, evaluation, and confirmation. In fact, if we are to believe many "new ecologists," a literal reading of that maxim is about as scientifically respectable as a literal interpretation of Genesis. Gone is the easy assurance of "the integrity and stability of nature." Even "community," that cornerstone of the Leopoldian land ethic, is in disrepute. The "beauty" of nature, a concept saturated with subjectivism and evaluation, has never cut much scientific ice. "Balance" and "equilibrium" are rarely heard today in respectable eco-scientific circles, and according to some radical critics of classical ecology even the *system* of "ecosystem" is suspect.

Attacks on the once-cherished concepts of "ecological stability," "equilibrium," "balance," and "integrity" come from both within and beyond the ranks of biological science. For example, the biologist Michael Soulé writes: "[T]he idea that species live in integrated communities is a myth. . . . Living nature is not equilibrial—at least not on a scale that is relevant to the persistence of species."[2]

One of the most carefully articulated and thoroughgoing critiques of "classical ecology" is by philosopher Mark Sagoff and was published in the March 1997 issue of the *College of William and Mary Law Review*.[3] Given the importance of this paper, and because Sagoff is a valued and respected member of the Global Integrity Project, the primary burden of our critical attention will be directed to that paper.[4]

Sagoff's Critique of "Theoretical Ecology"

In Sagoff's lengthy and scrupulously argued critique, the following eight points are conspicuous:

1. The principles of theoretical ecologists cannot predict and are not falsifiable. Thus, by implication, they are not confirmable and thus are devoid of scientific significance. (p. 888)

2. "Ecosystems" are, in fact, devoid of "system." Put bluntly, "the terms 'eco' and 'system,' when conjoined, constitute an oxymoron" (p. 923). This is because "the ecosystem as an object of scientific inquiry is just a pointless hodgepodge of constantly changing associations of organisms and environments." (p. 901)

3. Nature is in constant change. In support of this claim, Sagoff quotes the biologist Daniel Botkin: "Wherever we seek to find constancy, we discover change. . . . [We find] that nature undisturbed is not constant in form, structure, or proportion, but changes at every scale of time and space."[5]

4. Ecology lacks a classification system. "If the term 'ecosystem' or 'community' [is] to be predicated on a collection of objects over time, there must be a way of telling when this collection is the same community or ecosystem and when it has evolved or changed into a different one. After all, ecosystems never die; they just fade into other ecosystems." (p. 894)

5. Ecology lacks baselines. There are no norms from which to assess deviations. (p. 900)

6. "There are no general truths about ecosystem organization. Anything is possible consistent with the laws of physics in nature. If ecosystems are unstructured, transitory, and accidental in nature, it would seem to follow that no general economic or utilitarian grounds exist for protecting them from change." (p. 931–32)

7. Ecosystems are unaffected by organic evolution. "Ecosystems could not possibly have acquired [their allegedly] wonderful organization through evolutionary processes. This is because natural selection operates only on creatures that breed true, that is, creatures that enjoy genetic inher-

itance. Ecosystems do not reproduce, possess genomes, or breed true; heredity is nothing to them." (p. 957)

8. Value is grounded in individual organisms and (at most) species, not ecosystems. "It is the unlikelihood, not the perfection, of the living world that amazes us; the improbability of every plant and animal leads us to treasure its existence. Species, even those not yet named, command our moral attention because they have emerged through a billion-year-old toil of evolution." (p. 966)

The implications of "the new ecology" for public environmental policy are profound. Gone is a justification for wilderness preservation, much less of wilderness restoration. For if ecosystems are in constant but aimless flux, then attempts to "preserve" (i.e., protect from change) an allegedly "pristine" state are "contrary to nature."[6] And proposals to "restore" wilderness raise the question, Restore *to what condition?* If there is no definable "baseline" condition that describes "wilderness," then that question has no answer and thus "restoration" policy has no foundation or meaning. Finally, endangered species legislation loses its justification, for, according to Sagoff, extinction is of no great practical significance. After all, he writes, "[N]o extinction of any species in the United States seems thus far to have altered the capacity of the ecosystems to provide these services. The reason may be that for any species that is lost, tens, hundreds, or thousands of others are ready, willing, and able to perform the same functions and services valuable to human beings" (p. 904). And, human beings aside, "no prima facie, general, or theoretical reason can be given, then, to suppose that the extinction of species now feared will in any meaningful way harm nature, because nature, having neither design nor direction, is not the sort of thing that can suffer harm"[7] (p. 967).

To be sure, Sagoff is not indifferent to the loss of species, which, he insists, "commands our moral attention." (And thus I wrote, above, of extinction as having "no practical significance," though to Sagoff it would be of *moral* significance.) Accordingly, Sagoff endorses an "ethic of preservation," which "values every species as intrinsically marvelous and worthy of respect and admiration" (p. 966). How, then, are we to act in conformance to this "ethic of preservation"? By preserving habitats and ecosystems? Only if such preservation serves as effective means to the end of protecting the species. The ecosystems themselves, he assures us, have no intrinsic value. So if, for example, the California condor would be safer in a zoo or refuge than in its "natural" habitat, so be it. There remains no further objection to bringing in the bulldozers and "developing" the Los Padres National Forest.[8]

The Ecologist's Rebuttal

So what remains of ecology, and is it enough to lend comfort to those still attracted to the Leopoldian land ethic or, for that matter, an ethic of "integrity"? I believe there is. But while I believe much of value can be salvaged from the older notion of "nature as community," it would be a mistake to assume that this older view can be rescued intact from these critics. Ecology will never be the same—nor should it be.

I offer six fundamental points of rebuttal to the new critics in general, and to Sagoff in particular:

1. "Constant change" is unproblematic to theoretical ecologists.

2. Some of the challenges are plainly false: in particular, the charge that ecological theory is nonfalsifiable, nonpredictive, and devoid of an operational classification system.

3. Ecosystems are, in fact, *systems.*

4. Ecosystems are sensitive to natural selection among their components, and thus exhibit the kind of systemic structure, integrity, and resilience that is found among organisms.

5. Ecosystems *can* be evaluated, in some nonnormative sense, as "healthier" or "less healthy" than others. Thus there may well be good reason to prefer "natural" ecosystems to those "cultivated" by human societies.

6. The ultimate inscrutability of ecosystems suggested by the deconstructionists serves to strengthen, rather than undermine, ecological morality.

"Constant Change" Is Unproblematic to Theoretical Ecologists

"Wherever we seek to find constancy," writes Daniel Botkin, "we discover change." Perfect equilibrium and balance are nowhere to be found in nature. "Nature is in constant flux."[9]

But of course nature is in constant flux. What self-respecting biologist would deny this! It's called "evolution." But this does not preclude us from recognizing significant differences in the *scale* of change. After all, species change through evolution. But this does not forbid biologists from utilizing the concept of species, nor from developing a taxonomy of species. In fact, without that taxonomy, the theory of evolution might never have been developed.

The issue deserves closer scrutiny. And so we return to Botkin—in particular, his summary of his outstanding study of the biotic history of the Boundary Waters region of northern Minnesota and southern Ontario.

Botkin points out that following the ice age, the region was characterized, in turn, by tundra, then spruce, then pine, then birch and alder (indicating a warmer climate), then a return to spruce and pine. "Thus," he reports, "every thousand years a substantial change occurred in the vegetation of the forest, reflecting in part changes in the climate and in part the arrival of species that had been driven south during the ice age and were slowly returning."[10]

Botkin then asks, rhetorically, "which of these forests represents *the* natural state," as if to suggest that, due to the multiplicity of states thus described, there is no so-called natural state. But this very passage suggests a nonrhetorical rebuttal: "*the* natural state" is that which is brought about by the climatic (and other) conditions that prevail at the time. That "state" is established by (relatively) undisturbed nature, and then is succeeded when natural circumstances change.

Put bluntly, I suggest that a critical examination of this passage will yield us less here than meets the eye, and less than Botkin intended. For what is Botkin asserting that any informed "equilibrium model ecologist" such as Odum or Leopold would deny? All these ecologists are well aware that North America undergoes periodic recurrences of ice ages and other climatic changes, measured in tens of thousands of years. But "balance," "equilibrium," and "resilience" are conditions posited *within* stable abiotic (e.g., climatic) conditions—or as the popular phrase has it, "all else being equal." Granted, "all else" is *never* completely "equal," and so classical ecologists write of "tendencies" toward balance, equilibrium, and resilience. Still, these ecosystemic concepts are quite enough to supply us with explanations of the past and predictions for the future.

To illustrate this point, let us shift our attention from the Boundary Waters to the Pacific Northwest.

About 10 years ago, on a flight from Los Angeles to Seattle, I looked out the window upon an unforgettable scene of utter devastation. It was, of course, the area immediately north of Mount St. Helens. On that vast mantle of tan pumice and fallen logs there was no apparent sign of life. And yet, a layperson might surmise, and a professional historical-ecologist would confirm, that in another five hundred years (absent climate change or massive human intervention), the area would look very much as it did on that early morning of May 18, 1980, moments before the north face of the mountain exploded. Through known stages of ecological succession, it will once again become what it was before: a northern conifer rain forest—not a tundra, or a tropical rain forest, or a prairie, or a Sonoran desert.

How would we know this? We know by studying neighboring areas up and down the Cascade Range, where other volcanoes, at determined dates in the geologically recent past, caused similar devastation. There we find, at this moment, the various stages of succession and recovery. And in those regions untouched by a recent eruption or fire or logging, we encounter an identifiable "type" of integrated life community—an *ecosystem*—very much as one would have encountered two-, three-, or four-hundred years ago. This is what ecologists correctly call a "climax stage."

No one suggests that "balance, equilibrium, and resilience" are ever perfectly exemplified in nature. Nor is a "climax community" ever completely static. These concepts, after all, describe "tendencies." But surely, these concepts are scientifically useful, as they describe significant conditions and differences. True, there is no "perfect balance and equilibrium" in nature. Still, there is a significant difference between the "imbalance and disequilibrium" of the Pacific Northwest forests of, say, four hundred years ago, and that of the same forest today as it is assaulted by Weyerhaeuser's chain saws. The former is measured on a time scale of millennia, while the latter is measured in years.[11]

To ignore such contrast in scale would be comparable to dismissing the concept of "disease" in medicine with such an argument as this: "You say that so-called disease causes changes in the organism? Well, so too does aging. So what's the difference?" Similarly, "the biodiversity crisis" is casually dismissed with the remark, "why worry about extinction? After all, extinction is a natural process." In all these cases the difference is degree and scale—and it is a difference that is ignored at the peril of both the patient and a civilization.[12]

No doubt, the concepts of ecological balance and stability have been exaggerated in the hands and heads of some uncritical writers and activists, and some unfounded ideology has emerged from these abuses. We are thus indebted to Daniel Botkin and others for supplying a much-needed antidote. But is it not possible that Mark Sagoff has taken an overdose of that antidote, as he proclaims that the term "ecosystem" is "oxymoronic," and that so-called natural communities are merely "random, accidental, contingent and purposeless collections of biological flotsam and jetsam" (p. 931n)?

Some of the Challenges Are Plainly Groundless
In fact, ecological theory is falsifiable and predictive, and it contains an operational system. Consider first the criterion of *falsifiability*.

Sagoff correctly points out that scientific hypotheses and theories must be *falsifiable*: that is, they must describe a world that is identifiably different from what the world would be like if the scientific claim were false (p. 949). Thus a scientifically sound theory yields predictions that, by implication, "rule out" alternative but conceivable states of affairs.

For example, there are numerous imaginable fossil depositions, or DNA sequences, or anatomical structures, and so forth that, if discovered, would refute organic evolution. Exhaustive field and laboratory research has failed to find any of these.

In contrast, consider two creationist "theories" of the origin of fossils that I was taught as a child: (a) God placed them in the ground to test our faith, and (b) Satan placed them in the ground to lead us astray. Each theory is nonfalsifiable, since, no matter what we might find in nature, we can assume, a priori, that God or Satan (take your pick) has superior capabilities to "test" or "deceive," as the case may be. Put another way, neither of these "theories" "explain" fossils; rather, they attempt to "explain them away." Presumably, Sagoff's complaint against "theoretical ecologists" is that reports of failure to find "integrity" in ecosystems are routinely followed by the retort, "well, you just haven't looked hard enough"—i.e., that these ecologists give no hint of what it would be like for their theories to be false, and thus they interpret this self-defined "failure" to refute as confirmation of their theory.

Contra Sagoff, it appears, in numerous cases, that ecological theory is quite falsifiable—i.e., that it describes a world that could readily be found to be otherwise if the theory were false. Consider for example, "succession theory." Any time someone returns, contrary to that theory, with a confirmable report of a meadow being replaced, first by shade-tolerant conifers, then by shrubs and "junk wood" such as aspens and birches—at such a time, standard succession theory will have been falsified and refuted.

Or consider Liebig's law of "limiting factors." One can describe a Julian Simon–type world in which an ecosystem, or a species population within, having utilized all available amounts of a necessary nutrient, then goes about finding some suitable "substitute resource." Nature can readily be shown not to work that way.

Finally, there are all kinds of ways that energy flowing through ecosystems might be imagined to violate fundamental thermodynamic laws. If, for example, these laws did not apply to ecosystems, the numbers or the biomass of predators in proportion to their prey would be found to be different than they in fact are.

The *predictability* of ecological assertions follows directly from their accordance with the falsifiability criterion. Thus we can correctly predict the succession of tree communities in a clear-cut or burnt-over forest. And, once we have ascertained that oxygen is the limiting factor in an aquatic ecosystem, we can predict the consequences of oxygen deprivation.

Finally, classificatory systems: Sagoff points out that "in order to predicate properties of ecosystems, we must have a classification scheme that allows us to determine when the object of study remains the same ecosystem even though its qualities change, and when an ecosystem of another kind replaces it" (p. 894).

In this criticism of "the old ecology," Sagoff is employing "the spectrum argument" (also known as "the argument of the beard"[13]); namely, the argument that from the absence of clear lines of demarcation along a continuum, one concludes that there is no difference in extremes in that continuum. Applied to the case at hand, it is admittedly true that absent catastrophic events such as fires, floods, or volcanic eruptions, ecosystems change gradually. Thus, the "boundary lines" (if any) between ecosystemic types are indistinct and somewhat arbitrary. However, it does not follow from this that an ecological classification scheme is unattainable. The ecological application of the "spectrum" fallacy is compelling: When settlers find a forest, and then clear-cut it to make way for monocultural fields, at which particular tree-felling does the ecosystem change from forest to field? None? Then, the argument goes, there is no difference between a forest and a field. Clearly a fallacy.

In point of fact, ecology does have a classification scheme. The distinction between producers, consumers, and decomposers is as secure in ecology as the distinction between igneous, sedimentary, and metamorphic rocks in geology—and as fundamental to the structure of the science. In addition, it is noteworthy that these concepts are defined in terms of *functions* within a system—the *ecosystem*. And while Daniel Botkin might disagree, there is also a less firm but nonetheless essential classificatory distinction between transitional and climax communities. The former are characterized by internal mechanisms of relatively rapid change often following sudden catastrophic interventions (such as fire or volcanic eruption), while the latter are characterized by slow change brought on by moderate external perturbations. However, as the "new ecologists" never tire of reminding us (while few of the "old" have ever disagreed), so-called climax communities are never totally static.

Notwithstanding all this, Sagoff insists that ecology is a quasi science since "there are no universal patterns or determinate relationships among the typical constructs of ecological theory" (p. 949). Really? What about the universal pattern that describes the relationship between producers, consumers, and decomposers? What about the unidirectional flow of energy and nutrients "up" the trophic pyramid? Wolves "universally" hunt; they never graze—even when there is no game to hunt, in which case they starve. Why is this? Because of the digestive system of canids, which has evolved to its state due to the ecological niche that the organisms have come to occupy. The ecosystem has shaped the genome of the wolf, which, reciprocally, has implications for the system. All this is described by rules and concepts of ecology that are falsifiable—i.e., might be recognizably false in a world differently ordered (e.g., a *Star Trek* world of "shape-shifter" and "genome-shifter" organisms—a conceivable world, but not our world).

Ecosystems Are, in Fact, Systems

Perturbations to parts of an ecosystem affect most other parts. As Garrett Hardin famously observed, "you can't do just one thing." Yet Sagoff would have us believe that "the terms 'eco' and 'system,' when conjoined, constitute an oxymoron" (p. 923).

If we are to determine whether or not ecosystems are "systemic," we must first define "system." I propose the following definition: "a system is a collection of identifiably separate entities acting in dynamic interaction to perform tasks in concert that cannot be accomplished separately." Accordingly, a watch and a computer are systems—also a football team, a thermostat and furnace, and, as I hope to demonstrate, an ecosystem.

Consider first a thermostat and furnace. Acting together, they constitute a simple "negative feedback system." We all know the "loop" mechanism: furnace on → heat rises → thermostat off → furnace off → heat falls → thermostat on → furnace on—thus the loop is closed, and the process continues *in perpetuo*, "all else being equal" (which it never is).

But take note of some properties of this simplest of systems. First of all, the temperature is constantly changing, and thus "unstable" and in "disequilibrium." We will call this "first-order instability." But the pattern and the outer limits of that change are constant ("all else equal"), providing what we shall call "second-order stability and equilibrium." However, "all else" is *not* equal, for the temperature outside the house fluctuates, so that when that temperature rises, the furnace-on phase is proportionately briefer until, past a certain point, the system shuts down.

But although the furnace–thermostat system undergoes constant "first-order" change, no one would deny that it constitutes a "system." A thermostat alone cannot heat the house, and a furnace alone will not provide a regulated temperature. Together, these components accomplish what each cannot do alone.

Consider next a biotic analogue to the thermostat–furnace system, namely the Canadian lynx–hare cycle, familiar to most beginning students of animal ecology. When the lynx population is low, the hare population soars, increasing the food supply for the lynx, causing an increase in the lynx population, causing a crash in the hare population, followed by a crash in the lynx population, once again opening an opportunity for the hares to do their rodent-thing—*da capo, perpetuo moto*. So much for the hypothesis. In fact, a two-hundred-year record from the Hudson's Bay Company confirms the hypothesis.[14]

Thus we are led to ask: if the thermostat–furnace interaction constitutes a "system," then why not the lynx–hare interaction? What do the lynxes and hares accomplish together that they might not accomplish alone? First of all, they have (at least in part) selected each other's genomes. Also, the "system" succeeds precisely because the lynx do *not* succeed in hunting down the last hare, for if they did, the ecosystem would collapse. Thus the hares "cooperate" by obligingly avoiding complete annihilation. More to the point, the ecosystem to which these two species belong—comprising climate, soils, and many additional species, including those that feed the hares—provides a "home" for all these species, which could not survive outside of such a system.[15]

In short, ecosystems are "systems" because the components are dynamically interactive. An organism receives its nutrients from other components, and in turn yields its nutrients to still others. A functional change in one component organism thus reverberates throughout the system. The literature of ecology is rich, even notorious, with examples of inscrutably complex interactions and "webs" in life communities, catastrophically disrupted by the introduction of exotic invaders—notably, the arrival of avian malaria to Hawaii, rabbits to Australia, zebra mussels to the Great Lakes, feral goats to the Channel Islands off California, and so on.

None of this impresses Sagoff, as he assures us that there is "no prima facie reason to believe that changes we humans inflict on nature . . . must go badly for us." For if, as Sagoff has argued, "ecological systems and communities are just random, accidental, contingent, and purposeless collections of biological flotsam and jetsam, then there is no general instrumental reason to preserve them" (p. 931).

On the contrary, it seems that Sagoff's allegedly random, chaotic hodgepodge of life forms cannot be duplicated by any available amount of human ingenuity. This fact was vividly demonstrated by that spectacularly failed experiment, Biosphere 2. This $200 million project attempted to establish a totally isolated and enclosed ecosystem that, like natural systems, could sustain the eight "ecospherians" indefinitely. Instead, report Paul Ehrlich and associates, "[T]he experiment ended early in failure. . . . Not even heroic efforts on the part of the system's desperate inhabitants could suffice to make the system viable."[16] Biosphere 2, it seems, reiterates J. B. S. Haldane's reflection that nature is more strange than we know or can even imagine.[17] More to the point, it seems to tell us, contra Sagoff, that not just any collection of aggregated life forms is sustainable—still worse, we seem quite incapable of assembling any group of organisms into a system that *is* sustainable without our constant surveillance and management.

Ecosystems Are Sensitive to Natural Selection among Their Components
Sagoff contends that while organisms exhibit systemic structure (logos) and goal-oriented activity (telos), these traits are the result of evolution. However, he argues, none of this applies to ecosystems, for "natural selection

operates only on creatures that breed true, that is, creatures that enjoy genetic inheritance. Ecosystems do not reproduce, possess genomes, or breed true; heredity is nothing to them. Accordingly, they are not subject to evolution. We should have to account for any order, design, harmony, or structure we impute to ecosystems by appealing to some cause other than evolution" (p. 957).

On the contrary, far from being irrelevant to ecosystems, evolution is the source and sustenance of these integrated life communities, and thus evolution suffices to account for any and all "design, harmony, or structure we impute to ecosystems." This is so, simply because the integration of the organism with its ecosystem is essential and inalienable, to both organism and ecosystem. Thus organisms evolve as they do because of the contingencies in the environment—which is to say, because of conditions in the ecosystem of which the organisms are components. And this is a reciprocal and dynamic interaction: adaptations to the organism due to the environing ecosystem cause changes in the ecosystem, which subsequently affect the organism, and so on.

If this is so, then Sagoff is wrong to deny an "order of design" in ecosystems while affirming the same in organisms. As Darwin suggests in the case of organisms and species, ecosystems display an "order of design" grounded in efficient causes. Since Darwin's time, we have recognized that the eagle's eye, the bee's dance, and the deer's alertness are all traits "designed" (better, "selected") to enhance the prospects for survival of the organisms. Why, then, do critics like Sagoff have such difficulty acknowledging that these survival traits "fit," one to another, into larger patterns of mutually accommodating arrangements? Any student of biology recognizes such arrangements when they exist between two species; they are called symbioses, of which the cooperative arrangement between the bee and the blossom is the paradigm example. The bee evolves better to find the blossom, as the blossom evolves better to attract the bee. Thus emerges a subsystem of the larger ecosystem. Further investigation reveals that these interactions are not only binary, but also triadic, quadratic, n-atic—i.e., systemic. In other words, the number of species with which an organism interacts and that determines its genome far exceeds the number of species that it eats and by which it is eaten. Just to begin to extend that list, we must include those that eat and are eaten by their prey and their predators, and the many species that regulate the soils and climate, and still others that perform symbiotic services—and so on, ad infinitum.

And when there is a tear in the fabric of the system, does not the system react in a manner that is least traumatic to the component members, for no other reason than that those members are designed to respond "conservatively," which is to say, within the capacities of their genomes? There is no mysterious telic "design" at work here, nor does the ecologist need to hypothesize such a design.

With evolution brought back into the ecosystemic picture, the integrated and "self-organizing" structure of ecosystems ceases to be an unexplained mystery. For organisms must have *some* (albeit not total) order and stability in the environment if they are to survive in a niche. Natural selection is simply too slow to allow any macroorganisms to survive in the sort of chaotic nonsystem that Sagoff describes. In fact, a Sagovian chaos describes precisely what is wrong with thoughtless human intervention into nature; after a clear-cut or the planting of a monocultural grainfield, there are few niches remaining that can be occupied by any species, save the managed species (e.g., corn or red pine) and, of course, short-lived organisms and rapidly adapting species such as insect and microbial pests, which must, in turn, be "managed."

In sum: natural ecosystems are "self-organizing" simply because the component species require some order and stability if they are to survive— that is simple genetics. And if no ordered stability, then no ecosystem—or at best, a simple and desolate system, such as a desert.

Thus far, we have suggested how ecosystemic evolution reflects and reciprocates the evolution of the component species. However, there is an even more direct "natural selection" of ecosystems that takes place even though, as Sagoff reminds us, ecosystems do not reproduce, lack genomes, and do not breed true. The basis of this "natural selection" is the simple fact that most combinations of coexisting life forms are not sustainable.

Consider the implications of two laboratory studies. Botkin reports G. F. Gause's experiment involving two protist species, a predator (*didinium*) and a prey (*paramecium*). They did not follow the "Lotka-Volterra model" of predator–prey oscillation, such as that which takes place between the lynx and the hare. Instead, the predator *didinium* devoured the very last *paramecium*, following which, of course, the predators starved. A similar, and quite familiar, experiment involves fruit flies confined to a jar and an abundant supply of food. The population soars, and then drops to zero as the flies consume all their food, or alternatively are poisoned by their own waste before the food is gone. (This phenomenon precisely describes why naturally fermented wine achieves no more than 12 percent alcohol content. At that concentration, the alcohol, a waste product of the yeast's metabolism, destroys the yeast cells.)

These are two laboratory examples of failed ecosystems. No doubt there are, in nature, many comparable failures. In the case of the Canadian lynxes and hares, if the lynxes could manage to hunt out the very last hare, and no hares were to migrate in, then that ecosystem would collapse. The external perturbations and internal mutations, of which the "new ecologists" are fond of reminding us, constantly "throw up" new arrangements, most of which presumably fail. Those that succeed do so (through no prearranged or "thought-out" design) because they happen to come up with sustainable patterns of nutrient recycling, energy flow, population control, and other essential services that characterize a stable ecosystem. Established ecosystems of which we are aware are necessarily systems that have thus succeeded. The failed systems, per hypothesis, are not available for study, unless of course we happen to find them as they collapse.

This is how "natural selection" operates "on the ecosystem level." As with evolving organisms, "ecosystemic evolution" is not planned, but it is *selected,* resulting in systems that are intricately structured, robust, resilient— in a word, hospitable, to the species they comprise.

The falsifiable implications of the ecological theory that I have sketched here are easily articulated and, moreover, are widely discovered in nature. A catastrophic intervention in the system, such as a fire or a drought, creates conditions that are no longer viable for the organisms that are specialized or higher in the trophic pyramid. The system suffers what is called a "crash," leading not just to "some other" community, but rather to a community that is simpler (less diverse), less productive (of biomass), and more entropic (ergo more probable). And so we find the desert that follows the forest and the prairie.

In short, while it is true that "ecosystems do not reproduce, possess genomes, or breed true" (p. 956), the biotic components of ecosystems do all these things! And thus, ecosystems evolve as their components evolve. ("Fallacy of Composition," you say? However, not all composition arguments are fallacies. Ask any chef.) Or, putting it another way, the component species of ecosystems evolve concomitantly, selecting strategies of survival in their environment. And since that environment provides both food sources and threats, this means that those "strategies of survival" must be attuned to the evolving natures of the other species in the system. The deer owes its alertness and fleetness to the wolf, which selected those traits, as the wolf owes its keen olfactory sense to the deer, which selected that trait— and thus they evolve together, two adjoining parts of a complex system, the parts and interactions of which can never be fully enumerated, but which include earthworms, dung beetles, intestinal bacteria, and all the other "little things that run the world," which, as E. O. Wilson reminds us, we need but do not need us.

To Sagoff, nature is wonderful enough without what he considers the ill-founded baggage of ecology. He writes that "the unlikelihood—not the perfection—of the living world amazes us; the improbability of every plant and animal leads us to treasure its existence. Species, even those not yet named, command our moral attention because they have emerged through a billion-year-old toil of evolution" (p. 966).

Eloquent and commendable sentiments. But note what is omitted. "Toil of evolution" *through what!* Through the interactive company of other species, of course, the vast majority of which have passed into extinction. And these surviving species and their lineal predecessors have prevailed because, throughout that billion-year history, they have functioned in ecological niches from which they have secured nourishment and defense sufficiently adequate to keep this biotic line intact. Any sudden break in that constant condition, and that species would not now be available for Sagoff's and our admiration. Not just any arbitrary and chaotic "hodgepodge" of aggregated coexisting life forms can accomplish this—only a moderately (though not perfectly) stable and integrated "community" of life forms.

Sagoff's view of nature reminds me of the Bronx Zoo that I visited as a child. There I encountered, in adjacent and isolated cages and boxes, one species, and then another, and then another. But as Sagoff knows full well, that is not how nature "works." What else but a complex "community" of dynamically interacting life forms, in the context of favorable physical and chemical conditions, could possibly account for the evolution of that abundance of life, with all its beauty, mystery, and wonder, that Sagoff treasures, along with the rest of us? Yet, somehow, I find in his de-ecologized nature much less to wonder at.

Ecosystems Can Be Evaluated as "Healthier" or "Less Healthy" than Others; Moreover, There May Well Be Good Reasons to Prefer "Natural" Ecosystems to Those "Cultivated" by Human Societies.

The essential difference, I contend, between (relatively) "natural" and artificial ecosystems is that undisturbed nature is "self-managing"—i.e., absent significant perturbations from the outside, in the "climax" stage of succession, it remains pretty much as it is. In contradistinction, "artificialized" ecosystems (e.g., farms) must be "managed." And even so, they tend to lose even their anthropocentrically defined "values," as, for example, topsoil is lost or soil nutrients of the forest are "exported" in the form of lumber. Sagoff insists that there are no "constant states" in natural ecosystems—that "all is flux." Granted, perfect constancy is a myth—an "ideal type," if for no other reason than that no ecosystems are entirely "closed," and thus outside forces (migrations, climate changes, etc.) keep "bumping" the system. Moreover, mutations are constantly occurring within the system. But here is the essential point: the heraclitean "flux" in natural ecosystems that so captivates the attention of the "new ecologists" is a very slow and self-healing process, while anthropogenic effects are sudden and disruptive.

Another difference between natural ecosystems and artificial "extractive systems" is that the latter require the importation of labor and nutrients if they are to be sustained, and even so, their life cycle is numbered in decades or even years, while natural systems persist for millennia (though not forever, as Botkin reminds us) on nothing more than the importation of solar energy. However, human habitation can be prolonged if nature is successfully "imitated" and not overpowered. A couple of years ago, while in the Tuscany region of Italy, I looked across a broad valley in constant production since the days of the Etruscans over three thousand years ago—three thousand years of "inefficient," solar-driven, organic agriculture. But will the bounty of that magical soil continue for another three millennia, after the soils have been "improved" with artificial fertilizer and bioengineered organisms? Don't count on it.

The barren hills of Lebanon, where the cedars once stood; the deserts of Iran, where Darius could once ride in constant shade from Persephelus to the sea; the deserts of north Africa, once the granaries and orchards of the Roman Empire—all these testify to the ultimate consequences of careless human intervention with natural systems.

Are we now to conclude that there are no noteworthy differences between the fertile ecosystems of ancient Lebanon, Persia, and Algeria, and their barren remnants of today? Clearly they are different from the point of view of human purposes. Are they now "just another kind of ecosystem, no better or worse than before"? There are noteworthy differences—just to begin, diversity of species and productivity of biomass.

The Ultimate Inscrutability of Ecosystems Serves to Strengthen, Rather than Undermine, Ecological Morality

How has this criticism of "the old ecology" eroded the scientific foundations of such ecological moralities as Aldo Leopold's land ethic? Arguably, not very much.

We owe a debt to Mark Sagoff, along with Soulé, Botkin, Shrader-Fréchette, and other critics of traditional ecology, for indicating how the "pop ecology" of the activists and the New-Agers has wandered far beyond the characteristic skepticism and qualifications of the scientists. "Natural communities," the new ecologists remind us, are far more complex and inscrutable than we may have imagined. But this is exactly what such ecomoralists as Aldo Leopold have been saying all along: the complexity and inscrutability of nature mandate policies of careful restraint and respect. Nor is traditional ecomorality seriously compromised by an acknowledgment that the concepts of "balance" and "equilibrium" have been oversimplified, since "constant gradual change within limits" is a concept quite congenial with ecological morality.

If "the new ecology" retains four essential concepts of the old, then, I think, this will be foundation enough for a sound ecological morality and policy. These are: (1) that life communities are *systems* of organisms in dynamic interaction, (2) that ecosystems can be meaningfully distinguished and graded in terms of biodiversity, productivity, relative stability, and negentropy, (3) that differences in the *scale* and *pace* of change are significant, and (4) that the complexity of natural systems is beyond our understanding, and perhaps even our imagination—a fact that mandates respect and caution as we intervene in nature.

As for "ecological science," that discipline utilizes productive and discriminable concepts, and it does provide falsifiable hypotheses and predictions, although, as numerous critics have correctly pointed out, there is vast room for improvement in this regard.

Sagoff demurs, as he dismisses ecology with the suggestion that "the only nontheological tenable position" is "that nature is just a pointless hodgepodge of constantly changing associations of organisms and environments" (p. 901).

I submit that the answer to this charge is quite simple and straightforward. We need only ask:

- Does the study of ecology have anything to tell us about resource or population policies—or, for that matter, such applied biological sciences as forestry, fisheries, and agriculture?

- Would anyone, having learned the allegedly "vacuous" theories and concepts of ecology, look at the world more "realistically" than, say, an adherent of "creation science"?

If the theories and concepts of ecology constitute authentic knowledge, then the application of such knowledge should have predictable and discriminable consequences—it should, so to speak, "make a difference." I submit that it has: in agriculture, forestry, and Leopold's field of wildlife management.

Because significant and enduring patterns do exist among that seeming "hodge podge of constantly changing associations," we should continue our inquiries in ecological science. And we would be well advised to pay attention to the traditional ecologists, while keeping a critical eye on their rhetorical excesses.

NOTES

1. Aldo Leopold, *A Sand County Almanac,* New York: Oxford University Press, 1989, pp. 224–25.
2. Michael Soulé, "The Social Siege of Nature," in *Reinventing Nature,* ed. Michael E. Soulé and Gary Lease, Washington, DC: Island Press, 1995, p. 143.
3. Mark Sagoff, "Muddle or Muddle Through? Takings Jurisprudence Meets the Endangered Species Act," *College of William and Mary Law Review,* 38:3 (March 1997), pp. 825–993. Sagoff's critique of theoretical ecology is found primarily in Sections IV and V (pp. 877–968). Because of the large number of citations from this work, subsequent references thereto will be found in parentheses in the text.
4. I must note that my personal and professional debt to Mark Sagoff is beyond measure. His critique of the economization of public environmental policy is brilliant and devastating, and I have utilized his work in my classes and writing to great effect. I am so much impressed and convinced by his work in this field that I have been much concerned that I might become a Sagovian disciple— and discipleship is most unbecoming a philosopher. After reading his work on ecology, however, this concern about impending disciplehood has been considerably diminished.
5. Daniel Botkin, *Discordant Harmonies,* New York: Oxford University Press, 1990, p. 62.
6. "If ecosystems are unstructured, transitory, and accidental in nature, it would seem to follow that no general economic or utilitarian grounds exist for protecting them from change." And, "If ecological systems and communities are just random, accidental, contingent, and purposeless collections of biological flotsam and jetsam, then there is no general instrumental reason to preserve them." Sagoff, "Muddle or Muddle Through?" pp. 931–32, 931n.
7. Regarding the biodiversity crisis, Sagoff parts company with most of the "new ecologists," who are as alarmed and appalled as most biologists at the current "extinction spasm."
8. Once again, I would separate this position from that of most of the "new ecologists." From 1980 to 1982, I was a visiting professor of environmental studies at the University of California, Santa Barbara. The chairman of the program was Daniel Botkin. I vividly recall how, at that time, he supported the "habitat strategy" of preserving the California condor—in other words, the "ecosystemic approach." As we shall discover later in this chapter, Botkin, while notoriously opposed to "equilibrium" and "stability" models of ecology, nonetheless asserts that ecosystems are in fact *systems* (Botkin, *Discordant Harmonies,* p. 7).
9. Botkin, *Discordant Harmonies,* p. 6.
10. Botkin, *Discordant Harmonies,* pp. 58–59.
11. Mark Woods concurs: "[N]o ecologist has held the view that nature is static and completely unchanging. Rather, as proponents of [the new ecology, such as Botkin and Budiansky] would have us believe, when ecologists have spoken

of 'stability' in nature usually they have meant that all the variables of any population, community, ecosystem, etc. will return to equilibrium conditions after they have been displaced or disturbed. In other words, in spite of disturbances (variables) in nature, the structures and compositions of nature remain or return to the same.

"Has anyone really held this view? In his equilibrium theory of succession leading to climax communities, Clements (organismic model) stressed that such an equilibrium was a *dynamic* equilibrium: 'Even the most stable association is never in complete equilibrium, nor is it free from disturbed areas in which secondary succession is evident.' Elton (community model) claimed: 'The "balance of nature" does not exist and perhaps never has existed.'" Woods, "Upsetting the Balance of Nature: Can Wilderness Preservation Survive the New Ecology?" Paper presented at a meeting of the International Society for Environmental Ethics, March 1998, Los Angeles, pp. 22–23.

12. For an excellent treatment of "the scale issue," see J. Baird Callicott, "Do Deconstructive Ecology and Sociobiology Undermine Leopold's Land Ethic?" *Environmental Ethics* 18:4 (Winter 1996), pp. 369–72 (the final two sections of the paper).

13. If you pull whiskers, one by one, from a beard, which particular whisker "removes" the beard? *Answer: no* particular whisker. *Ergo,* there is no difference between a bearded and a clean-shaven face. *Variant:* At what particular day after a full shave does a beard appear? *Answer:* at *no* particular day. *Ergo:* no beard ever appears. *Some applications:* "At what point in prehistory did human beings appear?" (employed as an argument against human evolution). "At what day does a child become an adult—or learn a language?" And most notoriously, "at what point in time does human life begin?"

14. W.S. Allee, A.E. Emerson, O. Park, T. Park, and K.P. Schmidt, *Principles of Animal Ecology,* Philadelphia: Saunders, 1949. Cited by Botkin, *Discordant Harmonies,* p. 46.

15. Predictably, Daniel Botkin (from whose book I have borrowed these citations), sees things differently. He points out that the "Lotka-Volterra equations" that describe a perfectly "symmetric, out-of-phase oscillation between predator and prey" do not exactly describe the empirical data brought back from the field. "Predators," he concludes, "do not seem to control the abundance of their prey in an exact sense." The operative word here is "exact." But for such "exact control" to be operative—i.e., for there to be a "perfect" and constant "balance"of nature—all other factors (e.g., climate, migrations, etc.) would have to be constant, and mutations would have to cease. And no biologist has ever defended such a concept of "stability" and "equilibrium." All agree that "all else" is *not* "equal." Botkin denies "stability" in the "first-order sense," as he rhetorically asks: if "a pilot guaranteed that an airplane was stable and very constant in flight, but its path through the air traced out the curve of the lynx's population . . . Who would want to call that airplane stable?" But that analogy is faulty, for it is the "second-order stability" that interests the ecologists. And the data on lynx population that Botkin supplies displays a sustainable pattern

of fluctuations—a "second-order stability." (Botkin, *Discordant Harmonies,* pp. 38, 47, 48).

16. Paul Ehrlich, Gretchen Daily, Scott Daily, Norman Myers, and James Salzman, "No Middle Way on the Environment," *Atlantic Monthly* (December 1997), p. 101.

17. The exact quotation: "Now my own suspicion is that the Universe is not only queerer than we suppose, but queerer than we can suppose." *Possible Worlds and Other Essays,* London: Chatto and Windus, 1930.

Toward the Measurement of Ecological Integrity

Robert E. Ulanowicz

The notion of ecosystem integrity has repeatedly appeared in the legislation of Canada and the United States in the absence of serious consideration as to exactly what the term means. The charge to the Global Integrity Project has been to give concrete definition to "ecological integrity" and to suggest how the concept might be implemented (Westra 1994).

Accordingly, the Project has identified the concept of ecological integrity with at least four attributes: (1) system "health," that is, the continued successful functioning of the community; (2) the capacity to withstand stress; (3) an undiminished "optimum capacity" for the greatest possible ongoing developmental options; and (4) the continued ability for ongoing change and development, unconstrained by human interruptions.

The main question to be considered here is whether these attributes can be anchored in sound ecological theory. By addressing this issue, I also hope to address the larger controversy of whether the current body of ecological theory is indeed sound—for critics of the concept of ecological integrity in particular, and ecosystem theory in general, are indeed numerous and highly articulate. Shrader-Fréchette and McCoy (1993), for example, maintain that "[e]cology is not a science enough to provide testable laws." Furthermore, Shrader-Fréchette asserts that "[i]ntegrity is stipulative" and therefore possesses no phenomenological or operational character (personal communication to L. Westra).

Similarly, Mark Sagoff (chapter 4, this volume) contends that "[s]cience is too changeable, insecure and internally conflicted to be able to provide any guidance for environmental morality or public policy." Both Shrader-Fréchette and Sagoff take their cues from Peters (1991), who in his *Critique for Ecology* chided ecologists for indulging in theory that is (1) not operational, (2) tautologous and therefore nontestable, and (3) not predictive.

These are serious charges leveled by respected individuals and are not to be taken lightly. Most will acknowledge that there are credible reasons for such misgivings. But is ecology actually in such dire straits that the best its practitioners can do is to stipulate characteristics that cannot be quantified or made elements of testable theory? The majority of those who make up the Global Integrity Project are not so pessimistic, but it remains to respond to these challenges in a succinct but convincing manner. We offer three points by way of apology:

1. Many critics of ecology theory *assume an unnecessary dichotomy between determinism and stochasticity* as these characteristics pertain to ecology. Indeed, this "error of the excluded middle" is widespread throughout science in general. Most practicing scientists believe that strict Newtonian causality prevails over macroscopic phenomena, and that indeterminacy, if it exists at all, is confined to the netherworld of molecular and quantum phenomena. Philosophers, such as Charles Saunders Peirce and Karl Popper, however, believe the world to be causally open at all levels of the hierarchy. Furthermore, Popper (1990) warns that we will never achieve an "evolutionary theory of knowledge" unless we first revise our views on basic causality. He advocates a shift from the Newtonian notion of "force" to a more general concept that he calls "propensity." Elsewhere, I have attempted to elaborate a new view of causation in living systems (Ulanowicz 1997, 1999) and have suggested ways to make the idea of propensity operational in ecology and the other life sciences (Ulanowicz 1996).

2. Many detractors of ecology cling to an *unwarranted refusal to admit directionality into ecological discourse.* The ambiguities surrounding whether directionality is admissible into evolutionary theory are somehow thought to be universal. This extrapolation, of course, is consistent with the modernist view that only material and efficient causes exist in nature—whence any perceived directionality must be epiphenomenal or illusory. According to this viewpoint, to admit of essential direction anywhere in the living realm is to take the first, irreversible step down the slippery slope into the depths of teleology! Mayr (1992), among others, countered by asserting that biology without directionality is puerile. Again, it is the "error of the excluded middle" not to consider directionalities, like Mayr's "teleonomy," that are distinctly nonteleological in essence. Elsewhere, I have posited the existence of a "telos" in ecosystem development as a weak form of final cause that falls far short of teleology (Ulanowicz 1997).

3. Skeptics are not convinced that *ecological integrity can become an operational tool.* They choose to ignore the obvious successes that quantitative indices, such as Karr's (1986) index of biological integrity (IBI), have

contributed to ecological management. Perhaps they disregard IBI as being "stipulative" because they feel that its connections with basic science are not as explicit as might be desired. But other quantitative assessments of ecological integrity exhibit strong links to the corpus of accepted science and phenomenology (e.g., Svirezhev and Svirejeva-Hopkins 1998, Jorgensen 1997).

Space does not permit a full exposition of all three apologies, and the reader interested in either of the first two counterassertions is urged to consult the references cited. The remainder of this chapter will bear upon the final point, and, in particular, will elaborate current efforts to invoke the theories of networks, information, and economics to identify tools that will give palpable quantitative form to all four aspects of ecological integrity.

Quantifying Ecosystem Performance

As defined above, ecological integrity explicitly subsumes the notion of "health." Costanza (1992) identifies the health of an ecosystem as its ability to sustain its structure and function over time in the face of external stress (Mageau et al. 1995). The function, or vigor, of a system relates to its overall level of activity in processing material and energy. Its structure, or organization, refers to how effectively its various processes are linked to each other. Together vigor and organization specify the system's level of performance as pertains to aspect 1 under the definition of ecological integrity. The third point, resilience to perturbation, corresponds to aspect 2.

The task now before us is to quantify the levels of vigor, organization, and potential for resilience exhibited by any arbitrary ecosystem. Toward this end we will assume that these attributes are identifiable properties of the network of trophic exchanges of material or energy that occur within the system. Inevitably, some will object that the magnitudes of palpable flows do not make explicit the multitude of signs and intricate behaviors that influence and guide those flows. This is true; however, such detailed phenomena do function as implicit constraints that modulate and direct the perceived exchanges. It will be argued here how the effective magnitudes of these constraints can be measured in the absence of any knowledge of their explicit details.

We begin by identifying four different types of exchanges that occur in an ecosystem (Figure 6.1). The rate at which taxon i contributes as prey to the sustenance of predator j will be denoted by T_{ij}, where $i,j = 1,2,3, \ldots n$. The large majority of transfers in an ecosystem usually consist of such intrasystem exchanges, but all ecosystems also are open to the external

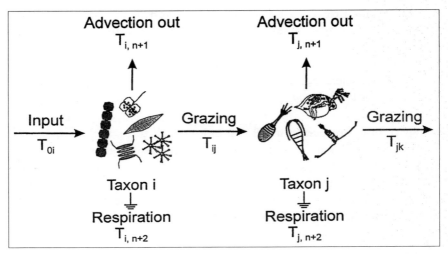

FIGURE 6.1

The four types of exchanges used to quantify ecosystem flow networks. (T_{ij}) Internal flow from arbitrary compartment i to any other taxon, j, of an n-compartment system. (T_{0i}) External inputs to the arbitrary compartment i. ($T_{i,n+1}$) Export of usable resources from unit i. ($T_{i,n+2}$) Dissipation of resources from system element i.

world. There are three categories of exogenous exchanges: (1) inputs from the external world, signified by T_{0i}, (2) exports of medium that can be used by systems of similar size, denoted by $T_{i,\,n+1}$, and (3) dissipation of medium into a form that is useless or of marginal value elsewhere, signified by $T_{i,\,n+2}$.

Once all four types of flows pertaining to all the important taxa of an ecosystem have been measured, the values may be either arrayed into matrices and vectors or depicted in schematic form as "box and arrow" diagrams. Figure 6.2 is a schematic example of the trophic exchanges of carbon (in mgC/m²/y) among the 36 most significant taxa of the mesohaline (moderately salty) ecosystem of Chesapeake Bay (Baird and Ulanowicz 1989). Sets of such measurements allow one to quantify the degrees of vigor, organization, and resilience inherent in the prototype ecosystems.

Of the three attributes, vigor is easiest to quantify. One measure of system vigor would be the simple sum of all the individual exchanges that occur in the system—a quantity known in economic theory as the "total system throughput," T, where

$$T = \sum_{i,j} T_{ij}$$

The total system throughput is related to (but not identical to) the ubiquitous "gross domestic product" that is a common item in the daily news.

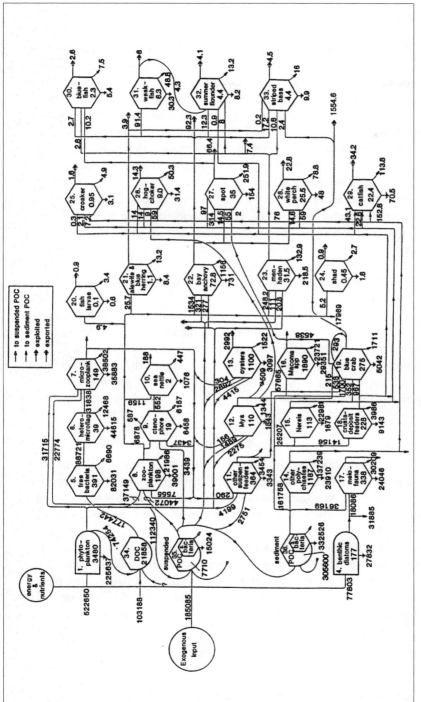

FIGURE 6.2

Estimated flows of carbon (mg/m²/y) among the 36 principal components of the mesohaline Chesapeake Bay ecosystem (Baird and Ulanowicz 1989). Circles represent autotrophic system elements (plants); hexagons, heterotrophic taxa (fauna); and "birdhouses," nonliving storages. Numbers inside each box are the standing stocks in mg/m².

Organization requires somewhat more effort to quantify. We take as a working definition of organization, "the degree of constraint that guides a typical flow in the system." That is, medium leaving a particular taxon does not flow arbitrarily to just any other taxon. Only a limited number of other taxa are capable of consuming a given source. The actual distributions of flow from various prey to their specific predators are the outcomes of organism morphologies and behaviors. As a result, when the system is viewed on the whole, certain pathways will tend to dominate the network of exchanges. Constraints that channel flows along these major routes usually are the outcomes of interspecific competitions and/or indirect mutualisms (autocatalysis) among the participating taxa.

Autocatalysis as an agency that drives ecosystem development (the increase of organization) deserves more attention than can be paid it here. Suffice it to mention that, when autocatalysis acts against a background of indeterminate kinetics, it comes to exhibit properties that are decidedly nonmechanical in nature (Ulanowicz 1997). Among other traits, autocatalysis is a source for what physicists call "symmetry-breaking" that establishes the direction in which the system will develop.

How, then, to quantify the constraints that engender system organization? As with so many approaches in mathematics, one first considers the opposite of what is being defined, namely, freedom or indeterminacy. Thus information theory, as pioneered by Boltzmann (1872) and Shannon (1948), begins by postulating that the indeterminacy of phenomenon A_i is related to the probability of its occurring, $p(A_i)$, through the expression

$$\left[-k \log p\left(A_i\right) \right]$$

where k is a scalar constant, and the base of the logarithm is taken to be 2. Because $p(A_i)$ is a number between 0 and 1, the indeterminacy is sure to be a positive quantity (the logarithm of a fraction is a negative number), and it becomes very large when A_i is rare or very small when the outcome is almost certainly A_i.

In writing $p(A_i)$, we do not take explicit account of any constraints upon the occurrence of A_i. If, however, A_i happens to be in proximity to some other event, B_j, and the effect of B_j is to constrain, to a degree, the probability of A_i, then the conditional probability of A_i under the influence of B_j is written $p(A_i | B_j)$. The revised indeterminacy thus becomes,

$$\left[-k \log p\left(A_i | B_j\right) \right]$$

On average, the indeterminacy of unconstrained A_i should exceed its indeterminacy when under the constraint of B_j, so that the difference,

$$\left[-k \, \log \, p\left(A_i\right)\right] - \left[-k \, \log \, p\left(A_i | B_j\right)\right]$$

should measure the degree of constraint that B_j exerts upon A_i. Because the difference between two logarithms may be expressed as the logarithm of the quotient, this last expression may be rewritten,

$$k \, \log\left(\frac{p\left(A_i | B_j\right)}{p\left(A_i\right)}\right)$$

Those familiar with probabilities will recognize that this last expression is related via Bayes' theorem to the (symmetrical) joint probability that A_i and B_j will co-occur:

$$\frac{p\left(A_i | B_j\right)}{p\left(A_i\right)} = \frac{p\left(A_i, B_j\right)}{p\left(A_i\right)p\left(B_j\right)} = \frac{p\left(B_j | A_i\right)}{p\left(B_j\right)}$$

Whence, the measure of the constraint of B_j upon A_i is equal to that which A_i exerts upon B_j. One thus may speak of the mutual constraint that A_i and B_j exert upon each other, as given by the expression,

$$k \, \log\left(\frac{p\left(A_i, B_j\right)}{p\left(A_i\right)p\left(B_j\right)}\right)$$

This last expression pertains to any arbitrary pair of events A_i and B_j. We are more concerned, however, with the overall degree of constraint present in the system as a whole. Accordingly, we calculate the average mutual constraint by multiplying each pairwise mutual constraint by the probability of its occurrence $[p(A_i, B_j)]$ and summing the products over all combinations of i and j. Because constraint is operationally indistinguishable from information, we call the result of this averaging process the average mutual information (AMI) and write it as

$$\text{AMI} = k \sum_{i,j} p\left(A_i, B_j\right) \log\left[\frac{p\left(A_i, B_j\right)}{p(A_i)p\left(B_j\right)}\right]$$

It remains to specify how A_i and B_j might relate to a network of trophic exchanges. We therefore identify A_i with the event, "a quantum of medium leaves taxon i" and B_j with "a quantum of medium enters taxon j." This allows us to estimate all the probabilities constituting AMI in terms of the intercompartmental flows, T_{ij}, and the total system throughput, T, as follows:

$$p\left(A_i, B_j\right) \approx \frac{T_{ij}}{T}$$

$$p\left(A_i\right) \approx \left(\frac{\sum\limits_{j} T_{ij}}{T}\right)$$

$$p\left(B_j\right) \approx \left(\frac{\sum\limits_{i} T_{ij}}{T}\right)$$

and

$$p\left(B_j|A_i\right) \approx \frac{T_{ij}}{\sum\limits_{q} T_{iq}}$$

Substituting these estimators into the expression for AMI yields the formula

$$\text{AMI} = k\sum_{i=0}^{n}\sum_{j=1}^{n+2}\left(\frac{T_{ji}}{T}\right)\log\left[\frac{T_{ji}T}{\sum\limits_{k} T_{kj}\sum\limits_{q} T_{iq}}\right]$$

Information theory guarantees that AMI ≥ 0.

It bears repeating that whenever all the T_{ij} are known from the network of trophic exchanges, it then becomes a straightforward task to calculate an AMI for the system. That this measure does indeed quantify the degree of constraint in a system can be seen from Figure 6.3. All three networks of four "taxa" have identical total system throughputs (96 units). In Figure 6.3a, however, there is minimal constraint about where medium currently in a particular box will flow next. It is equally likely to flow to any of the three other taxa, or to remain where it is. The AMI of this configuration is identically zero. In Figure 6.3b outputs from any box are constrained to flow to only two other boxes. The measure of this constraint is $1k$ bits. (A "bit" is the unit associated with the resolution of a single binary indeterminacy [fork].) In Figure 6.3c the system is maximally constrained. Medium leaving any taxon may flow to only one other taxon. The AMI rises to $2k$ bits.

It is awkward to express the values of AMI in terms of multiples of the scalar constant, k. The usual practice in information theory is to choose a base for the logarithms (2, e, or 10), set $k = 1$, and call the resultant units "bits," "nats," or "hartleys," respectively. By retaining the scalar constant, however, we wish to emphasize that it can be used to impart physical units to the information index that it multiplies (Tribus and McIrvine 1971). Accordingly, we choose to normalize AMI in a very natural way by setting $k = T$, i.e., we use the system vigor to scale its corresponding measure of

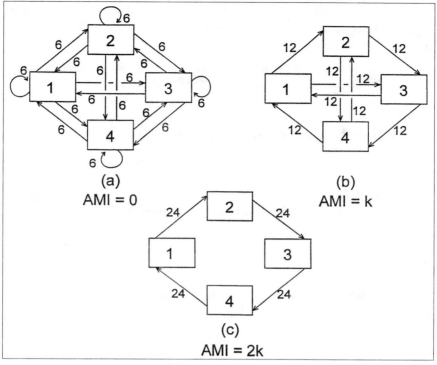

FIGURE 6.3

(a) The most equivocal distribution of 96 units of transfer among four system components. (b) A more constrained distribution of the same total flow. (c) The maximally constrained pattern of 96 units of transfer involving all four components.

organization. To highlight that the resultant product is a physical measure, we rename it the system ascendency (Ulanowicz 1980) and denote it simply by A. In the ascendency we have incorporated both aspects of system performance,

$$A = T \times \sum_{i,j} \left(\frac{T_{ij}}{T} \right) \log \left(\frac{T_{ij}T}{\sum_k T_{kj} \sum_q T_{iq}} \right)$$

or

Ascendency = Vigor × Organization

It can be demonstrated that the magnitude of system ascendency is abetted by greater speciation, more specialization, further internalization, and increased cycling (Ulanowicz 1980). These four attributes represent groupings of the 24 system properties that Eugene Odum (1969) identified with more highly developed ecosystems. We arrive, then, at the following phenomenological principle:

> In the absence of major perturbations, ecosystems exhibit a propensity toward configurations of ever greater ascendency.

Quantifying Potential for Resilience

It was noted above how the AMI was maximal for the configuration depicted in Figure 6.3c. Such a statement was possible, because information theory reveals that the AMI possesses an upper bound. Without going into detail (see Ulanowicz and Norden 1990), an appropriate upper bound on the ascendency may be taken as

$$C = -\sum_i \sum_j T_{ij} \log\left(\frac{T_{ij}}{T}\right)$$

where C is termed the system capacity. Information theory guarantees that $C \geq A \geq 0$. This allows one to define a systems overhead as $\Phi = C - A$, where $\Phi \geq 0$. In terms of the system flows, the overhead works out to be

$$\Phi = -\sum_{i,j} T_{ij} \log\left(\frac{T_{ij}^2}{\sum_k T_{kj} \sum_q T_{iq}}\right)$$

The system overhead is complementary to the ascendency. Whereas ascendency gauges how well the internal constraints cause the system to perform, the system overhead gauges all the inchoate, inefficient, and redundant degrees of freedom that the system retains.

To recapitulate what has just been accomplished, the system capacity can be parsed into two distinct and complementary components—the ascendency and the overhead (Figure 6.4). Whenever external conditions are relatively benign, there is a propensity for the system ascendency to grow at the expense of its overhead, i.e., the ecosystem "ratchets" itself toward ever higher and more efficient performance.

The real world is never so benign, however. External perturbations always arise, and a system with very high performance is "brittle" and subject to collapse (Holling 1986). It can successfully adapt to novel perturbation only if it retains a sufficient repertoire of degrees of freedom. That is, overhead, which is inimical to performance under undisturbed conditions, becomes essential if the system is to recover from trauma. Overhead becomes a prerequisite for system resilience, creativity, and persistence (Ulanowicz

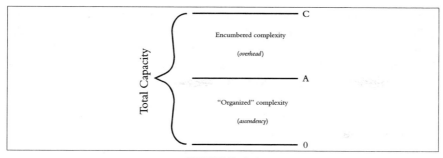

FIGURE 6.4

Graphical representation of the segregation of development capacity (complexity) into dis-ordered and organized components (overhead and ascendency, respectively).

1980, 1997). Engineers have always been cognizant of the antagonism be-tween efficiency and reliability, and that complementarity is given quantita-tive form in the relationship between ascendency and overhead.

Quantifying Integrity

The countervailing attributes of ascendency and overhead nonetheless sum to yield the system capacity. In other words, the capacity subsumes the system's capabilities to perform well, to be resilient, and to develop in a creative fashion. We recall points 3 and 4 in the definition of integrity: an undiminished "optimum capacity" for the greatest possible ongoing de-velopmental options, and the continued ability for ongoing change and de-velopment, unconstrained by human interruptions. We recognize, therefore, in the decomposition of the capacity, all four elements of ecosystem integrity, namely,

$$C \quad = \quad A \quad + \quad \Phi$$

$$\begin{pmatrix} Capacity \\ for \\ development \end{pmatrix} = \begin{pmatrix} Healthy \\ Performance \end{pmatrix} + \begin{pmatrix} Resilience \\ and \\ creativity \end{pmatrix}$$

$$(3 \text{ and } 4) \qquad (1) \qquad (2)$$

If one has access to sufficient data to assemble a network of trophic in-teractions, one is equipped to assess ecosystem integrity in a quantitative way. Wulff and Ulanowicz (1989), for example, constructed networks of the ecosystems of the Baltic Sea and the Chesapeake Bay, respectively, with the intention of using the networks to compare their relative trophic status. The picture that emerged from the exercise was somewhat surprising. Despite being much more vigorous (T in Chesapeake is about fourfold that of the Baltic), the Chesapeake showed visible signs of heavy impact. The flow diversity (C/T) remained higher in the Baltic ecosystem, which also exhibited a higher relative proportion of ascendency (A/C). The evidence for impact on the Chesapeake ecosystem was no surprise to those who study and manage its resources, but the fact that the oligohaline Baltic seemed to have more integrity than the mesohaline Chesapeake raised numerous eyebrows among the Baltic Sea research community.

A final observation on capacity: The diversity of exchanges that make up the system capacity obviously is limited by the diversity of the participating taxa. Hence, any decrement in the biodiversity is likely to have detrimental consequences for the system capacity, i.e., its integrity. Ascendency theory, therefore, provides a theoretical link between the preservation of biodiversity and the maintenance of biotic integrity (which in its turn encompasses both system functioning and sustainability).

Summary and Conclusions

Despite the protests of its detractors, ecosystem integrity has already become an operational concept. The IBI is currently being used to evaluate the integrity of numerous aquatic ecosystems, and plans are afoot to extend the measure to cover marine, estuarine, and terrestrial communities.

Ecosystem ascendency and its related measures derive quite naturally from a mix of disciplines, tightly weaving the concept into the existing web of phenomenological sciences—most especially, thermodynamics. Ascendency measures have already been employed to assess the relative integrities of real systems, and one can anticipate many more such comparisons as new software makes the task of assembling trophic networks ever easier (Christensen and Pauly 1997).

That ascendency variables fit the notion of ecosystem integrity hand-in-glove derives in part from a certain overlap in the goals of those who developed both concepts. The correspondence between the capacity and its components and the several aspects of ecological integrity permits one to assess quantitatively how the aspects of integrity stand in relation to one another in any particular system.

The foregoing considerations on the relationship between ascendency and integrity did not include a riposte to the criticism that ecological theory deals only in tautologies and does not provide testable predictions. Ascendency as described above is a highly aggregated measure. In order to apply the concept to more specific hypotheses, the notion must be elaborated along several lines. Toward this end, ascendency has recently been extended to apply to systems that vary in time (Pahl-Wostl 1992) and space (Ulanowicz 2000). Furthermore, ascendency has been revised to incorporate species stocks in a natural way (Ulanowicz and Abarca 1997).

This latter advance has allowed the use of the ascendency formula to investigate problems of nutrient limitation and control. For example, if B_{ik} is the amount of mass of element k in taxon i, and T_{ijk} is the amount of k flowing from i to j, then one may calculate the sensitivities of the ascendency with respect to either of these variables in the hope that such sensitivities will provide clues in the search for limiting nutrients and processes (Ulanowicz and Baird 1999).

In particular, when one calculates

$$\left(\frac{\partial A}{\partial B_{ik}} \right)$$

the derivative of the ascendency with respect to each nutrient stock, the nutrient that is present in least proportion in each taxon emerges as the one with the greatest sensitivity. That is, the ascendency principle can be shown to *subsume* Liebig's Law of the Minimum. Demonstrating that a general principle encompasses a more specific, acknowledged law is certainly a point in favor of the covering law. But there is more.

Liebig's Law provides no clue as to what the limiting source of a limiting element might be. By calculating the sensitivity

$$\left(\frac{\partial A}{\partial T_{ijk}} \right)$$

one is able to identify the limiting source as the one that is being depleted at the fastest relative rate. Often, this source is not identical to the one that is supplying the limiting element at the fastest rate (Ulanowicz and Baird 1999). Thus the identification of the limiting source is a "prediction" of the ascendency principle that can be tested experimentally.

So long as one is careful to build new theory with identifiable connections to the existing body of science, the likelihood remains good that progress will not become mired in untestable tautologies. In view of what has been reported here, the prospect for a robust ecosystems theory no longer should be regarded with pessimism, but rather with hope.

ACKNOWLEDGMENTS

The author wishes to acknowledge partial support for this work from the U.S. Environmental Protection Agency Multiscale Experimental Ecosystem

Research Center (Contract R819640) and the U.S. Geological Survey Program for Across Trophic Levels System Simulation (Contract 1445CAO9950093).

REFERENCES

Baird, D. and R. Ulanowicz. 1989. The seasonal dynamics of the Chesapeake Bay ecosystem. *Ecological Monographs* 59:329–364.

Boltzmann, L. 1872. Weitere Studien ueber das Waermegleichtgewicht unter Gasmolekuelen. *Wiener Berichte* 6:275–370.

Christensen, V. and D. Pauly. 1997. *Ecopath with EcoSim, Vers. 4.0 Alpha: A Software for Analysis and Management of Aquatic Ecosystems.* International Center for Living Aquatic Resources Management, Manila.

Costanza, R. 1992. Toward an operational definition of ecosystem health. Pp. 239–256 in R. Costanza, B.G. Norton, and B.D. Haskell, eds., *Ecosystem Health: New Goals for Environmental Management.* Island Press, Washington, DC. 269 p.

Holling, C.S. 1986. The resilience of terrestrial ecosystems: Local surprise and global change. Pp. 292–317 in W.C. Clark and R.E. Munn, eds., *Sustainable Development of the Biosphere.* Cambridge University Press, Cambridge.

Jorgensen, S.E. 1997. *Integration of Ecosystem Theories: A Pattern.* Second Revised Edition. Kluwer, Dordrecht. 388 p.

Karr, J.R. 1986. *Assessment of Biological Integrity in Running Water: A Method and Its Rationale.* Illinois Natural History Survey, Publication 5, Champaign, IL.

Mageau, M.T., R. Costanza, and R.E. Ulanowicz. 1995. The development, testing and application of a quantitative assessment of ecosystem health. *Ecosystem Health* 1(4):201–213.

Mayr, E. 1992. The idea of teleology. *Journal of History of Ideas* 53(1):117–177.

Odum, E.P. 1969. The strategy of ecosystem development. *Science* 164:262–270.

Pahl-Wostl, C. 1992. Information theoretical analysis of functional temporal and spatial organization in flow networks. *Mathematical and Computer Modelling* 16(3): 35–52.

Peters, R.H. 1991. *A Critique for Ecology.* Cambridge University Press, Cambridge. 366 p.

Popper, K.R. 1990. *A World of Propensities.* Thoemmes, Bristol. 51 p.

Shannon, C.E. 1948. A mathematical theory of communication. *Bell System Technical Journal* 27:379–423.

Shrader-Fréchette, K.S. and E.D. McCoy. 1993. *Method in Ecology: Strategies for Conservation.* Cambridge University Press, Cambridge. 328 p.

Svirezhev, Y.M., and A. Svirejeva-Hopkins. 1998. Sustainable biosphere: Critical overview of the basic concept of sustainability. *Ecological Modelling* 106:47–61.

Tribus, M. and E.C. McIrvine. 1971. Energy and information. *Scientific American* 225:179–188.

Ulanowicz, R.E. 1980. An hypothesis on the development of natural communities. *Journal of Theoretical Biology* 85:223–245.

Ulanowicz, R.E. 1996. The propensities of evolving systems. Pp. 217–233 in E. Khalil, ed., *Evolution, Order, and Complexity.* Routledge, London.

Ulanowicz, R.E. 1997. *Ecology, the Ascendent Perspective.* Columbia University Press, New York. 201 p.

Ulanowicz, R.E. 1999. Life after Newton: An ecological metaphysic. *BioSystems* 50:127–142.

Ulanowicz, R.E. 2000. Quantifying constraints upon trophic and migratory transfers in landscapes. Pp. 113–142 in J. Sanderson and L.D. Harris, eds., *Landscape Ecology: A Top-Down Approach.* Lewis Publishers, Boca Raton, FL.

Ulanowicz, R.E. and L.G. Abarca. 1997. An informational synthesis of ecosystem structure and function. *Ecological Modelling* 95:1–10.

Ulanowicz, R.E. and D. Baird. 1999. Nutrient controls on ecosystem dynamics: The Chesapeake mesohaline community. *Journal of Marine Systems* 19:159–172.

Ulanowicz, R.E. and J. Norden. 1990. Symmetrical overhead in flow networks. *International Journal of Systems Science* 21(2):429–437.

Westra, L. 1994. *An Environmental Proposal for Ethics: The Principle of Integrity.* Rowman & Littlefield, Lanham, MD. 237 p.

Wulff, F. and R.E. Ulanowicz. 1989. A comparative anatomy of the Baltic Sea and Chesapeake Bay ecosystems. Pp. 232–256 in F. Wulff, J.G. Field, and K.H. Mann, eds., *Flow Analysis of Marine Ecosystems.* Springer-Verlag, Berlin.

PART III

The Sustainability and Integrity of Natural Resource Systems

In chapter 6, Robert Ulanowicz presented a method for measuring ecosystem integrity. Part III continues to explore what needs to be done to measure ecosystem integrity. It also examines the efficacy of government-created protected areas in safeguarding ecological integrity and explores policy issues relating to agricultural practices and fisheries. This part also describes some of the causes of current unsustainable practices that are degrading global ecological integrity.

In chapter 7, "Environmental Sustainability and Integrity in the Agriculture Sector," Robert Goodland and David Pimentel examine the environmental sustainability of agricultural practices after reviewing the concepts of environmental, social, and economic sustainability. Next, the authors examine the appropriate use of renewable and nonrenewable resources in agricultural practices, how to match emissions from agriculture to the assimilative capacity of ecosystems, and how to sustainably increase food supply. Lastly, the authors discuss enlightened water and chemical pollution policy, water and air pollution problems, the relationship between population and human disease, the degradation of land resources, the need for sustainable energy, and concerns about biotechnology.

In chapter 8, "Patch Disturbance, Ecofootprints, and Biological Integrity: Revisiting the Limits to Growth," William E. Rees argues that there is an unavoidable conflict between ecological integrity and current growth-oriented economic development practices. In this chapter, Rees examines human behavior relating to the natural world from a thermodynamic point of view. He starts by noting that like all animals, humans are patch disturbers. Humans have always affected the ecosystems in which they live, but now the patches that they affect go far beyond the local ecosystems in which they find themselves. Rees then goes on to explain why there is virtually no possibility for an industrial society of 6 to 10 billion people using prevailing or anticipated technologies to live sustainably on the Earth. Rees also notes that further growth of the human enterprise necessarily compromises prospects for preserving biodiversity, maintaining ecosystem integrity, and ensuring an enduring period of geopolitical stability. Because of this, Rees argues that humans must depend less on managing the environment and more on managing themselves. Rees is particularly concerned with the fact that the wealthiest fifth of the population now consumes over 80 percent of the global economic output and has unwittingly claimed the entire sustainable biophysical output of the ecosphere for themselves.

In chapter 9, "Can Canadian Approaches to Sustainable Forest Management Maintain Ecological Integrity?," Peter Miller and James W. Ehnes examine the concept of ecological integrity in the context of Canadian forests and forest policy. Recent visionary policy, as found in the 1992 Canada Forest Accord, sets a forest management goal that approximates integrity. Successful implementation of that goal awaits conceptual clarification, new adaptive management strategies linked to forest research, and a means to measure and monitor ecological integrity.

In response to these challenges, Miller and Ehnes propose the concept of maintaining "biosocial regional integrity" to accommodate some human exploitation of ecosystems while maintaining a form of integrity at the regional scale. In practice, this policy requires combining a strategy that protects representative areas and features of the landscape with forest management that is ecosystem based and tries to fit human exploitation of forests within the natural ranges of variability of those forests.

Next Miller and Ehnes explain the importance of establishing a set of criteria and indicators for setting more specific management goals and determining whether the new forest management strategies are capable of protecting the ecological integrity of Manitoba's forests. To develop appropriate indicators, they adopt a multiscale, multimetric approach that builds on James Karr's index of biological integrity. Miller and Ehnes show graphically how forest conditions of original integrity, health, and sustainability can be defined by such measures and thus provide targets for forest managers. In particular, their recommended management goal of maintaining biosocial regional integrity (i.e., "living in integrity") can be specified by this means. Because a detailed, research-based set of validated criteria and indicators does not yet exist, we cannot now say whether recent Canadian approaches to forest management will be successful in maintaining ecological integrity across forested landscapes. However, we do understand how that question could be answered.

In chapter 10, "Pattern of Forest Integrity in the Eastern United States and Canada: Measuring Loss and Recovery," Orie L. Loucks examines the ecological integrity of forests by looking primarily at ecosystem functions. Loucks is interested in measuring the functioning of forests to show how anthropogenic stresses can decrease forest function. He begins by describing why certain parameters of forest function are important candidates for measurement of forest ecological integrity. These parameters include net primary production, secondary production, hydrologic pumping/evapotransporation, biomass decomposition, and nutrient/mineral recycling. Loucks proposes the use of mean functional integrity (MFI), a system that combines functional parameters as the way to measure forest ecological integrity. Like Karr's index of biological integrity, Loucks's method would measure integrity through direct measurements of ecosystem parameters. But for forests, Loucks believes measuring function is preferable to measuring other biological indicators because forests are dominated by long-lived organisms that express change in abundance rather slowly. After a discussion of the theoretical issues, Loucks presents some case studies to demonstrate the usefulness and application of MFI.

In chapter 11, "Maintaining the Ecological Integrity of Landscapes and Ecoregions," Reed Noss describes how to protect the integrity of landscapes and ecoregions. He suggests that the appropriate scale of concern for protection of landscape integrity is the ecoregion. Noss reviews the amount of degradation to ecosystems worldwide and concludes that most landscapes have been degraded by human action. He states that appropriate goals for conservation of landscapes are: (1) representing all kinds of ecosystems, across their natural range of variation, in protected areas; (2) maintaining viable populations of all native species in natural patterns of abundance and distribution; (3) sustaining ecological and evolutionary processes within their natural range of variability; and (4) building a conservation network that is adaptable to environmental change.

Noss next concludes that most protected areas are too small to remain viable over the long run unless they are buffered and connected. To answer the question of how much additional protected area is needed, Noss argues that the answer must be developed empirically, case by case. Nevertheless, most estimates of the area needed in reserves in order to attain well-accepted conservation goals range from 25 to 75 percent of an ecoregion.

This discussion is followed by a description of the criteria for selecting protected areas. The criteria are identified as: (1) protection of special elements; (2) representation of all habitats; and (3) meeting the needs of focal species. Noss states that recent analyses of protected areas lead to the conclusion that the most important habitat lies outside of protected areas. Noss goes on to identify principles of protected reserve design that need to be examined upon their application. These principles are: (1) species well distributed across their native range are less susceptible to extinction than species confined to small portions of their range; (2) large blocks of habitat, containing large populations, are better than small blocks with small populations; (3) blocks of habitat, containing large populations, are better than blocks far apart; (4) habitat in contiguous blocks is better than fragmented habitat; (5) interconnected blocks of habitat are better than isolated blocks; and (6) blocks of habitat that are roadless or otherwise inaccessible to humans are better than roaded and accessible habitat blocks. Finally, Noss argues for the application of a management of ecosystems principle that incorporates the needs of nonhuman species into management assumptions while acknowledging human needs and desires.

In chapter 12, "Health, Integrity, and Biological Assessment: The Importance of Measuring Whole Things," James R. Karr reviews the concept of ecological health and argues that the use of the term "health" is grounded in science, yet acknowledges that ultimately the level of health that is acceptable is a societal value judgment. Karr argues for a definition of integrity as something that applies to conditions of places at one end of a continuum of human influence that supports biota, which is the product of evolutionary and biogeographical processes, with minimal influence from human society. Karr states his reasons for disagreeing with definitions of integrity that rely on the theoretical concepts of productivity, self-organization, and resilience. He chooses instead to measure integrity directly in terms of multimetric biological indices. These multimetric indices measure the biological condition and evaluate the results in terms of divergence from baseline biological conditions. Although Karr acknowledges natural variability in river systems, he believes that integrity can be measured through biological indicators because natural variation in rivers is trivial compared to the type of variation that one sees caused by row–crop agriculture, timber harvest, grazing, and urbanization. Society has, according to Karr, chronically undervalued the biological components of river systems. He states that success in protecting the health of rivers depends on realistic models of the interactions of landscapes, rivers, and human actions. In developing multimetric indices, Karr states that the following five tasks are critical: (1) classification to define homogeneous sets; (2) selection of appropriate metrics; (3) development of sampling protocols; (4) analysis of data to reveal biological patterns; and (5) communication of biological conditions.

In chapter 13, "Global Change, Fisheries, and the Integrity of Marine Ecosystems: The Future Has Already Begun," Daniel Pauly examines the future of marine fisheries. Pauly explores the effects of climate change on fisheries and concludes that science is not now capable of predicting the impact of changed climate on regional fisheries. He goes on to state that fisheries and the ecosystems supporting them are threatened by current fishing methods. Pauly identifies four processes that will continue to threaten fisheries. First, pressure from growing human populations will create demand that will exceed the supply and create incentives for humans to fish further down the food chain. Second, increased prices caused by increased demand will put even more pressure on the fisheries because increased prices will act like a subsidy. Third, fishing down the food chain will eventually result in species loss and degradation of supporting ecosystems. Last, scientists and others will forget that they are working on the remnants of a system that has been overexploited for decades. And, as a result, overexploitation will continue. To prevent worldwide ecosystem degradation, Pauly sees the need for decarbonization and dematerialization of the industrial economy, massive reforestation, and the transition to sustainable small-scale farming. To retain ecosystem integrity of marine ecosystems, Pauly recommends the abolition of subsidies for fishing, transition to small-scale fishing wherever possible, the establishment of large marine-protected areas, enforcement of limits, and rapid implementation of market-, community-, and ecology-based mitigation measures.

Environmental Sustainability and Integrity in the Agriculture Sector

Robert Goodland and David Pimentel

This chapter outlines parts of the huge and complex field of sustainability and integrity in agriculture (Brown 1997a). Sustainability is a vast field in itself, so this chapter focuses only on one of the three main types of sustainability, namely environmental sustainability (ES). Broadly, ES is discussed in connection with (1) agricultural production, (2) consumption of agricultural products, and (3) food policy. Significant parts of the agricultural sector are omitted, such as the role of sewage, annuals vs. perennials, agricultural transport, and the energy implications of fertilizers and biocides. We define environmental sustainability as "the maintenance of natural capital, or the maintenance of environmental source and sink capacities or rates," which is amplified in Box 7.1.

Soil fertility depletion, erosion, and soil regeneration rates are of paramount importance. Investments are needed to combat soil erosion and restore fertility, such as by fallowing. Regeneration rates are one hundred years or so in the case of trees, and five hundred years to form 25 mm of topsoil. Services from biodiversity (pollination, recycling, natural pest control) should not be impaired. As most agricultural production exceeds regeneration rates, the rates of depletion of natural capital need to be accounted for.

The gap between depletion and regeneration is partly narrowed by artificial inputs (e.g., fertilizer, energy), so the sustainability of input supply (e.g., nutrients and energy to extract and transport them) is included in the definition. Where modern inputs are not affordable, ES seeks to foster production without depletion, such as by reducing depletion first, then by increasing regeneration or fallow, which reduces needs of inputs.

It is impossible to make a nonrenewable stock resource totally sustainable, but El Serafy's rule (1993, 1996) promotes quasi sustainability (Box 7.2). El Serafy's rule holds that a fraction of nonrenewable liquidation proceeds should be invested in renewable substitutes, so that when the nonre-

BOX 7.1

Definition of Environmental Sustainability

Output Rule

Waste emissions from a project or action being considered should be kept within the assimilative capacity of the local environment without unacceptable degradation of its future waste-absorptive capacity or other important services.

Input Rule

Renewables: Harvest rates of renewable resource inputs must be kept within regenerative capacities of the natural system that generates them.

Nonrenewables: Depletion rates of nonrenewable resource inputs should be set below the historical rate at which renewable substitutes were developed by human invention and investment according to the Serafian quasi-sustainability rule (Box 7.2). An easily calculable portion of the proceeds from liquidating nonrenewables should be allocated to the attainment of sustainable substitutes.

Source: Daly 1996, 1999; Daly and Cobb 1994; see Goodland 1999, Goodland and Daly 1998.

BOX 7.2

Serafian Quasi Sustainability of Nonrenewables

The Serafian rule pertains to nonrenewable resources, such as fossil fuels and other minerals, but also to renewables to the extent they are being "mined." It states that their owners may enjoy part of the proceeds from their liquidation as income, which they can devote to consumption. The remainder, a user cost, should be reinvested to produce income that would continue after the resource has been exhausted. This method essentially estimates income from sales of an exhaustible resource. It has been used as a normative rule for quasi sustainability, whereby the user cost should be reinvested, not in any asset that would produce future income, but specifically to produce renewable substitutes for the asset being depleted. The user cost from depletable resources has to be invested specifically in replacements for what is being depleted in order to reach sustainability, and must not be invested in any other venture—no matter how profitable. The future acceptable rate of extraction of the nonrenewable resource should be based on the historic rate at which improved efficiency, substitution, and reuse became available. These calculations show the folly of relying on technological optimism, rather than on some historic track record.

Source: El Serafy 1993, 1996; Daly and Cobb 1994.

newable is exhausted, the substitute is sustainable. The renewable substitute has to be in the same sector as the nonrenewable factor that is being depleted. For instance, if irrigation depends on diesel pumps, proceeds from diesel depletion should be invested in renewable pumping such as solar or wind pumps (not in, for example, school education, however worthy that may be). The depletion of fossil water aquifers is a special case. First, the use of this water should be reduced to the lowest possible by boosting efficiency and reducing demand. Then such water should be accounted for and paid for—at "full cost," user cost, or the cost of substitution or backstop technology. Ultimately, the rate of water extraction needs to be balanced with either replenishment rate or the rate of development of a substitute. Most (87 percent) of the world's fresh water is used by the agriculture sector. The issues of oil prices, oil depletion, and the energy consumption of individual agricultural processes are crucial to sustainability in the agriculture sector.

We fully acknowledge that sustainable agriculture will often yield less per area than today's high-input and depleting agriculture in the short term, so demand management (involving such activities as controlling population and stabilizing living standards) are essential to achieving sustainability. It is impossible to overemphasize population control and stabilizing living standards, but they are outside the focus of this chapter.

Trade-offs

Environmental sustainability in the agriculture sector creates many trade-offs—e.g., the trade-off between food production (and cooking fuel) and nonfood agricultural production (fibers, building materials, tobacco, alcoholic beverages) (Brown 1997b). There will be competition between essential food crops and cooking fuels on the one hand, and nonfood agricultural production on the other. Sustainability demands that these rarely recognized trade-offs be addressed.

The trade-off between manufactured fibers (nonrenewable, oil-based nylon, polyester) and renewable agricultural fibers (wood, cotton) is recognized, although the differential environmental impacts are unclear. There is a sharp trade-off between growing cotton versus growing food crops in areas suitable for growing cotton.

Given that the impacts of producing cooking fuel can exceed the impacts of producing food, what should the balance be between the two? When biomass energy is used for cooking, approximately 2 kcal of biomass are used for each kcal food cooked in efficient stoves. Cooking efficiencies can vary widely depending on whether items such as agricultural "wastes" for fuel, improved stoves, pressure cookers, microwaves, and solar cookers are used, so such items bear greatly on sustainability.

In the race between food consumption and population growth, what is the optimal allocation of investments? The emphasis globally seems severely skewed, with much more focus on agricultural production than on slowing population growth, which may be the only long-term solution. Despite intensification in agricultural production, agricultural land ratios per capita are already unsustainably low in many countries, which therefore depend on imported grain. Sustainability means seeking a balance between investments in reducing population pressures on the one hand, and investments in increasing agricultural production on the other hand.

Agricultural Production
Extensification versus Intensification

Possibly the biggest debate over the means to increase production of food devolves on the balance between intensification and extensification of agricultural production. Extensification, the cultivation of hitherto uncultivated lands, creates massive environmental impacts, not the least of which is biodiversity loss. Most (c. 70 percent) of forest loss is due to agricultural extensification. The majority of extensified land has much lower productivity than today's average. Most new land is too erosion-prone, dry, steep, or infertile to match the average yields of existing lands. In view of such large environmental costs and modest yields, the balance between extensification and intensification is inching toward the latter.

Intensification is greatly preferable to extensification for any approach to sustainability. The sustainability of intensification depends on issues such as eutrophication, water use, agricultural runoff, the sustainability of fertilizer supply, and sources of energy and raw materials (e.g., oil). The key question is the balance between, on the one hand, the current heavy use of nonrenewable fertilizer to make up for soil erosion and fertility degradation and, on the other hand, replacing crop product nutrient export out of the agroecosystem with renewables through the improved use of agricultural "wastes."

Climate

A stable climate is also necessary for ES. If climate change intensifies, the risks to agriculture vastly outweigh any conceivable gains. Even where the climate actually improves, the soils and water regime may not follow, so yields may not increase. Since practically all agriculture depends on stable climates, practically all climate change will harm agriculture. To what extent should the agricultural sector invest in promoting climate stability?

These factors are exceptionally important, but are excluded from further treatment in this chapter.

Balancing Self-Sufficiency with Exports

ES demands careful balance between self-sufficiency in certain products, and trade and trickle-down effects. How should one reach a balance between some measure of self-sufficiency and export crop production? Or between home gardens, agroforestry, and monoculture export cropping? Now that self-sufficiency is no longer the dirty word that it was until very recently, what is the sustainable balance?

ES requires balancing the export of raw materials against the value added by domestic processing. For example, in the case of timber, the transport costs when timber is exported need to be internalized; and once that is done, there is a clear choice to be made between exporting crude logs and exporting door frames and windows. Repealing national log export bans may improve processing efficiency in Japan, but it postpones development in the timber-supplying country. In Mozambique, there was a controversy over the desire to boost employment by processing cashews domestically, roasting the nuts and producing jelly, wine, and other conserved cashew products. The alternative was to export crude cashews to India, which would then capture all the value added through processing. ES requires balancing investments in direct alleviation of poverty, hunger, and malnutrition with investments that "trickle down" to the poor, by following the comparative advantage of the export crop model (e.g., in the cases of coffee, cocoa, strawberries, and carnations).

What are the prospects, in the future, for less developed countries to import internationally traded grain bought with their export crop production? Fewer and fewer countries are net exporters of grain (presently, only the United States, Canada, Brazil, Australia, and Argentina are); therefore, the crunch seems inevitable, just a question of timing. If the U.S. population doubles in the next 70 years, the country will not have any grain left for export, assuming production remains the same.

Energy Resources

One or another form of energy is used by humans to provide them with their food and other needs. Over many centuries, humans relied on their own energy, animal power, wind, and waterpower. They have gradually turned to wood, coal, gas, and oil for fuel and power. About 385 quads from all energy sources per year are used worldwide. Currently, energy expenditure and the associated environmental degradation are directly related to the rapid growth in the world population.

Although worldwide about 50 percent of all solar energy captured by photosynthesis is used by humans, this is inadequate to meet their needs for food and forest products. To make up the shortfall, about 321 quads (1015 BTU or 337 × 1018 joules) of fossil energy are utilized worldwide each year. Of this, 81 quads are consumed just in the United States. American consumption of fossil fuel is about three times the 28 quads of solar energy harvested as crop and forest products each year. Thus the U.S. population consumes 40 percent more fossil energy than all the solar energy captured by U.S. vegetation each year.

In agriculture and forestry, fossil fuels are used to run machinery, pump water, and supply fertilizers and pesticides. Fossil energy is used to fuel a wide array of other human activities including industrial production; fuel for automobiles, trains, and trucks; highway construction; heating and cooling of buildings; and packaging of goods.

Developed nations annually consume about 80 percent of the fossil energy worldwide, while developing nations, which have about 75 percent of the world's population, consume only 20 percent. The United States consumes about 25 percent of the world's fossil energy output annually (Pimentel 1993). Fossil energy use in different U.S. economic sectors has increased 20- to 1,000-fold in the past three to four decades, attesting to America's heavy reliance on this finite energy resource to support its affluent lifestyle (Pimentel and Pimentel 1996).

Some developing nations that have high rates of population growth are increasing their use of fossil fuels to augment their agricultural production of food and fiber. In China, as mentioned, there has been a 100-fold increase in the use of fossil energy in agriculture since 1955. This increase has been mainly for fertilizers, pesticides, and irrigation.

The world supply of oil is projected to last for about 50 years at current pumping rates. The supply of natural gas is adequate for 20 to 35 years, and the coal supply for about 100 years. However, these estimates are based on current consumption rates and current population numbers. If all people in the world enjoyed a standard of living and energy consumption similar to that of the U.S. average and the world population continued to grow at a rate of 1.5 percent, the world's fossil fuel reserves would last a mere 15 years. At present, transportation represents 40 percent and electricity represents about 34 percent of total U.S. energy consumption, with nuclear energy contributing 18 percent of electricity needs.

Land Resources
More than 99 percent of human food comes from the terrestrial environment, and the remaining small percentage comes from the oceans, lakes, and other aquatic ecosystems. Worldwide, food and fiber crops are grown

on 12 percent of the Earth's total land area. Another 24 percent of the land is used as pasture to graze livestock that provide meat and milk products, while forests cover an additional 31 percent. The small percentage of forest and grassland set aside as protected national parks to conserve biological diversity amounts to only 3 percent of the total terrestrial ecosystem. Most of the remaining one-third of land area is unsuitable for crops, pasture, and forests because it is too cold, dry, steep, stony, or wet, or the soil is too infertile or shallow to support plant growth.

To provide a diverse nutritious diet (including feed grains), about 0.5 ha of cropland per capita is needed. At present, the United States has slightly more than this amount. In China, however, only 0.08 ha of cropland is available to feed the people, and the present land availability is rapidly declining because of continuing population growth, urbanization, road building, and rapid land degradation. The world cropland average is only 0.27 ha available per capita, or nearly one-half of the required amount. This shortage of productive cropland is, in part, the cause of the food shortages and poverty that many humans are experiencing today.

Currently, a total of 1,481 kg of agricultural products (including feed and grains) are produced annually to feed each American, while China's food supply averages only 476 kg/capita/year. The world average value is 614 kg/capita/year. The low number for China correlates with a vegetarian diet—and indeed, most people in China eat essentially a vegetarian diet. By all measurements, the Chinese have reached the carrying capacity of their agricultural system. China is now the world's biggest importer of grains, and is planning for huge imports of grains in the future. China's reliance on large inputs of fossil-based fertilizers and other inputs to compensate for severely eroded soils suggests that serious problems will arise in the future.

Most crop and pastureland throughout the world is presently threatened by at least one type of degradation. The major types of degradation include rainfall and wind erosion, and the salinization and waterlogging of irrigated soils (Kendall and Pimentel 1994). Worldwide, more than 10 million ha of productive arable land are severely degraded and abandoned each year. Moreover, each year an additional 5 million ha of new land must be put into production to feed the 80 million humans added yearly to the world population. Most of the total of 15 million ha needed for both replacement and expansion is coming from the world's forests. The urgent need for more agricultural land accounts for more than 60 percent of the deforestation now occurring worldwide.

Soil erosion by wind and water is the single most serious cause of soil loss and degradation. Erosion rates are greater than ever before in history, averaging about 30 t/ha/year worldwide. Soil erosion on cropland ranges from about 13 t/ha/year in the United States to 40 t/ha/year in China (Wen

1993). In Africa, the rate of soil loss has increased 20 times during the past 30 years. Wind erosion is so serious in China that Chinese soil can be detected in the Hawaiian atmosphere when planting starts in China. Similarly in 1992, soil eroded from Africa was detected in Florida and Brazil. Worldwide, soil erosion is about 30 t/ha/year.

The current erosion rate throughout the world is of particular concern because of the slow pace of topsoil formation; it takes approximately five hundred years for 2.5 cm (1 inch) of topsoil to form under agricultural conditions. Thus, topsoil is being lost 13 to 40 times faster than it is being replaced, or 13 to 40 times above the sustainable rate.

Erosion adversely affects crop productivity by reducing the water-holding capacity of the soil, soil nutrients, soil organic matter, and soil depth—all factors that depress crop plant growth. Estimates are that agricultural land degradation can be expected to depress world food production between 15 and 30 percent during the next 25-year period, unless new production strategies are used to curtail this loss and improve the sustainability of crop soils.

Water Resources

The present and future availability of adequate supplies of fresh water is frequently taken for granted. Natural collectors of water such as rivers and lakes vary in distribution throughout the world and are frequently shared within and between countries. All surface water supplies, but especially those in arid regions, are diminished by evaporation. For instance, reservoir water experiences an average yearly loss of about 24 percent.

All vegetation requires and transpires massive amounts of water during the growing season. For example, a corn crop that produces about 7,500 kg/ha of grain will take up and transpire about 5 million liters/ha of water during the growing season. To supply this much water to the crop, not only must 8 million liters (800 mm) of rain fall per hectare, but also a significant portion must fall during the growing season. Different crops require different amounts of water (Table 7.1). High-yield "green revolution" crops require more water than lower-yield crops. This is one reason why the worldwide demand for water has tripled in the last two decades.

Perhaps the greatest threat to maintaining freshwater supplies is overdraft of surface and groundwater resources used to supply the needs of the rapidly growing human population and the agriculture that provides its food. Agricultural production "consumes" more fresh water than any other human activity. Worldwide, about 82 percent of the fresh water that is pumped is "consumed" (so that it is nonrecoverable) by agriculture (Postel 1999). In the United States, this figure is about 85 percent. All people require nearly 3 liters/day per capita of water, including the water in milk and other foods,

TABLE 7.1
Liters of Water Required to
Produce 1 Kilogram of
Food

Potatoes	500
Wheat	900
Alfalfa	900
Sorghum	1,110
Maize	1,400
Rice	1,910
Soybeans	2,000
Chicken	3,500
Beef	100,000

Source: Pimentel et al. 1997.

but need a minimum of 90 liters/day for cooking, washing, and other do-mestic needs. Each American uses about 400 liters/day for domestic needs. About 80 nations in the world are already experiencing significant water shortages. For instance, in China, more than three hundred cities are short of water and the problem is intensifying.

Surface water in rivers and lakes and groundwater provide the freshwater supply for the world. Groundwater resources are renewed at various rates but usually at the extremely slow rate of 0.1-0.3 percent per year. Because of their slow recharge rate, groundwater resources must be carefully man-aged to prevent overdraft. Yet humans are not effectively conserving groundwater resources, and their overdraft is now a serious problem in many parts of the world. For example, in Tamil Nadu, India, groundwater levels declined 25 to 30 meters during the 1970s because of excessive, but needed, pumping for irrigation. In Beijing, China, the groundwater table is diminishing at a rate of 1 to 2 m/year, while in Tianjin, China, it drops 4.4 m/year. In the United States, aquifer overdraft averages 25 percent higher than replacement rates. But in the vast U.S. Ogallala aquifer, annual over-draft is 130 to 160 percent above the replacement level. If this continues, this vital aquifer is expected to become nonproductive in about 40 years. High consumption of surface and groundwater resources is beginning to limit the option of irrigating arid regions. Furthermore, per capita irriga-tion area is also declining because of salinization and waterlogging, both deleterious effects of continual irrigation (Postel 1999).

Urban water demand is outcompeting agricultural water needs. There-fore, ES in agriculture depends on reducing urban water demand, or re-dressing the imbalance in some other way. An important solution would be to cease financing sewerage and invest instead in source waste separation. If human effluent were converted into valuable agricultural fertilizer input, the energy balance would be improved, and the need for artificial fertilizer would be reduced.

Developing countries discharge approximately 95 percent of their untreated urban sewage directly into surface waters. Of India's 3,119 towns and cities, just 209 have partial treatment facilities and only 8 have full wastewater treatment facilities. A total of 114 cities dump untreated sewage and partially cremated bodies directly into the sacred Ganges River. Downstream, the untreated water is used for drinking, bathing, and washing. In China, an estimated 80 percent of industrial and domestic wastes are discharged untreated into river systems.

Role of Fish and Aquaculture

Overall, less than 1 percent of global food comes from oceans or fresh water. Nevertheless, small but critical quantities of animal protein can make a big difference to the starchy diets of the world's poor. Accordingly, the production of protein through aquaculture might be desirable if it could be achieved at a cost low enough for the poor. However, most aquaculture production is presently achieved only at high cost.

At present, fish and other aquatic resources provide about 0.6 percent of the food calories consumed by the world's population and about 5 percent of the protein (Pimentel et al. 1996). The subset of aquatic resources provided by aquaculture constitutes less than 0.1 percent of the world's food calories—and it is doubtful that it ever will be much greater than 0.1 percent, because aquaculture is much more feed- and energy-intensive than is terrestrial agriculture. Aquaculture also contrasts with fish growing in natural settings, many of which eat plankton, which in turn feeds on sunlight and water.

There are a number of serious environmental concerns in aquaculture. Cultured fish have to be fed grain (as well as animal wastes), and this is expensive in terms of dollar costs and energy. In addition, large amounts of energy are used in aquaculture to pump water and keep it aerated and free of disease organisms. To produce catfish, one of the most profitable fish in culture, about 34 kcal of fossil energy are required to produce 1 kcal of catfish protein, more than three times the energy cost of producing broiler chicken protein. Oysters have been produced through aquaculture, but the costs were enormous, with more than 600 kcal of fossil energy required to produce 1 kcal of oyster protein. About 25 percent of shrimps are farmed, many from converted mangroves, resulting in major adverse environmental impacts, including impacts that decrease offshore fish catches. The main factor constraining the expansion of aquaculture is often the lack of sufficient amounts of clean water.

Most major ocean and freshwater fisheries are in decline. Catch sizes in most major fisheries have been exceeding regeneration rates for a number of years. Estuaries, mangroves, wetlands, and other fish habitats have been polluted and many destroyed. Seafood consumption per person probably peaked in 1989. While seafood was once eaten mainly by the poor, prices are now so high that it has become a food for the rich, and this trend looks likely to accelerate in the future. From now on fish consumption, because of human population growth and overfishing, seems likely to decline from 19 kg/person to about half that in the next couple of decades.

Aquaculture has two extremes. Low-productivity and low-impact aquaculture depends on autotrophs (green plants, plankton, algae) for nutrients. No nutrients are added; harvests are low in amount and in impact. High-productivity and high-impact aquaculture depends on inputs of feed (including agricultural residues, by-catch fishmeal, hog manure, and sewage). The higher productivity is achieved at the expense of the environmental impacts involved in providing the feed, diesel, pumps, transport, and so on. Even so, aquaculture can be more productive than raising livestock and can have less environmental impact. Some species of fish need only 2 kg of feed per kg of liveweight gain, compared with 7 kg for beef. Aquaculture, a $30 billion industry worldwide, is valuable in producing protein and recycling waste. For long-term sustainability, fish ponds recycling sewage into protein should be encouraged.

In the worldwide effort to increase food production, aquaculture merits more attention than raising grain-fed cattle. Many food fish are actually carnivores or piscivores (eating other fish). About two-thirds of aquaculture is in freshwater rivers, lakes, ponds, and tanks; the rest is coastal mariculture, for which there is a lot of room for expansion. Today's global aquaculture of 16 million tons could meet 40 percent of world fish demand within 15 years (Brown et al. 1998).

Chemical and Biological Pollution and Disease

Intensifying environmental degradation contributes to chemical and biological pollution of food, air, water, and soil; malnutrition; increased ultraviolet radiation; and pathogenic microbe explosions. These pollution and associated disease problems will be compounded further as the world population expands from 6 billion to 12 billion in the next 50 years, and as the U.S. population doubles during the next 60 years to 520 million, if current growth rates are maintained.

Since the advent of DDT use for crop protection in 1945, global growth of pesticide use in agriculture has been phenomenal. In 1945, about 50 million kg of pesticides were applied worldwide. Exhibiting an approximate

50-fold increase, global usage is currently at about 2.5 billion kg per year. In the United States, the use of synthetic pesticides since 1945 has grown 33-fold to about 0.5 billion kg. Unfortunately, the increase in hazards is even greater than it might appear because the toxicity of modern pesticides has increased more than 10-fold when compared to those used in the early 1950s.

Biotechnology

Many hoped that biotechnology would be the new green revolution, but this has not been the case. The green revolution focused on using fossil energy to increase fertilizer and pesticide use as well as to provide power to supply irrigation water. With suitable short-stature plants, the application of fertilizers, pesticides, and irrigation could be achieved relatively rapidly over a 10-year period.

The achievements in biotechnology have not been significant despite the last 20 years of research. Biotechnology research has increased crop yields only in small increments (Paoletti and Pimentel 1996). Partly this has been due to the difficulty of the task, and partly it has been due to the focus of biotechnology research. For example, most of the research (more than 40 percent) has been focused on developing herbicide-resistant plants. Developing herbicide-resistant plants helps the chemical companies sell more herbicides, but it does not increase crop yields. Of course, the heavy use of herbicides increases environmental pollution.

Little has been accomplished either in developing crops that are resistant to insects and plant pathogens or in having grain plants like corn fix their own nitrogen. There has been talk by some that drought-resistant crops could be developed. However, this approach has not progressed far because water use by a crop is essential to its photosynthetic activity. Some plant physiologists doubt that anything above a 5 percent reduction in water use can be achieved by biotechnology in crop plants because of the vital role that water plays in plant physiology.

Consumption of Agricultural Products

This section focuses on the consumption of food, rather than other agricultural products such as cotton. With regard to food consumption, meeting the conditions for ES threatens to become more and more difficult—because of population growth. The first and absolutely essential prerequisite for ES is a stable human population (a constant or declining number of consumers). ES will become practically impossible unless the human population of the region or country stabilizes.

Demand Management

Reducing demand for food is half of the equation (just as insulation is half of the energy conservation equation). Demand can be reduced in part by reducing losses through the use of conventional methods such as control of insects, rodents, birds, and molds; improved storage; and breeding resistance.

Reducing demand can also be achieved by eating more efficiently on the food chain. Diet matters; ES can be brought about by reducing feeding inefficiencies, such as those existing in producing grain-fed livestock, and encouraging more efficient diets, such as plant-based ones. A balance needs to be achieved between investments in food and investments in food additives, such as micronutrients (e.g., iodine in salt, and iron in flour) and vitamins.

Diet and the Food Chain

The acceptability of plant-based diets is a matter of degree. Human societies differ in what diet they find comfortable. Among those who restrict their consumption of animal-based foods, there is a continuum from eschewing red meat, then "white" meat (poultry), then mammals or all terrestrial animals (Box 7.3). Some people draw the line between eating warm-blooded animals and cold-blooded animals. In other words, some people eat fish, but not rabbits or chickens. Another stage on the continuum involves eating only invertebrates, such as shrimp and shellfish. Ovo-lacto-vegetarians eat eggs, milk, and cheese, but not the animal itself. Vegans eat no animal products of any kind. Ethicists try to interpret people's behavior, but people often are neither strictly logical nor consistent in their diets. Nor need they be. Flexibility and opportunism in diet are valuable, especially for the poor.

The issue is to produce food more sustainably, and at lower environmental, social, and economic costs. People should always be allowed to choose the diet that they want, but the full costs of their choices should be reflected in the price that they pay for their diet.

Richer people eat higher on the food chain than poor people do. When people get richer, they tend to move up the food chain and eat more meat. This partly explains why the world is hurtling away from sustainability. For sustainability to increase, and to help reduce hunger in poorer societies, incentives are needed to encourage people to descend the food chain, eat less meat, and move toward plant-based diets. The most needed transition is toward eating mainly autotrophs (green plants) and saprophytes, and fewer heterotroph products, especially homeotherms. This would buy valuable time to implement other prudential measures on the transition to a sustainable society.

We do not advocate that everyone should adopt strictly plant-based diets. On the contrary, a world in which scarcity and overpopulation did not force choices between more carnivory on the one hand, or more grain-based diets on the other, would be preferable. We prefer a world in which there is plenty of room for solitude, ample space for all species, and wildlands for all to enjoy. Lamentably, we do not have the luxury of that choice any longer. Overpopulation, resource scarcity, and consumption far above sufficiency now largely preclude such choices.

The choice to go for a full world has foreclosed many wonderful options. Most people no longer can practice hunting and gathering, few can practice slash-and-burn, and even small-scale self-sufficient communities can be practiced only by the very few. The other agony of having let overpopulation and resource scarcity dictate our choices is that even in the unlikely event that all people suddenly elect to become vegan aesthetes, the problem would be postponed only temporarily.

The main need is the internalization of the costs of dietary preferences. If one chooses to eat high-impact food, one should pay the full costs of such a choice. This is consonant with the "polluter pays" principle. Encouragingly, a powerful trend to eat lower on the food chain has started. For example, annual U.S. beef consumption peaked in 1976 at 95 pounds per person; in the 1990s it has stagnated around 66 pounds. U.S. beef consumption grew at only 1 percent between 1990 and 1995. European and especially U.K. beef consumption never reached those levels, but is falling faster than in the United States. European Union consumption of beef and veal fell 6 percent between 1990 and 1995. The countervailing trend is for people to eat more meat as they become richer, however. China's pork consumption, for example, jumped 14 percent in 1995 alone (Brown et al. 1998). Meat demand in developing countries will increase by a staggering 160 percent by 2020.

Clearly, those seeking to reduce poverty should phase out of investing in livestock production, especially grain-fed livestock, and leave it to the private sector. (Natural range–fed meat, the family pig, and scrap-fed chickens could be exceptions.) Such groups should ensure that good economics prevail, including accounting for full environmental and social costs.

In the United States, beef sales are the single-largest revenue source within the whole agriculture sector. Only four meatpackers in the United States hold 82 percent of the market, suggesting a low-cost place to tax. Incentive methodology could address taxing feedlots, ranchers, or slaughterhouses. The 104-million-strong cattle herd is the country's largest single user of grain, mainly in the form of winter feed cakes or pellets. Possibly that can be taxed. In some counties, livestock account for half the tax base. Presumably taxes on livestock could be increased. Or a land-use intensity tax could be designed to foster intensification, where appropriate, and demote extensification, such as ranching.

BOX 7.3

Environmental Sustainability and Food Chain Ranking

↑ WORST

Most Impact/Least Efficient/Least Healthy
—To Be Taxed Highest—

1. Mammals: Swine/Cattle/Goats/Sheep
Rodents/Lagomorphs/Camelids/Deer
[Eggs/Cheese/Milk/Butter]

2. Birds: Chickens/Geese/Ducks/Pigeons/Turkeys

Homeotherms (Warm-Blooded)

Poikilotherms (Cold-Blooded)

3. Other Vertebrates: Fish/Reptiles/Amphibians

4. Invertebrates: Crustaceans/Insects/[Honey/Propolis]/Annelids/Mollusks

Carnivores

Heterotrophs

Vegans

5. Saprophytes: Fungi/Yeasts/Other Microbes

6. Autotrophs: Legumes/Grains/Vegetables/Starch Crops/Fruits/Nuts/Algae

↓ BEST

Least Impact/Most Efficient/Healthiest
—Zero Tax—

Source: After Goodland 1997.

Conclusion

In summary, in order to achieve long-term sustainability and integrity in agriculture, the following three circumstances are envisaged: (1) most people of the world—those already at the efficient, low-impact end of the food chain—would stay at the low end of the chain, but would diversify their diet; (2) affluent people now eating at the top of the food chain would pay full costs or elect to consume more efficiently lower down the food chain; and (3) people starting to move up the food chain (e.g., in China and India) would be encouraged to stop where they are—and to consider moving back down the chain.

Incentives are needed to promote grain-based diets by applying good economics and good environmental management to food and agriculture.

In particular, conversion efficiency and "polluter pays" principles should be used in setting full-price policies, which internalizes environmental and social costs. On the lower end of the scale, natural range–fed sheep and cattle can produce milk and meat while making the most of vegetation inedible for humans. On the higher end of the scale, cattle feedlots and slaughterhouses consume much water and generate much highly polluting waste. Wastes often are not efficiently reused but are instead disposed of in the nearest watercourse. Feed and forage production consume even more water. This needs to be internalized.

The highest taxes would fall on the least efficient converters, namely hogs and cattle. Slightly lower taxes would be assessed on sheep and those cattle grazing natural grassland more than do feedlot cattle. Taxes would be lower on free-range poultry recycling household wastes than on cattle— and even lower on rodents and lagomorphs, which eat wastes or are not fed. The family cow may not be entirely discouraged, as it may facilitate manure recycling and help in grain production.

If such sustainability and poverty-alleviating measures become widely adopted, mammalian flesh consumption would decline and would consist mainly of males not needed for draught. Hogs and poultry would be kept mainly to recycle wastes; their meat would be an occasional by-product. Ruminants would be restricted to natural range unusable for more intensive production.

No taxes would be paid on grains (rice, maize, wheat, buckwheat), starches (potatoes, cassava), and legumes (soy, pulses, beans, peas, peanuts). Modest subsidies on coarse grains (millet, pearl millet, sorghum) would alleviate hunger and are unlikely to be abused (as the rich usually won't eat such foods).

Encouragement for domestic or village-scale beneficiation, such as of peanuts to peanut butter and cashew fruits to roasted nuts, often doubles or triples the profit to the grower. Peanut butter and cornflakes were invented expressly to increase the consumption of those low-impact foods at the bottom of the food chain. Adoption of such policies will not solve world hunger overnight, but it will certainly help.

REFERENCES

Brown, L.R. 1995. *Who Will Feed China? Wake-up Call for a Small Planet*. New York: W.W. Norton.

Brown, L.R. 1997a. The agricultural link: How environmental deterioration could disrupt economic progress. Washington, DC: Worldwatch Institute, Paper 136.

Brown, L.R. 1997b. *Tough Choices: Facing the Challenge of Food Scarcity*. New York:

W.W. Norton.

Brown, L.R., M. Renner, and C.C. Flavin. 1998. *Vital Signs 1998: The Environmental Trends That Are Shaping Our Future.* Washington, DC: Worldwatch Institute.

Daly, H.E. 1996. *Beyond Growth: The Economics of Sustainable Development.* Boston: Beacon Press.

Daly, H.E. 1999. *Ecological Economics and the Ecology of Economics.* Cheltenham: Edward Elgar.

Daly, H.E. and J. Cobb, 1994. *For the Common Good.* (2nd ed.) Boston: Beacon Press.

El Serafy, S. 1993. Country macroeconomic work and natural resources. Environmental Working Paper 58. Washington, DC: The World Bank.

El Serafy, S. 1996. Natural resources and national accounting: Impact on macroeconomic policy. *Environment, Taxation and Accounting,* Parts 1 and 2: 27–47, 39–59.

Goodland, R. 1997. "Agricultural sustainability: Diet matters." *Ecological Economics* 23(3): 189–200.

Goodland, R. 1999. "The biophysical basis of environmental sustainability." In *Handbook of Environmental Economics,* edited by J.C.J.M. van den Bergh. London: E. Elgar Press.

Goodland, R. and H.E. Daly. 1998. "Imperatives for environmental sustainability: Decrease overconsumption and stabilize population." In *Population and Global Security,* edited by N. Polunin, 117–132. New York: Cambridge University Press.

Kendall, H.W. and D. Pimentel. 1994. "Constraints on the expansion of the global food supply." *Ambio* 23(3): 198–205.

Paoletti, M.G. and D. Pimentel. 1996. "Genetic engineering in agriculture and the environment." *BioScience* 46(9): 665–673.

Pimentel, D., ed. 1993. *World Soil Erosion and Conservation.* New York: Cambridge University Press.

Pimentel, D. and M. Pimentel. 1996. *Food, Energy and Society.* Niwot: University Press of Colorado.

Pimentel, D., R.E Shanks, and J.C. Rylander. 1996. "Bioethics of fish production: Energy and the environment." *Journal of Agricultural and Environmental Ethics* 9(2): 144–164.

Pimentel, D., J. Houser, E. Preiss, O. White, H. Fang, L. Mesnick, T. Barsky, S. Tariche, J. Schreck, and S. Alpert. 1997. "Water resources: Agriculture, the environment, and society." *BioScience* 47(2): 97–106.

Postel, S. 1999. *Pillar of Sand: Can the Irrigation Miracle Last?* Washington, DC: Worldwatch Institute, W.W. Norton.

Wen, D. 1993. "Soil erosion and conservation in China." In *World Soil Erosion and Conservation,* edited by D. Pimentel, 63–86. New York: Cambridge University Press.

Patch Disturbance, Ecofootprints, and Biological Integrity: Revisiting the Limits to Growth (or Why Industrial Society Is Inherently Unsustainable)

William E. Rees

Global Change and Human Ecology

Greenhouse gas accumulation, ozone depletion, fisheries collapse, soils degradation, endocrine disruption, accelerating species loss—these and related trends, both local and global, are symptoms of a fundamental imbalance in the relationship between the human enterprise and "the environment." Many technical analysts and ordinary people alike have therefore come to believe that the current global development path is fundamentally unsustainable. The continuous growth in energy and material "throughput" required to feed aggregate human demand has created a genuine global ecological crisis (Daly 1991a, Goodland 1991).

Despite increasing awareness of the danger, human pressure on the planet is increasing relentlessly. The human population reached 6 billion in 1999 and is growing by 84 million per year; by the end of the decade (and millennium), it had almost doubled twice in this century.[1] All these people, rich and poor alike, have rising material expectations sustained by an economic system that assumes the latter are insatiable. Little wonder that the global economy has expanded fivefold in half a century.

That the benefits of this economic explosion have been unevenly distributed is a major complicating factor. While 20 percent of the world's population enjoy an unprecedented level of material well-being, another 20 percent remain in abject poverty. This situation is clearly morally intolerable. However, rather than contemplate mechanisms to redistribute the

world's wealth, mainstream governments and international institutions have
determined to abolish poverty through *another* five- to tenfold increase in
industrial activity (see WCED 1987). In theory, if the economic pie is big
enough, even the relatively poor should enjoy adequate material well-being
(thus easing political pressure for redistributive policies).

Unfortunately, there is no indication that this approach will relieve the
moral dilemma or the sociopolitical tensions associated with the income
gap anytime soon. In 1960, the fraction of global income enjoyed by the
richest 20 percent of people was "only" 30 times greater than the share
received by the poorest 20 percent; by 1990 this ratio had increased to 60
to 1 (UNDP 1994). In short, the income gap actually doubled in 30 years
of continuous global growth!

Not surprisingly, society at large is deeply divided on both the problem
and its solutions.[2] A minority, mainly ecocentric and community-oriented
groups, see the growth ethic and rampant consumerism as the main concern. They argue that beyond a certain point (long past in richer countries)
there is no evident relationship between income and perceived well-being.
Further growth may therefore be unnecessary. Rather, the solution lies in
policies to ensure more equitable distribution of the world's present economic output and in changing consumer behavior. The majority, however,
including many humanists, techno-optimists, and mainstream policymakers, remain dedicated to growth and consumer ideals. They see freer
markets and a new efficiency revolution as the only politically feasible solution to both global ecological decline (wealth can purchase a "cleaner"
environment) and the problems caused by persistent material inequity.

Environmentalism Is Not Human Ecology

Whatever their proposed solutions, almost everyone in the mainstream
shares the perception that we are confronting an "environmental" crisis
rather than a human ecological crisis. This distinction is not a trivial one.
The former term externalizes the problem, effectively blaming it on an environment gone wrong or on defective resource systems that need to be
fixed. By contrast, the latter term places blame squarely where it belongs, on
the nature and behavior of people themselves, and suggests that it is human
wants which should be better controlled.

This chapter starts from the premise that the current dilemma is at least
partly rooted in this perceptual tension. The Cartesian dualism that underpins Western scientific culture has created a psychological barrier between
humans and the rest of nature, a barrier that prevents us from understanding
ourselves as ecological beings. The difficulty for sustainability is that "no
amount of ethical axiology, or legal, policy, and technological engineering,
is going to solve problems that are misunderstood" (Drengson 1989).

My overall purpose, therefore, is to reanalyze the so-called environmental crisis—the erosion of global ecological integrity—as a problem of human ecological dysfunction. This requires acceptance of two unconventional interpretations of human material reality. First, I adopt an ecological perspective that sees people as components of, and participants in, most of the world's major ecosystems. In this light, material economic activity is really the expression of human ecological relationships, and the economy is seen as an inextricably integrated, completely contained, and wholly dependent growing subsystem of a nongrowing ecosphere (Daly 1992, Rees 1995a).

Second, we must recognize that whatever else it implies, human economic activity (like the economic activity of any other real-world species) requires continuous energy and material transformations and that such irreversible transformations are ultimately subject to constraints imposed by the second law of thermodynamics (Georgescu-Roegen 1971; Daly 1991b,c; Rees 1999).

In its simplest form, the second law states that any isolated system[3] will always tend toward equilibrium; alternately, the "entropy" of any isolated system always increases. This means that available energy spontaneously dissipates, concentrations disperse, gradients disappear. An isolated system thus becomes increasingly unstructured in an inexorable slide toward thermodynamic equilibrium. This is a state of maximum entropy in which "nothing happens or can happen" (Ayres 1994, p. 3).

Early formulations of the second law referred strictly to simple isolated systems close to equilibrium. We now recognize, however, that all systems, whether or not isolated and near equilibrium, are subject to the same forces of entropic decay. *Any* differentiated far-from-equilibrium system has a natural tendency to erode and unravel.

But not all of them do. Many biophysical systems, from individual fetuses to the entire ecosphere, actually gain in mass or organizational complexity over time (i.e., they actually *increase* their distance from equilibrium). This seemingly paradoxical behavior can nevertheless be reconciled with the second law. Biophysical systems exist in a loose, nested hierarchy, each component system being contained by the next level up and itself comprising a chain of linked subsystems at lower levels (Kay 1991).[4] Living systems are thus able to import available energy and material (essergy) from their host environments and use it, in the face of entropic decay, to maintain their internal integrity and to grow. They also export the resultant waste (entropy) back into their hosts. Because such systems continuously degrade and dissipate available energy and matter, they are called "dissipative structures" (see Prigogine 1997).

In effect, modern formulations of the second law posit that all highly ordered systems develop and grow (increase their internal order) "at the expense of increasing disorder at higher levels in the systems hierarchy" (Schneider and Kay 1994). The quasi-parasitic hierarchical relationship between the human enterprise and nature thus ensures that continuous material economic growth will inevitably become a problem.

This human ecological perspective contrasts sharply with the dominant worldview. The latter assumes that the human enterprise is more or less independent of nature and that the "environment" therefore poses no significant constraints on the economy. In effect, conventional economic theory sees humans as free to act as if economic production/consumption were somehow exempt from thermodynamic and other critical natural laws. It is this ecologically empty vision that drives the current global development paradigm and has generated the sustainability conundrum. The following sections make the case that understanding the human niche is a prerequisite for restoring biological integrity and achieving sustainability.

Humans as "Patch Disturbers"

Human ecology begins with recognition that the mere existence of people in a given habitat implies significant effects on local ecosystems' structure and function. This is the inevitable consequence of two simple biological realities: first, human beings are big animals with correspondingly large individual energy and material requirements; and second, humans are social beings who live in extended groups. The invasion of any previously "stable" ecosystem by people therefore invariably produces changes in established energy and material pathways. There will be a reallocation of resources among species in the system to the benefit of some and the detriment of others. To this extent at least, people invariably perturb or "disturb" the systems of which they are a part.

These basic facts of human ecology, together with food productivity data for typical terrestrial ecosystems, would be enough for an alien ecologist to advance the following hypothesis:

> In most of the potential habitats on Earth, groups of human hunter-gatherers will sooner or later overwhelm their local ecosystems and be forced to ramble farther afield in search of sustenance.

Indeed, the productivity of most unaltered ecosystems is inadequate to support more than a few people for long in the immediate vicinity of a temporary camp. Thus, in preagricultural times, when a group of human foragers had hunted out and picked over a given area, they had to move on.

This would enable the abandoned site to recover, perhaps to be revisited in a few years or decades. By moving among favored habitat sites, exploiting one, allowing others to recover, early humans could exist in an overall dynamic equilibrium with the ecosystems that sustained them, albeit across their total home ranges. Hunting-gathering and closely related swidden (slash-and-burn) agriculture, with their long fallow periods after episodes of intensive use, may well be the most nearly sustainable lifestyles ever adopted by humans (see Kleinman et al. 1995, 1996).

Such quasi steady-state systems, established after long periods of human habitation, were quite different from the systems that would have existed in the same areas in the absence of people. Perhaps the most dramatic evidence of this is the systemic changes that occur when humans first invade and settle a new habitat or land mass. Some of these changes are permanent. The recent paleoecological, anthropological, and archaeological literature tells a convincing story of the extinctions of large mammals and birds that accompanied first contact and settlement of their habitats by human beings (Ponting 1991, Diamond 1992, Flannery 1994, Pimm et al. 1995, Tuxill 1998). "For every area of the world that paleontologists have studied and that humans first reached within the last fifty thousand years, human arrival approximately coincided with massive prehistoric extinctions" (Diamond 1992, p. 355). The species so extirpated include not only those upon which humans preyed, but also various other predators to whom humans proved to be competitively superior (Table 8.1). In North America, South America, and Australia, about 72, 80, and 86 percent, respectively, of large mammal genera became extinct after human arrival (Diamond 1992, p. 357). Pimm et al. (1995, p. 348) estimate "that with only Stone Age technology, the Polynesians exterminated >2000 bird species, some ~15% of the world total."

Upping the Impact Ante

As noted, prehistoric humans eventually came to live in more or less stable dynamic equilibrium (or steady state) within their altered ecosystems, often for thousands of years. However, in subsequent millennia, with the development of complex language and improvements in tools and weapons, these long-term stable relationships have broken down. Human hunter-gatherers seem to have been instrumental in the eventual extinction of various large animals with which they had long coexisted in many parts of the world. These species include giant deer and mammoths in Eurasia, giant buffalo, antelopes, and horses in Africa, and bears, wolves, and beavers in Britain (Diamond 1992, p. 356). In short, the slow spread of preagricultural humanity across the face of the Earth, accelerated by the diffusion of more advanced hunting technologies and the inexorable expansion of human

TABLE 8.1

Examples of Areas Where Large-Scale Extinctions Are Thought to Have
Accompanied Human Occupation

Geographic Area	Species Extinguished by Humans (in last 50,000 years)
Africa	giant buffalo, giant hartebeest, giant horse
Australia	diprotodonts (marsupial equivalent of cows and rhinos), giant wombat, giant kangaroo
Crete and Cyprus	pygmy hippos and giant tortoises, dwarf elephants and deer
Europe	European rhino, cave-bear, long-tusked elephant, hippopotamus, Irish elk, woolly mammoth, woolly rhino
Hawaii	flightless geese and ibises, 50 species of small birds
Henderson Island	three large pigeons, one small pigeon, three seabirds
Madagascar	half-dozen species of giant flightless "elephant" birds, two giant land tortoises, a dozen species of large lemurs, pygmy hippo, large mongoose-like carnivore
New Zealand	moas, giant duck, goose, coot, raven, eagle, pelican, swan, numerous small songbirds and mammals, frogs, snails, giant insects
North and South America, Australia	numerous large mammals
West Indies	several monkeys; ground sloths; bear-sized rodent; several owls— normal, colossal, and titanic

Sources: Diamond 1992, 1997; Flannery 1994; Ponting 1991.

numbers, seems, invariably, to have been accompanied by significant, permanent modifications in ecosystem structure at all spatial scales.

The already significant impact of humans on ecosystems escalated dramatically with the shift away from the hunter-gatherer lifestyle. With the dawn of agriculture ten thousand years ago and the much larger human populations it could support, people acquired the capacity to permanently alter entire landscapes. Increased food production also enabled the establishment of permanent settlements, the division of labor, the evolution of class structure, the development of government including bureaucracies and armies, and other manifestations of civilization. As Diamond has argued, "the adoption of food production exemplifies what is termed an autocatalytic process—one that catalyses itself in a positive feedback cycle, going faster and faster once it has started" (Diamond 1998, p. 110). More food made higher population densities possible, enabled large permanent settlements with the specialized skills and inventiveness this implies, and shortened the time-spacing between children. This, in turn, enabled the higher populations to produce still more people, which increased both the demand for food and the technical and organizational capacity to produce it. Pressure on the land and ecosystems increased accordingly and, in the process, ended even the possibility of returning to a hunter-gatherer lifestyle for the majority of people.

Patch Disturbance and Biological Integrity

All this is to emphasize that humans are, by nature, a typical patch-disturbance species, a distinction we share with other large mammals ranging from beavers to elephants (see *BioScience* 1988).[5] The fact is that "large animals, due to their size, longevity, and food and habitat requirements, tend to have a substantial impact on ecosystems" (Naiman 1988). Thus, a patch-disturbance species may be defined as any organism that, usually by central place foraging, degrades a small "central place" greatly and disturbs a much larger area away from the central core to a lesser extent (definition revised from Logan 1996).

The fact that humans are patch disturbers by nature is problematic when it comes to defining biological or ecological integrity. As noted, there can be little question that the species composition and developmental trajectory of an ecosystem inhabited by even preagricultural humans will be different from the trajectory it would follow without them. However, the same statement could be made about many other ecosystems with reference to their respective keystone species. For example, the extirpation of large predators (jaguars, cougars, and harpy eagles) on Barro Colorado Island in Panama was followed by a ripple effect that saw major increases in the relative abundance of smaller predators and medium-sized seed-eaters. This, in turn, led to the extinction of little antbirds and several similar species, as well as to a large-scale shift in forest tree composition (Diamond 1992). Similarly, the early decline in passerine birds in eastern North American rural and forest ecosystems may be the direct result of an increase in small predators (including domestic and feral cats), but the distal cause may well be the elimination of cougars and wolves from the system. In short, the presence of any large predator may significantly affect the structure of its entire ecosystem, a fact that may not be fully appreciated until its removal appears to disrupt the established order of things.

Now, biological integrity is sometimes defined as a property of near-pristine ecosystems, i.e., ecosystems not significantly modified by human intervention (see Karr, chapter 12, this volume). But this begs the question of why ecosystem modification by humans should be treated differently from that induced by other species like jaguars and cougars. After all, the presence of these large cats results in a climax system different from that which develops in their absence. Yet few people would argue that Central American forests naturally populated by jaguars and cougars lack biointegrity because of the unseen structural effects of their presence.

In fact, I argue that there *is* a major difference, i.e., that the quality of human "patch disturbance" *should* be distinguished from that of other species. However, the distinguishing feature is not related to the simple structural impacts of early "man" (which may be comparable to those of other species), but rather derives from longer-term system dynamics. Because human knowledge and technology are uniquely cumulative, human patch disturbance, unlike that of other species, has tended over the millennia to diverge in surges from previously established dynamic equilibria. We have already noted that humanity's drift from a steady state with nature has been accelerating since the Neolithic. It received a major boost with agriculture, and really broke free with the use of fossil fuels and the industrial revolution.[6] The loss of ecosystems integrity associated with human beings is thus best measured by persistent or accelerating trends (e.g., greenhouse gas accumulation, soil degradation, nutrient leakage, biodiversity loss) and increasing variability (loss of stability and resilience). Both signal the potential for irreversible catastrophic change in ecosystem function.

In effect, I am arguing that the makings of the ecological crisis are programmed into the ecology and sociobiology of our species. We are naturally a patch-disturbance species, whose capacity to disrupt the ecosphere is steadily augmented by cumulative learning and behavioral plasticity. In short, despite — or because of — the marvels of modern technology, little has changed in the nature of human–ecosystems interaction but the scale of the "patches" we disturb, the intensity of the disturbance, and the risk to our own survival.

The Invisible Foot of the Economy

This can be shown graphically using "ecological footprint analysis," a tool my students and I have developed to estimate human demands on nature in terms of "appropriated" ecosystem area (Rees and Wackernagel 1994; Wackernagel and Rees 1996; Rees 1996, 1997; Wackernagel et al. 1997, 1999). Given adequate data, we can calculate an ecological footprint for any designated population—an individual, a city, or an entire country.

Ecological footprinting starts from the premise that human beings are integral components of the ecosystems that support them. The method builds on traditional trophic ecology by constructing what is, in effect, an elaborate "food web" for the study population. This requires quantifying the material and energy flows supporting the population and identifying corresponding significant sources of resources and sinks for wastes. Of course, the human food web differs significantly from those of other species. In addition to the material and energy required to satisfy the metabolic requirements of our bodies, a human food web must also account for our industrial metabolism (Ayres and Simonis 1994).

Ecofootprinting is further based on the fact that many material and energy flows (resource consumption and waste production) can be converted into land- and water-area equivalents. These are the ecosystem areas required to produce the biophysical goods and services used by the study population. Thus

> the ecological footprint of a specified population is the area of land/water required to produce the resources consumed, and to assimilate the wastes generated by that population, on a continuous basis, wherever on Earth the relevant land may be located.[7]

It therefore includes both the area "appropriated" through commodity trade and the area needed to provide the referent population's share of certain free land- and water-based services of nature (e.g., the carbon sink function). In effect, ecological footprint analysis measures the extended patch (productive habitat) occupied ecologically by contemporary populations.[8]

People are so psychologically distanced from nature that very few have ever asked themselves the most fundamental personal ecological question: How much of the Earth's surface is dedicated to supporting just me in the style to which I am accustomed? Ecofootprint analysis provides an approximate answer to this question, and most people are astonished to learn the magnitude of their continuing dependence on the ecosphere. The latest estimates show that the residents of high-income countries typically require the biophysical output of 5 to 10 hectares (12–25 acres) to support their consumer lifestyles (Wackernagel et al. 1999).

The Ecofootprints of Modern Cities

Consider the implications of this dependence in an increasingly urban world. As ecologist Eugene Odum wrote almost 30 years ago, "Great cities are planned and grow without any regard for the fact that they are parasites on the countryside which must somehow supply food, water, air, and degrade huge quantities of wastes" (1971, p. 233). Ecofootprinting enables us to quantify the extent of this urban parasitism. For example, let's assume the residents of my home city, Vancouver, are typical Canadians with an average per capita ecological footprint of 7.7 hectares.[9] The 472,000 residents of this city, which has a political area of just 11,400 hectares, therefore actually use the biophysical output of about 3.6 million hectares. This is 318 times the size of the city. Most of this ecosystem area is located at great distance from the people it sustains; indeed, it is scattered all over the planet.

This situation is characteristic of high-income cities (Rees 1997). In a particularly comprehensive analysis, Folke et al. (1997) estimate that the 29 largest cities of Baltic Europe appropriate for their resource consumption and waste assimilation an area of forest, agricultural, marine, and wetland ecosystems 565 to 1,130 times larger than the areas of the cities themselves.

A more limited study by the International Institute for Environment and Development shows that the biophysical demands of London alone appropriate an area elsewhere on Earth the size of the entire United Kingdom (IIED 1995).

It is true, of course, that rural areas benefit from the economic vitality and inventiveness of cities, that the rural–urban relationship is a reciprocal one. Nevertheless, while the countryside could survive without the city, the city's dependence on the countryside is absolute. This reality raises at least one troubling question: How secure are the populations of the world's cities, great and small, if vital resource flows are disrupted by resource depletion, accelerating ecological change, and resultant civil or international strife?

Extending the Human Patch

Ecofootprinting emphasizes that modern humans remain inherent patch disturbers. Both the scale of our collective patches and the intensity of disturbance have dramatically increased through commercial trade and the use of advanced exploitation technologies, both heavily subsidized by fossil fuel. Thus, the built-up areas of cities are the modern equivalent of the highly degraded "central place" of our foraging, patch-disturbing ancestors. The rest of our urban ecological footprints—more than 99 percent of the total area—represents the less disturbed but often fully exploited areas further afield.

One thing has changed, however. Unlike hunter-gatherers, modern humans no longer move around their home ranges as they deplete local patches nor migrate seasonally among productive habitats. Rather, we moderns live largely "in place," depending on trade to bring the products of our many distant functional habitats to us. The spatial separation of production from consumption creates the illusion of increasing independence from nature, even as trade, technology, and rising material expectations combine to extend our ecological footprints globally. Worse, because of technology and trade, urbanites have little incentive to conserve productive landscapes near their home cities, are blind to the degradation caused at a distance by imported consumption, and remain unconscious of their increasing dependence on a deteriorating global resource base (Rees 1994, Rees and Wackernagel 1994).

Given the vast ecohinterlands of cities, and the large volume of low-entropy energy/matter they dissipate in their own vicinities (cities too are far from equilibrium-dissipative structures), it is little wonder that urban areas are often characterized by locally dangerous levels of air, water, and soil pollutants. However, as important from the perspective of ecosystems integrity, cities disrupt natural biogeochemical cycles of vital nutrients and other chemical resources. Removing people and livestock far from the land that supports them—cattle are often fattened in feedlots near urban markets—prevents the economic recycling of phosphorus, nitrogen, other nutrients, and organic matter back onto farm- and forestland. As a consequence of urbanization, local, essentially closed, cyclically integrated ecological production systems have become global, open-ended, horizontally disintegrated throughput systems. Instead of being returned to the land, Vancouver's daily appropriation of Saskatchewan mineral nutrients goes straight out to sea. Agricultural soils are thus degraded—half or more of the natural nutrients and organic matter from much of Canada's once rich prairie soils have been lost in a century of mechanized export agriculture—and we are forced to substitute nonrenewable artificial fertilizer for the once renewable real thing (Rees and Wackernagel 1996).

In sum, from the ecological perspective, cities are entropic black holes, nodes of intensive consumption, sustained largely by biophysical processes occurring outside their political boundaries.[10] Cities not only destroy the bioproductivity of their built-over areas, but, as presently conceived and managed, they severely impair the biological integrity of their vast and scattered hinterlands. Urbanites would do well to remember that parasites that destroy the vitality of their hosts are inherently unsustainable.

None of this should be taken as an argument against cities. Nor does it deny their potential contribution to sustainability. Indeed, because of economies of scale and agglomeration economies, cities offer many opportunities for reducing personal and collective consumption (e.g., for materials recycling, multifamily dwelling, district heating, public transit, etc.) that would not be available to the same populations in more dispersed settlement patterns (Mitlin and Satterthwaite 1994, Rees and Wackernagel 1996). Rather, the intent here is to change the way we think about cities so that their potential contribution can, in fact, be realized. People must come to understand that long-term urban security and sustainability are dependent on our capacity to achieve rural ecological integrity and mutually beneficial urban–rural relationships. This, in turn, depends on our capacity to maintain geopolitical stability in the face of accelerating global ecological change and potential resource scarcity.

Global Overshoot

It is not just cities that overshoot the productive capacity of local ecosystems. Most high-income countries have an ecological footprint several times larger than their national territories. In effect, they are running massive ecological deficits with the rest of the world (Rees 1996, Wackernagel and Rees 1996,

Wackernagel et al. 1999). As a result of continuous population growth, rising material demand, and expanding trade, our extended ecological footprints treat the entire planet as the common patch of humankind.

And what is the capacity of the global patch? Ecofootprinting confirms that the entire ecosphere is not enough to sustain the aggregate demand of even the present human population, assuming prevailing technology. Wackernagel and Rees (1996) and Wackernagel et al. (1997) estimate that at present consumption levels, the existing world population exceeds global carrying capacity by up to one-third. In effect, the wealthy fifth of the world's population that now consumes over 80 percent of global economic output has unwittingly claimed the entire sustainable output of key biophysical processes for themselves. The human enterprise now grows, in part, by drawing down cumulative stocks of natural capital. Regrettably, unlike our ancestors, modern humans can no longer simply move on to greener pastures when our present planetary patch wears out.

This means that contrary to prevailing international development models, so-called First World material lifestyles are simply not sustainably extendible to the entire world population. (There are only about 2 hectares per capita of adequately productive ecosystems on Earth, compared to the 5 to 10 hectares appropriated by wealthy consumers.) Nevertheless, *and this is critical,* enticed by electronic images of wealthy consumer lifestyles, the great majority of humankind is justifiably determined to improve its material lot. In these circumstances, unprecedented changes in population policy, technology, consumer values, material expectations, and governance are required to avoid a future of ecological decline and geopolitical strife.

Discussion and Conclusions: Plotting the Way Ahead

Pressures on our life-support systems are rising at an unprecedented rate as a result of human ecological dysfunction. The global economy has expanded fivefold in the past 50 years and is expected to double and double again in the next 50. With the extension of humanity's ecological footprint—overharvesting, pollution, and habitat destruction—the world is seeing the greatest extinction episode since the natural catastrophes at the end of the Paleozoic and Mesozoic eras (Wilson 1988, Pimm et al. 1995). The current extirpation rate is a hundred to a thousand times prehuman levels as inferred from the fossil and paleontological record (Pimm et al. 1995). Eleven percent of the 4,400 mammal species extant today are endangered or critically endangered, and a quarter of all mammal species are on a path of decline that, if not halted, is likely to end in extinction (Tuxill 1998). Some analysts are calling this human-induced process the "sixth extinction."

Perhaps the most important lesson for conservation biology in all this is that if and where biological integrity is relatively intact, it is presently under siege. The battle is all but lost in settled regions as the pressures of growth appropriate ever more of the landscape to human purpose. The fact that each citizen of industrial societies today is the thermodynamic equivalent of a hundred or more Neolithic humans bodes ill for efforts to maintain even present levels of ecological well-being.

This makes the case for large set-asides as an emergency measure for biodiversity conservation. We need substantial areas where nature can evolve "unconstrained by human interruptions past and present" (Westra 1994). But what do we mean by substantial? Twelve percent or 30 percent of the land? Where and in what spatial configuration? Biologists and conservationists may prefer the 30 percent to 12, but both figures are arbitrary (and does putting some area in reserve mean we are free to deplete the rest of the landscape, as many seem to believe?). In any case, even 12 percent wilderness (the UN recommendation) is a stretch for densely populated and industrial countries that have vastly modified their landscapes to support human activity.

Perhaps, then, we should simply adopt the approach of David Pearce and colleagues. They argue that since remaining natural capital stocks maintain the life-support functions of the ecosphere, the risks associated with their depletion are unacceptable, and there may be no possibility for technological substitution, "*conserving what there is* could be a sound risk-averse strategy" (Pearce et al. 1990, p. 7 [emphasis added]). While even this most modest of goals remains a formidable challenge, it may not be enough. Remaining natural capital stocks may prove insufficient to satisfy anticipated demand for ecosystem goods and services, including basic life support. Regaining long-term global biological health will require a massive effort at ecosystems restoration (we are using 30 percent more planet than we have right now).

Whatever its goals and strategies, conservation policy cannot succeed in a vacuum. Establishing conservation reserves will ultimately be to no avail if population trends are not reversed and material demands moderated. When push comes to shove, set-asides will be reclaimed by desperate people to satisfy their immediate needs. Witness the growing pressure on national parks from urban development, forestry, and mining, even in wealthy Canada. What hope is there to preserve ecologically productive habitats in chronically impoverished but rapidly growing developing countries if people have no alternative means to satisfy basic physical and economic requirements?[11] How many thousands of species disappeared unrecorded in the wildfires of Borneo and Indonesia in 1997–98 as the rain forest was cleared for both subsistence agriculture and oil-palm plantations to supply a burgeoning export market?

In short, if important ecosystems are to "retain the ability to deal with outside interference, and, if necessary to regenerate," if they are to retain "optimum capacity" for development, or even to remain in a healthy steady state of diminished potential (all important criteria for biological integrity [Westra 1994]), then integrity advocates must confront both the growth ethic and the prevailing maldistribution of the world's economic output.

In the final analysis, therefore, it seems that the greatest contribution to global integrity may come, not from systems of ecoreserves or improved resource management, but rather from efforts to

- develop more materially efficient technologies

- promote simpler, less material-dependent lifestyles

- improve living conditions for the chronically impoverished

- reduce human populations almost everywhere

The first two steps are essential if we are to reduce material consumption, particularly in the wealthy countries. This, in turn, would create the "environmental space" required to permit increased consumption in the Third World (Carley and Spapens 1998), thus enabling us to address the third goal. Even the international Business Council for Sustainable Development has recognized that "[i]ndustrialised world reductions in material throughput, energy use, and environmental degradation of over 90 percent will be required by 2040 to meet the needs of a growing world population fairly within the planet's ecological means" (BCSD 1993, p. 10).[12]

Population pressure is the fourth major factor in the impact equation. If humanity is to avoid population control imposed by nature, we must implement a global strategy to reduce human populations in virtually all countries.

Indeed, all sovereign nations must assume responsibility for preserving their own ecological health and for reducing their load on the global commons. In this context, simpler lifestyles and reduced populations go hand in hand. For example, if the United States were to commit to a renewable-energy economy and the sustainable use of land, water, and biological resources, that country could support an optimal population of about 200 million at a fairly high material standard. This is significantly less than the present population of about 270 million (Pimentel et al. 1994).

The global challenge is even more formidable. Current projections anticipate a population of 8 to 10 billion by the middle of the twenty-first century. However, without significant wealth redistribution and more ecologically benign technologies, the sustainable human-carrying capacity of the Earth is probably less than 2 billion (assuming average European to American lifestyles).

Conclusion

I have argued that the global ecological crisis is an all-but-inevitable consequence of unique qualities of human ecology and behavior. The solution, however, must be sociopolitical. Can we deconstruct the consumer society and replace it with something gentler, both more humane and more ecocentric? Will we be able to convince the wealthy and powerful, those with the greatest interest in maintaining the status quo, that they have an even greater stake in an ecologically secure future for all? (Scientific data and analysis generally have little impact on policy unless change is in the interests of those who wield real political power in key areas of decisionmaking.)

If we succeed in reaching consensus on needed change, we should be cheered by the fact that our present consumer-based, throwaway society is itself a conscious exercise in social engineering. This provides hope that creating incentives for behavioral change and developing strategies to modify cultural values using all the power of modern electronic media may prove to be the most effective strategy for sustainability, particularly in the so-called advanced economies. "It is also the most ethically responsible strategy in many cases, since it demands that solutions to problems be located in their source: humans, their behavior, and their institutions" (Jamieson 1996).

NOTES

1. For a comprehensive treatment of human population dynamics and issues see Cohen (1995).
2. Many people are simply in denial. The same page of almost any newspaper can carry a story trumpeting the previous year's 4 percent increase in per capita GDP immediately beside another item reporting the increasing frequency of violent climate events causing billions of dollars in damage without a hint of the possible causal link between the two.
3. An isolated system can exchange neither energy nor matter with its environment.
4. For example, consider the following nested hierarchy of biological organization (from high to low): ecosystem, population, individual, organ-system, organ, tissue, cell, cellular microorganelles. Kay et al. (1999) define such complex hierarchic structures as "self-organizing holarchic open (SOHO) systems."
5. Predictably, with the exception of a passing reference to modern humans as "primary agents of environmental change," people are not included in this special issue of the journal on "How Animals Shape Their Ecosystems."
6. Cheap plentiful fossil fuels have enabled humans to accelerate the exploitation of everything else.
7. A population's ecological footprint can also be interpreted in second law terms as the photosynthetic area needed continuously to generate much of the free energy (essergy) and matter required to support that population. In effect, it is the solar collector powering the population. (Even fossil fuel "replacement" is represented in the carbon sink component of the ecofootprint.)

8. Ecofootprinting does not measure all significant ecological impacts. For example, such pollution phenomena as ozone depletion, toxic contamination, and endocrine mimicry are not readily convertible to land area equivalents.

9. This compares to an earlier estimate of the average Canadian's land and water ecofootprint (using less refined methods and data) of about 5 ha/capita (Rees 1996, Wackernagel and Rees 1996).

10. Contrast this with the usual economic perspective on cities as productive centers of civilization and the engines of national growth.

11. The recent illegal landings of several unregistered ships overloaded with desperate Chinese would-be immigrants on the Pacific coast of Canada, the United States, and Australia is a striking symptom of the general problem.

12. Achieving such massive reductions will require unprecedented socioeconomic restructuring and fiscal reform to stimulate a new efficiency revolution (von Weizsäcker and Jesinghaus 1992, Rees 1995a,b, Roodman 1997).

REFERENCES

Ayres, R.U. 1994. *Information, Entropy and Progress: A New Evolutionary Paradigm.* Woodbury, NY: AIP Press.

Ayres, R.U. and U. Simonis. 1994. *Industrial Metabolism: Restructuring for Sustainable Development.* New York: United Nations University Press.

BCSD. 1993. *Getting Eco-Efficient.* Report of the BCSD First Antwerp Eco-Efficiency Workshop, November 1993. Geneva: Business Council for Sustainable Development.

BioScience. 1988. Vol. 38, No. 11 (special issue on "How Animals Shape Their Ecosystems").

Carley, M. and P. Spapens. 1998 *Sharing the World: Sustainable Living and Global Equity in the 21st Century.* London: Earthscan Publications.

Cohen, J.E. 1995. *How Many People Can the Earth Support?* New York: W.W. Norton.

Daly, H.E. 1991a. "From empty world economics to full world economics: Recognizing an historic turning point in economic development." In *Environmentally Sustainable Economic Development: Building on Brundtland,* edited by R. Goodland, H. Daly, S. El Serafy, and B. Von Droste. Paris: UNESCO.

Daly, H.E. 1991b. "The concept of a steady-state economy." In *Steady-State Economics* (2nd ed.) by H. Daly. Washington, DC: Island Press.

Daly, H.E. 1991c. "The circular flow of exchange value and the linear throughput of matter-energy: A case of misplaced concreteness." In *Steady-State Economics* (2nd ed.) by H. Daly. Washington, DC: Island Press.

Daly, H.E. 1992. "Steady-state economics: Concepts, questions, policies." *Gaia* 6: 333–338.

Diamond, J. 1992. *The Third Chimpanzee.* New York: HarperCollins.

Diamond, J. 1997. *Guns, Germs, and Steel: The Fates of Human Societies.* New York: W.W. Norton.

Drengson, A. 1989. "Protecting the environment, protecting ourselves: Reflections on the philosophical dimension." In *Environmental Ethics* (Vol. 2), edited by R. Bradley and S. Duguid. Vancouver: Simon Fraser University.

Flannery, T.F. 1994. *The Future Eaters: An Ecological History of the Australasian Lands and Peoples.* Chatsworth, NSW: Reed Books.

Folke, C., A. Jansson, J. Larsson, and R. Costanza. 1997. "Ecosystem appropriation by cities." *Ambio* 26: 167–172.

Georgescu-Roegen, N. 1971. *The Entropy Law and the Economic Process.* Cambridge, MA: Harvard University Press.

Goodland, R. 1991. "The case that the world has reached limits." In *Environmentally Sustainable Economic Development: Building on Brundtland,* edited by R. Goodland, H. Daly, S. El Serafy, and B. Von Droste. Paris: UNESCO.

IIED. 1995. *Citizen Action to Lighten Britain's Ecological Footprint.* Report prepared by the International Institute for Environment and Development for the UK Department of the Environment. London: International Institute for Environment and Development.

Jamieson, D. 1996. "Ethics and intentional climate change." *Climatic Change* 33: 323–336.

Kay, J. 1991. "A nonequilibrium thermodynamic framework for discussing ecosystem integrity." *Environmental Management* 15: 483–495.

Kay, J., H. Regier, M. Boyle, and G. Francis. 1999. "An ecosystem approach for sustainability: Addressing the challenge of complexity." *Futures* 31(7): 721–742.

Kleinman, P.J.A., D. Pimentel, and R.B. Bryant. 1995. "The ecological sustainability of slash-and-burn agriculture." *Agriculture, Ecosystems, and Environment* 52: 235–249.

Kleinman, P.J.A., R.B. Bryant, and D. Pimentel. 1996. "Assessing Ecological Sustainability of slash-and-burn agriculture through soil fertility indicators." *Agronomy Journal* 88: 122–127.

Logan, J. 1996. "Patch disturbance and the human niche." Manuscript at <http://csf.Colorado.edu/authors/hanson/page78.htm> (also, pers. comm. 1997, e-mail exchanges with the author on patch disturbance).

Mitlin, D. and D. Satterthwaite. 1994. *Cities and Sustainable Development.* Background paper prepared for "Global Forum '94," Manchester, 24–28 June. London: International Institute for Environment and Development.

Naiman, R.J. 1988. "Animal influences on ecosystem dynamics." *BioScience* 38: 750–752.

Odum, E.P. 1971. *Fundamentals of Ecology* (3rd ed). Philadelphia: Saunders.

Pearce, D., E. Barbier, and A. Markandya. 1990. *Sustainable Development: Economics and Environment in the Third World.* Aldershot: Edward Elgar.

Pimentel, D., R. Harman, M. Pacenza, J. Pekarsky, and M. Pimentel. 1994. "Natural resources and an optimum human population." *Population and Environment* 15: 347–369.

Pimm, S.L., G.J. Russell, J.L. Gittleman, and T.M. Brooks. 1995. "The Future of Biodiversity." *Science* 296: 347–350.

Ponting, C. 1991. *A Green History of the World.* London: Sinclair-Stevenson.

Prigogine, I. 1997. *The End of Certainty.* New York: The Free Press.

Rees, W.E. 1994. "Pressing global limits: Trade as the appropriation of carrying capacity." In *Growth, Trade and Environmental Values,* edited by T. Schrecker and J.

Dalgleish. London, Ontario: Westminster Institute for Ethics and Human Values.

Rees, W.E. 1995a. "Achieving sustainability: Reform or transformation?" *Journal of Planning Literature* 9: 343–361.

Rees, W.E. 1995b. "More jobs, less damage: A framework for sustainability, growth and employment." *Alternatives* 21(4): 24–30.

Rees, W.E. 1996. "Revisiting carrying capacity: Area-based indicators of sustainability." *Population and Environment* 17: 195–215.

Rees, W.E. 1997. "Is 'sustainable city' an oxymoron?" *Local Environment* 2: 303–310.

Rees, W.E. 1999. "Consuming the earth: The biophysics of sustainability." *Ecological Economics* 29: 23–27.

Rees, W.E., and M. Wackernagel. 1994. "Ecological footprints and appropriated carrying capacity: Measuring the natural capital requirements of the human economy." In *Investing in Natural Capital: The Ecological Economics Approach to Sustainability*, edited by A.-M. Jansson, M. Hammer, C. Folke, and R. Costanza. Washington, DC: Island Press.

Rees, W.E. and M. Wackernagel. 1996. "Urban ecological footprints: Why cities cannot be sustainable and why they are a key to sustainability." *Environmental Impact Assessment Review* 16: 223–248.

Roodman, D.M. 1997. *Getting the Signals Straight: Tax Reform to Protect the Environment and the Economy*. Worldwatch Paper 134. Washington, DC: Worldwatch Institute.

Schneider, E. and J. Kay. 1994. "Life as a manifestation of the second law of thermodynamics." *Mathematical and Computer Modeling* 19: 6–8, 25–48.

Tuxill, J. 1998. *Losing Strands in the Web of Life: Vertebrate Declines and the Conservation of Biological Diversity*. Worldwatch Paper 141. Washington, DC: Worldwatch Institute.

UNDP. 1994. *Human Development Report*. New York: Oxford University Press (for United Nations Development Program).

Wackernagel, M. and W.E. Rees. 1996. *Our Ecological Footprint: Reducing Human Impact on the Earth*. Gabriola Island, BC and Philadelphia, PA: New Society.

Wackernagel, M., L. Onisto, A.C. Linares, I.S.L. Falfán, J.M. Garcia, A.I.S. Guerrero, and M.G.S. Guerrero. 1997. *Ecological Footprints of Nations*. Report to the Earth Council, Costa Rica.

Wackernagel, M., L. Onisto, P. Bello, A.C. Linares, I.S.L. Falfán, J.M. Garcia, A.I.S. Guerrero, and M.G.S. Guerrero. 1999. "National natural capital accounting with the ecological footprint concept." *Ecological Economics* 29: 375–390.

WCED. 1987. *Our Common Future*. New York: Oxford University Press for the UN World Commission on Environment and Development.

von Weizsäcker, E. and J. Jesinghaus. 1992. *Ecological Tax Reform: A Policy Proposal for Sustainable Development*. London: Zed Books.

Westra, L. 1994. *An Environmental Proposal for Ethics: The Principle of Integrity*. Lanham, MD: Rowman & Littlefield.

Wilson, E.O. 1988. "The current state of biological diversity." In *Biodiversity*, edited by E.O. Wilson. Washington, DC: National Academy Press.

Can Canadian Approaches to Sustainable Forest Management Maintain Ecological Integrity?

Peter Miller and James W. Ehnes

War, Peace, and Sustainable Forest Management

Canada is a forest nation. Over 40 percent of our landscape is publicly owned forests, valued as both a precious wilderness heritage and enormous timber resource supporting over three hundred communities, 830,000 jobs, and forest products worth $71.4 billion in 1995 (CCFM 1998, p. 1). The latter benefits arise from harvest, in direct conflict with the wilderness imperative to "Let it be!" That conflict is manifest in a sporadic "war in the woods" that includes blockades, court actions, mass arrests (e.g., seven hundred at once in British Columbia's Clayoquot Sound [Smyth 1993]), forest product boycotts, and endless lobbying and public relations campaigns.

Against this background of discord, Canada developed a "peace treaty," the *Canada Forest Accord* (CCFM 1992a), and a companion strategic document (CCFM 1992b, 1998), which together set out a program for Sustainable Forest Management in Canada (hereafter SFM). The 1992 *Accord* affirms the importance of forests, not only for socioeconomic benefits, but also for Canada's national identity; for wildlife, spiritual qualities, and inherent beauty; and even for the health of all life on Earth. The *Accord*'s summary goal "is to maintain and enhance the long-term health of our forest ecosystems, for the benefit of all living things both nationally and globally, while providing environmental, economic, social and cultural opportunities for the benefit of present and future generations" (CCFM 1992a).

In this chapter we examine the hypothesis that this visionary policy and related implementation strategies could maintain ecological integrity. Although our hypothesis has a Canadawide scope, we focus on the western half of the Canadian boreal forest in northwestern Ontario and the Prairie Provinces of Manitoba, Saskatchewan, and Alberta. This forest has several characteristics that combine to create the rare possibility to manage large areas as in vivo experiments to determine whether we can live in integrity. First, forest operations are conducted by private forest companies with timber harvesting rights and planning and management responsibilities on public lands. Second, forest companies require areas as large as a million hectares to furnish a modern pulp and paper mill due to the relatively slow growth rates of trees. Third, if ecological integrity is defined to incorporate the condition of a forest in advance of industrial impacts, a large portion of the western Canadian boreal forest is in such a state, since large-scale forest industry is fairly recent and most of the forest still unharvested. It is also up-wind of major industrial sources of pollution that affect forests in the Great Lakes region (Loucks, chapter 10 this volume), although of course it is still subject to ubiquitous indirect influences such as elevated ultraviolet radiation and greenhouse effects.

Given these conditions, we ask, can western Canadian boreal forests be maintained in a condition approximating integrity as timber harvest continues and expands? If "living in integrity" is an ethical goal, can "timber harvesting in integrity" be a component of that life? Like it or not, forestry in Canada, under SFM policies, is committed to large scale in vivo experiments to answer questions like these. If these challenges cannot be addressed in a relatively unimpacted region, how can we hope to do so in more densely populated ones?

Since the in vivo experiments have barely begun, no definitive answer to our title question is possible. Instead we focus on three auxiliary questions:

1. On the basis of current knowledge, what forest management prescriptions are more likely to maintain ecological integrity, or at least manage human uses of forests sustainably?

2. How can we know if we succeed or fail at achieving conditions of integrity or sustainability? That is, how can we measure forest condition relative to a condition of integrity?

3. Using eastern Manitoba as a case study, what evidence is there that past timber harvest practices have maintained integrity?

Maintaining Integrity: A Complex Goal

To answer questions like these, we must specify the meaning of "ecological integrity." After reviewing several approaches, we conclude that a landscape-level concept, which we call Biosocial Regional Integrity, is needed to encompass both forest ecosystem dynamics and human use.

Three Approaches to Ecological Integrity

Within the Global Integrity Project, at least three distinct approaches to specifying integrity emerge: the "original integrity" of James Karr, Reed Noss, and perhaps Orie Loucks; the "systemic integrity" of Robert Ulanowicz and William Rees; and the "socially defined integrity" of Mark Sagoff and James Kay.

Original integrity takes wild nature as a baseline to define integrity. It thus includes the full complement of native biodiversity and ecological processes within their ranges of natural variability (Noss 1995, Karr and Chu 1999, Loucks, chapter 10 this volume).

Systemic integrity, on the other hand, is defined in terms of several abstract characteristics of ecosystems. For Robert Ulanowicz integrity is a function of a system's vigor, organization, and resilience. An area with integrity possesses these properties in high degree regardless of whether or not it is wild, although he believes in most cases original integrity will correspond with high systemic integrity (chapter 6 this volume). William Rees adds the importance of complexity, chaos, catastrophe, and hierarchy for understanding ecological reality (chapter 8 this volume).

Other authors, like Sagoff (chapter 4 this volume), Kay and Schneider (1995), and De Leo and Levin (1997), deny that integrity can be defined independently of social values. Integrity then becomes a condition of an ecosystem judged to be socially and culturally desirable. The social approach reminds us that concepts like integrity arise in an arena of public deliberation, not merely scientific investigation. However, unconstrained social preferences should not supplant an ecological understanding of the world in defining integrity, since that tendency is arguably at the root of our ecological crises. For example, an expressed social preference to keep golf courses dandelion-free should not lead us to call that condition ecological integrity, because a weed-free golf course is not self-organizing or resilient, but maintained by chemical extirpation of wild species in favor of exotics.

Our Approach Builds on James Karr's Index of Biological Integrity

Our own point of departure is the approach of James Karr's multimetric index of biological integrity (IBI) for aquatic sites (Karr 1981, Karr and Chu 1999). Karr (1996) defines biological integrity as "the ability to support and maintain a balanced, integrated, adaptive biological system having the full range of elements (genes, species, and assemblages) and processes (mutation, demography, biotic interactions, nutrient and energy dynamics, and metapopulation processes) expected in the natural habitat of a region."

Integrity is, roughly, a "natural" condition of a place as measured against a relatively pristine baseline by collecting samples for a variety of biological attributes, including species composition and abundance, trophic organization, health of organisms, and other factors. Degradation of integrity is defined as human-induced positive or negative divergence from this baseline (e.g., both species loss and introduced exotics mark deviations from integrity). The baseline for the IBI "is the condition at a site with a biota that is the product of evolutionary and biogeographic processes in the relative absence of the effects of modern human activity" (Karr 1997). Biological integrity is the most important component of ecological integrity, defined as "[t]he summation of chemical, physical and biological integrity" (Karr and Dudley 1981, p. 56).

Ecological health, on the other hand, is a norm that applies to sites modified by human activity. It incorporates two criteria: "no degradation of the site for future use," and "no degradation of areas beyond that site" (Karr and Chu 1995). It is thus a standard for ecologically sustainable development.

Our task is twofold: propose a conceptual framework for assessing the impacts of human activities on boreal forest integrity, and use the framework to construct a multimetric index of integrity for terrestrial ecosystems. We modify Karr's approach using a hierarchical or multiscalar conception of ecosystems in a regional framework incorporating the natural variability and ecosystem cycling that characterize the boreal forest.

Hierarchy and Integrity in Biological Systems: Individuals, Sites, and Regions

Integrity is valuable unimpaired wholeness; loss of integrity signifies a loss of value stemming from impairment to the whole. An individual organism is an obvious form of biological whole. Debilitating diseases and injuries are impairments that signal some loss of capacity to flourish. The organism's death is a more complete and final loss of integrity. As long as the organism can grow, develop, act, and reproduce in ways characteristic of its species, it retains its organismic integrity.

Now shift attention from individual organisms to a forested site following wildfire. A typical boreal wildfire kills the above-ground parts of plants and drives most vertebrate life from the area. Hence there has been a considerable negative impact on plant and vertebrate diversity, on biomass, and on many of the functions the affected organisms used to perform. The ecosystem specific to that site has been drastically altered; it has apparently lost integrity.

Of course fire does not spell an end to life at the site. Most soil organisms, root systems, and seeds survive and regenerate quickly. Other organisms colonize the site from adjacent unburned areas. Establishment, growth, and vegetation succession follow, until the next fire occurs. In pre-European times, a particular site in the Canadian boreal forest experienced wildfire about once every hundred years on average (Payette 1992), with dry areas burning more frequently and wet areas less frequently.

Wildfire-driven cycling of vegetation and animals creates the mosaic of vegetation types seen from the air. Boreal plant species are adapted to frequent disturbance by fire. In fact, some species such as jack pine or Bicknell's geranium require some of fire's effects to maintain their distribution on the landscape. Fire stimulates seed dispersal or germination, enhances the seedbed, and eliminates competition (Rowe 1983). Fire also rejuvenates soil fertility by altering chemical properties and releasing nutrients locked up in the vegetation and the forest floor (MacLean et al. 1983).

Stepping back from a particular site to consider the surrounding landscape as the relevant whole, a different description emerges. Fires do not destroy but maintain regional integrity (i.e., the full complement of species and processes operating at natural rates) by creating a mosaic of vegetation types of different ages and species composition. If anything is relatively stable in the same sense as a human with a normal temperature, it is measures taken across an area large enough to incorporate large wildfires of all ages—a region rather than a single site.

A description of natural processes and elements at spatial scales expanding from site to region provides a coherent way to characterize some complexities of ecological integrity without making it a universal feature of every entity or place in pristine nature. It is important to remember that integrity is a property of wholes, that wholes come in different sizes, that properties of wholes do not always characterize their parts, and vice versa, and that pristine nature is rife with forces that temporarily destroy particular forms of biological integrity. Integrity can be a property of regions even when it is not a property of every site or organism within the region, just as one's body remains alive even as large numbers of its cells die and are replaced.

Such a description resolves a basic dilemma that arises when integrity is adopted as an ecological ideal that is epitomized by wild nature yet supposed to govern a humanly inhabited world (Westra's [1998] ethics of "living in integrity"). The dilemma arises because wild nature is defined by the absence of the human impacts that human habitation and resource exploitation inevitably bring. But if the properties of wholes and parts differ, it is not an outright contradiction to set an objective of maintaining or restoring the ecological integrity of an inhabited, exploited region even if it contains local areas of disintegrity (e.g., cities and exploited areas). Thus we propose a broader concept of integrity that evaluates it at a spatial scale larger than a site and incorporates human use. We call this "biosocial regional integrity." It occurs when a region meets the following two conditions:

1. *Regional Original Integrity Condition.* Within the region, native biodiversity and ecological functions are maintained within their ranges of natural variability.

2. *Site Health and Sustainability Condition.* Human usage of a site is sustainable in the sense that current use neither degrades the site for future use nor degrades areas beyond the site (Karr and Chu 1995).

Thus, although it is impossible for members of an urbanized industrial society to "live in original integrity" at a site, it is possible, albeit difficult, for them to live in biosocial regional integrity: "biosocial" because the concept incorporates humans as part of the ecosystem, "regional" because integrity is assessed at the regional rather than at the local/site scale, and "integrity" because the condition approximates "original integrity."

Implementing SFM in Canada

Let us now ask, What are the prospects that the commitments of the *Canada Forest Accord* will maintain integrity? They will fail if (1) this policy direction is misconceived, or (2) insufficient will and commitment from government and industry are brought to bear, or (3) no effective strategies for implementing the visionary goals exist, even when the will is there. Of course we cannot know if strategies are effective without (4) a means to measure and monitor forest condition relative to ecological integrity. If the direction is right and the will is there to implement strategies that prove to be effective, we may reasonably hope integrity can be maintained, external conditions permitting. This last proviso is necessary because local conditions are part of an increasingly impacted global ecosphere, demanding a commitment to global integrity as well. Fortunately, Canadian visionary policies include such a global commitment.

Has Canada Made the Right Choices?

How do recent Canadian SFM initiatives measure up against the foregoing conditions for maintaining integrity?

1. Are the policy directions of the *Accord* misconceived? We think not, if sufficient emphasis is placed on the commitment to protect forest ecosystem health for all living things, specified with reference to humanly unimpacted natural forest conditions. Of course the policies contain other goals as well, including "a prosperous forest economy" and

supporting "the long-term competitive position of the forest sector" (CCFM 1992a), which might, in practice, rival the core commitment. We have argued in the preceding section that such exploitative goals are in principle compatible with biosocial regional integrity, but an enduring commitment to integrity in the face of potential conflicts is required.

2. Is there the will to implement practices conducive to maintaining integrity? Critics may agree with Greenpeace (1997) that there are many "broken promises." The continuing struggle between visionary policy and entrenched practices deserves its own analysis; its outcome is undetermined at this time (Miller 1998).

3. Are there plausible and feasible strategies to implement a form of SFM that maintains ecological integrity? In Canada, two broad, complementary, and interlinked approaches are under development: a protected areas strategy and ecosystem-based SFM for harvested forests. Whether these initiatives will be effective or not rests on the ability to specify management objectives and measure ecological outcomes relative to a standard of integrity. We postpone that discussion to the next section.

Protected Areas Strategy

The 1992 Rio Convention on Biological Diversity commits Canada to establish a system of legally protected areas as a primary, but not exclusive, strategy for biodiversity conservation in situ. The specific goal of Canada's Endangered Spaces program, subscribed to by all federal, provincial, and territorial jurisdictions, is the "completion of a protected areas network that *represents* the ecological diversity in each of Canada's natural regions by the year 2000" (Kavanagh and Iacobelli 1995). Protected areas are to be based on principles of conservation biology and an analysis of enduring geoclimatic features of the landscape to determine which locations, sizes, and shapes of protected areas will best protect Canada's biodiversity (Noss 1992, 1995, chapter 11 this volume). Viable representation rather than 12 percent is the bottom line, although political realities are unlikely to permit representation much in excess of Brundtland's (WCED 1987) arbitrary 12 percent figure where there are competing uses for the land. We believe it is unlikely that a region will satisfy the biosocial regional integrity conditions without a network of protected areas.

Ecosystem-Based SFM of Harvested Forests

Recent policies have spawned new approaches to forest management, including both social and ecological dimensions. Ecological dimensions of SFM encompass a rapidly evolving suite of strategies within an emerging model called "ecosystem-based SFM." Manitoba's forest plan (KPMG 1995), Franklin et al. (1997), and Weyerhaeuser Saskatchewan Timberlands (www.weyerhaeuser.com/sask20year) provide descriptions and examples.

Two complementary strategies of this multifaceted approach are (1) approximating effects of natural disturbances in designing timber harvests and (2) using adaptive management to link operations to research and monitoring. Boutin (1997) summarizes the links between management and research in the following steps:

1. Compare fire and harvest impacts.

2. Document the differences.

3. Identify which differences are ecologically significant.

4. Modify harvest practices to reduce the ecologically significant differences.

This program requires a natural baseline to compare with harvest impacts and thus supports the protection of some lands from harvest (and fire suppression) for scientific reasons as well as insurance if harvests have unmitigable impacts.

Measuring and Managing Human Impacts on Forests

The transition from principles to practice is often difficult. We aim to operationalize the principles of biosocial regional integrity in regions characterized by large-scale, stand-replacing disturbances and relatively unimpacted by industrial activities. In a synthesis of causal and hierarchy theory (Saris and Stronkhorst 1984, Allen et al. 1987), our conceptual approach is based on the linkage between ecological outcomes and the processes and elements from which they arise at nested levels of space, time, and organization.

A Conceptual Approach to Ecosystem Responses to Human Use

Our approach is developed through an example that considers a general ecological outcome and underlying process: primary production and nutrient cycling. A portion of net primary productivity (NPP), measured as net plant biomass produced/ha/year, is usually the focus of forest management: timber supply. Forest ecosystem productivity is one of Canada's criteria of SFM (CCFM 1997). Nutrient cycling, measured as nutrient supply/ha/year, is a key determinant of NPP.

To develop the conceptual approach properly, key determinants of NPP other than nutrient cycling must be controlled or incorporated. These include light (i.e., total photosynthetically active radiation), water availability, disease, and herbivory. Light is relatively homogeneous within a region as defined. Disease and herbivory effects are not explicitly controlled for and are thus part of natural variability. Grouping sites that are ecologically similar in terms of their soil conditions—that is, by site type—controls for differences in water availability. This example focuses on one site type, thin mineral soils (depth to bedrock between 4 and 20 cm).

DEFINING A TYPICAL NATURAL STATE
ENVELOPE (ORIGINAL INTEGRITY)

NPP from thin soil sites throughout a region can be plotted against age, that is, time since last wildfire (Figure 9.1). Data points form a crescent-shaped cluster. NPP eventually declines due to increasing respirational demands of accumulating biomass and poor tree regeneration as trees that regenerated well after fire progressively die.

There usually are sites removed from the main cluster ("outliers" in Figure 9.1) because many factors in addition to nutrient supply influence NPP. Outlier sites often reflect unusual events. For example, NPP can be very low 10 years after a very severe fire. One way to deal with outlier sites is to decide that, say, 90 percent of sites represent what is typical for the age class and site type and then draw an envelope around all these sites (Figure 9.2). The region contained in the envelope is referred to as the typical nat-

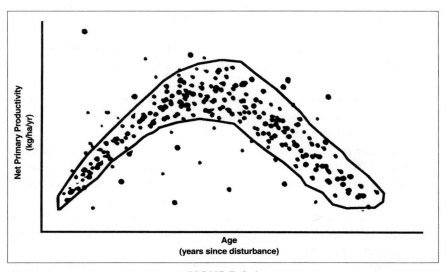

FIGURE 9.1

Net primary productivity by age on thin mineral soils. Envelope formed by the solid line contains the sites from each age group that fall between the 5th and 95th productivity percentile. (Data points in this figure are hypothetical based on the generalizations of other empirical research [Plonski 1981, Aber and Melillo 1991].)

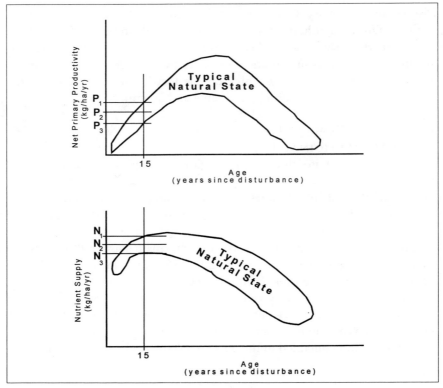

FIGURE 9.2

Typical natural state envelope for net primary productivity (*top*) and nutrient availability (*bottom*) by age on thin mineral soils.

ural state for this ecological function/outcome (Figure 9.2A). It identifies the typical successional pathway of NPP for the site type along with a measure of its natural variability.

We assume that all biological elements and processes are intact and operating at natural levels within the typical natural state envelope because the ecosystems represented by the data points are the products of a long history of coevolution (Karr and Chu 1995). This envelope is generally consistent with Karr's definition of integrity but differs in two important ways that reflect differences between streams and boreal forest ecosystems. First, the typical natural state envelope is inherently dynamic rather than static, being based on the successional pathway of NPP. What we expect to find at a particular site is a function of its age, i.e., time since disturbance. Second, by incorporating all sites within the region, the envelope assesses integrity at the regional rather than the site level.

Nutrient availability has a different-shaped natural state envelope (Figure 9.2B) than that of NPP. Nutrient availability shortly after wildfire (age 0) is determined by the interaction between fire characteristics and pre-fire conditions. In general, wildfire arrests the successional decline in nutrient availability. Wildfire also increases nutrient availability by releasing nutrients from vegetation and the forest floor and by creating conditions that accelerate decomposition (MacLean et al. 1983).

At any given age, typical sites exhibit a range of NPP (P_1 to P_3 at age 15 in Figure 9.2A). This is the natural variability that results from genetic variability, stochastic events, and minor variability within the factors used to group sites (e.g., water availability). A given level of productivity, say P_3 at age 15 in Figure 9.2A, is also associated with a range of nutrient availability, e.g., from N_2 to N_3 in Figure 9.2B.

REDUNDANCIES: DEFINING AN OUTCOME
MAINTENANCE ENVELOPE (HEALTH)

NPP at a site within the typical natural state region can remain unchanged, even if nutrient availability changes, due to redundancies. Redundancies give an ecosystem the inherent capacity to absorb some level of stress. A perennial plant that is not stressed usually responds to reduced nutrient availability by making better use of nutrients by, for example, removing a higher proportion of nutrients from leaves before they are shed. Conversely, an increase in nutrient availability at a site may have no effect on NPP because productivity is already limited by some other factor such as water availability. The ability of an ecosystem to maintain NPP despite a change in nutrient availability is referred to as a redundancy vis-à-vis productivity. In some types of ecosystems, not all species are required to maintain NPP (King 1993). Site integrity is maintained during human activities when they do not shift the outcome or underlying process outside their natural state envelopes.

Situations may occur where human activities push nutrient availability or species composition but not NPP outside its range of natural variability. This is illustrated in Figure 9.3B by the outcome maintenance region, which is between the intensive management and typical natural state envelopes. For example, the human-induced reduction in site nutrient availability from N_1 to N_2 in Figure 9.3B may not reduce NPP below P_3, the level defined by the typical natural state envelope. In this example, the site has lost its integrity because the rate of nutrient cycling has been altered outside its typical range of natural variability. Nevertheless, NPP is unimpaired because it has remained within its range of natural variability.

Unimpaired functions/outcomes can indicate freedom from stress so that

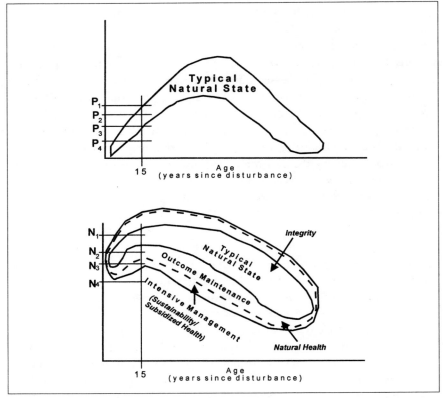

FIGURE 9.3

Envelopes identifying measurable states of outcomes (*top*) and underlying processes/elements (*bottom*) and their relationship to the concepts integrity, health, and sustainability. Nutrient availabilities represented by N_1 to N_3 represent various states where an initial net primary productivity (P_1) is maintained within its range of natural variability (P_1 to P_3) after industrial activity. N_1 approximates site integrity, N_2 = natural health but not integrity, N_3 = subsidized health but neither integrity nor natural health. N_4 is not sustainable.

this envelope is consistent with what some have termed ecosystem health. We call this state "natural health." A management goal that seeks to maintain natural health in terms of NPP seems ecologically achievable for some sites at least. Unfortunately, we do not know if any concomitant species replacements affect other ecological functions unless they are monitored. The safest goal, if it were feasible, is to maintain all outcomes, biological elements, and process rates within their ranges of natural variability during and after human use. This is impossible to achieve on all sites for some activities such as timber harvesting if they are to remain economically viable.

INPUTS: DEFINING AN INTENSIVE
MANAGEMENT ENVELOPE (SUSTAINABILITY)

If a human activity reduces nutrient availability below the level required to maintain NPP (i.e., causes nutrient availability to fall outside the outcome maintenance envelope, e.g., from N_1 to N_3 in Figure 9.3B), site health is impaired. It may be possible to prevent this effect by offsetting nutrient losses through imports from outside the site. Irrigation or fertilization are examples of imports. A third region, referred to as the intensive management envelope, identifies situations where an ecological outcome can be maintained within its range of natural variability only if humans import elements, energy, or matter to the site. The outer boundary of the intensive management region occurs where human imports become negated by interactions with other processes. For example, one experiment found that fertilization actually reduced nutrient availability due to unanticipated responses by fungi (Moore 1985).

Intensive human management is consistent with what some call sustainability if the interventions do not degrade the long-run productivity of a site. A site within this region may also be considered healthy if its nutrient supply rate returns within the outcome maintenance region once human use ceases and if use of the site does not shift other sites outside their outcome maintenance envelopes. The exact location of the intensive management envelope is speculative because it will take a long time to develop the understanding required to locate it. It may not even exist due to unintended feedback effects, in which case natural health will determine what is sustainable.

The region outside the intensive management envelope of the underlying process (e.g., N4 in Figure 9.3B) represents human impacts that shift an ecological outcome outside its range of natural variability (to P_4 in Figure 9.3A) and is, therefore, not sustainable. If too many sites are maintained outside the intensive management envelope, certain functions will be catastrophically affected at the regional level. Perhaps the collapse of the Atlantic cod fishery is an example of such an outcome.

A QUESTION OF SCALE: THE NEED TO
ESTABLISH TARGETS AT THE REGIONAL LEVEL

Sites within most regions exist on a continuum all the way from parking lots to pristine areas. If we wish to maintain the flow of goods, services, and values that we derive from forests, human use cannot push a large proportion of sites in a region outside the outcome maintenance envelope. The question for land management is not whether the integrity of the entire region is violated if it contains a single parking lot or clear-cut. Rather, we need to know how much of a region can be maintained in nonnatural states to satisfy human desires without compromising ecological functions or bio-diversity. Practically speaking, can we live in integrity?

With regard to timber harvesting, there are vast differences in the direct effects of wildfire and timber harvesting at the site scale. The most conspicuous difference is in the number of residual trees and snags. A management goal to maintain all sites within their natural state envelopes for all outcomes, elements, and processes is not feasible if timber harvesting is to be commercially viable. Neither can it be required since some areas are converted into states that are virtually nonproductive (e.g., roads). Consequently, management goals and evaluation of outcomes need to be applied to a large area, such as a region (e.g., an area of about 1 million ha), and meet the conditions for biosocial regional integrity.

Further elaboration of this conceptual approach and extensive regional data are required to identify regional outcome maintenance and intensive management envelopes. Such data are not available yet. Recognizing the need to take an immediate step forward, we leave complete elaboration of the conceptual approach for a future paper and take an ad hoc approach to specifying the regional range of natural variability. We assume that (1) the mean of randomly sampled site values in a relatively unimpacted region falls somewhere near the center of its range of natural variability, and (2) a conservative estimate of the range of regional natural variability is ±20 percent of the mean of those values. That is, if NPP is being considered, its post-harvest value should be between 80 and 120 percent of its comparable post-fire value.

A Partial Application of the Conceptual Approach: Timber Harvest in the Western Canadian Boreal Forest

A partial example of our approach is provided from eastern Manitoba. Ehnes (1998) assessed how well the vegetation of post-harvest communities was recovering using post-fire communities as the benchmark. Here we focus on plant communities on thin mineral soils. Mean total basal area is proportional to basal area increment per year and was used as an indicator of NPP. Tests for statistically significant differences between mean total basal area were made using nested analysis of variance (ANOVA) where age, site type, and disturbance type were treated as fixed effects and replicate as a random effect.

Total basal area in post-harvest communities at 13 and 37 years was much less than the 80 percent required to be within the regional range of natural variability ($\alpha = 5\%$: Table 9.1). Although the gap between post-fire and post-harvest communities apparently declined between 13 and 37 years, the change was not statistically significant.

Timber harvesting also affected species composition. The overstory

TABLE 9.1
Mean Total Basal Area in Post-Fire and Post-Harvest Communities

Age	Mean Total Basal Area (m²/ha)		Post-Harvest Basal Area as a Percentage of Post-Fire
	Post-Fire	Post-Harvest	
13 years	4.7	1.1	23
37 years	16.5	9.9	60

changed from one that was dominated by jack pine and/or black spruce to one that had less pine and spruce and more aspen and balsam fir. There were many differences in understory species composition. Ecosystem diversity is often assessed based on the area distribution of vegetation types. Thus harvesting (1) negatively affected the region's ecosystem diversity and (2) using understory species as indicators, had medium-term negative impacts on nutrient availability.

Ehnes (1998) discusses these and other effects on forest ecosystems in more detail. We emphasize that these results relate to winter harvesting with minimal ground disturbance and natural regeneration; they are not broad generalizations on the effects of timber harvesting. When comparing methods, some of the key characteristics to consider are season of cut, degree of ground disturbance, regeneration method, amount and location of residual material, post-disturbance weather, and effects on soils.

Conclusions and Recommendations

Can Canadian approaches to SFM maintain ecological integrity? In principle, forestry should be the most sustainable and ecologically friendly of extractive natural resource industries. Unlike mining, quarrying, and the petrochemical industries, forestry extracts a renewable resource. Unlike agriculture, it does not replace native with exotic vegetation and kill off everything else. And, unlike fishing, the biomass it appropriates need not create a net reduction in what is available to other creatures. Some suggest that, in the fire-prone boreal forests, fire suppression and timber harvesting are complementary activities that enable us to harvest fire's share and leave the rest behind as slash, snags, and clumps for the benefit of other living things. Perhaps this prima facie case for sustainability enabled the forest industry to subscribe to the *Canada Forest Accord* and pledge "to maintain and enhance the long-term health of our forest ecosystems, for the benefit of all living things" (CCFM 1992a). We accept this pledge as meeting the first requirement for maintaining ecological integrity: an appropriate policy commitment by governments and industry.

The next requirement is a resolve to persevere in that commitment in the face of contrary shorter-term economic incentives and entrenched practices that encourage the contrary. While there has been foot-dragging, there has also been movement, so we leave this political issue undecided.

Given a suitable commitment pursued with perseverance, two inter-linked requirements follow. Can we specify an operational goal and measure success or failure in achieving it? Are there feasible means to achieve the goal? We propose the maintenance of "biosocial regional integrity" as the most suitable overriding operational goal for SFM. That is, across the region, native biodiversity and selected ecological outcomes are maintained within their natural ranges of variability, and human usage of each site is sustainable, even though not every site will maintain all its attributes within natural ranges. This is our interpretation of what it means to "live in integrity" or to maintain forest health "for the benefit of all living things."

Ecosystem-based SFM is intended to provide feasible means to achieve SFM. Following the precautionary principle, an adequate management regime includes: (1) a protected areas network to contribute to regional integrity and serve as a baseline for identifying industrial impacts as well as for psychospiritual reasons and out of respect for "nature's legacy," (2) forest harvest operations designed to approximate the effects of the region's natural disturbance regimes, and (3) a process of adaptive management that requires (4) supporting research and (5) monitoring.

The retrospective look at eastern Manitoba shows that some historical harvesting practices were not equivalent to wildfire in their ecological effects. Thus we assume that a simple substitution of timber harvesting for fire will not, by itself, produce the desired outcome at any scale until the contrary is demonstrated and that the goal of maintaining integrity at every (or any) harvested site may be impossible to achieve.

Using the conceptual approach just described, designing forest harvest operations to maintain biosocial regional integrity by approximating the effects of natural disturbance means two things. First, practices at most harvested sites should maintain successional pathways for selected ecological outcomes within their natural state envelopes and maintain the underlying processes and elements of the selected ecological outcomes within their outcome maintenance envelopes. Second, the remaining harvested sites should be intensively managed to offset deviations from the typical natural state caused by infrastructure (e.g., roads) or by harvested sites where the first objective is not met. The less risky approach of maintaining both the outcome and its underlying processes and elements within their typical natural state envelopes seems unachievable due to existing political and financial commitments. If monitoring demonstrates that regional outcomes are being maintained by these operational goals, then incremental increases in the extent or intensity of use may be possible.

Even the best forest management possible cannot duplicate nature. As the collapse of the Atlantic cod fishery demonstrates, the economic and social costs of failure at the regional scale are substantial. Our fervent hope is that forest management which approximates the effects of a natural disturbance regime at the regional scale will maintain a state that approximates original integrity. Experimentation in management practices and scientific research will tell us whether this can be achieved. The conjectural nature of our proposed approach is unsettling. However, there are few other cautious alternatives that do not involve immediate and drastic reductions in human population and consumption.

REFERENCES

Aber, J.D. and Melillo, J.M. 1991. *Terrestrial Ecosystems.* Saunders College Publishing, Philadelphia.

Allen, T.F., O'Neill, R.V., and Hoekstra, T.W. 1987. Interlevel relations in ecological research and management: Some working principles from hierarchy theory. *Journal of Applied Systems Analysis,* 14:63–79.

Boutin, S. 1997. Presentation to Manitoba Model Forest workshop on emulating natural disturbance patterns. Winnipeg. October 28.

CCFM (Canadian Council of Forest Ministers). 1992a. *Canada Forest Accord.* Forestry Canada, Ottawa.

CCFM. 1992b. *Sustainable Forests: A Canadian Commitment.* Forestry Canada, Ottawa.

CCFM. 1997. *Criteria and Indicators of Sustainable Forest Management in Canada: Progress to date.* Natural Resources Canada, Canadian Forest Service, Ottawa.

CCFM. 1998. *National Forest Strategy 1998–2003—Sustainable Forests: A Canadian Commitment.* Natural Resources Canada, Canadian Forest Service, Ottawa.

De Leo, G.A. and Levin, S. 1997. The multifaceted aspects of ecosystem integrity. In *Conservation Ecology* [online] 1(1):3, www.consecol.org/vol1/iss1/art3.

Ehnes, J.W. 1998. The influences of site conditions, age and disturbance by wildfire or winter logging on the species composition of naturally regenerating boreal plant communities and some implications for community resilience. Ph.D. thesis, Univ. Manitoba.

Franklin, J.F., Berg, D.R., Thornburgh, D.A., and Tappeiner, J.C. 1997. Alternative silvicultural approaches to timber harvesting: Variable retention harvest systems. In K.A. Kohn and J.F. Franklin, eds. *Creating a Forestry for the 21st Century: The Science of Ecosystem Management.* Island Press, Washington, DC.

Greenpeace. 1997. Broken promises: The truth about what's happening to British Columbia's forests, www.greenpeace.org/~comms/97/forest/biglie.html.

Karr, J.R. 1981. Assessment of biotic integrity using fish communities. *Fisheries* 6(6):21–27.

Karr, J.R. 1996. Ecological integrity and ecological health are not the same. In P. Schulze, ed. *Engineering within Ecological Constraints.* Washington, DC: National Academy Press. 97–109.

Karr, J.R. 1997. Measuring biological integrity. In G.K. Meffe and C.R. Carroll, eds. *Principles of Conservation Biology.* Sinauer Associates, Sunderland, MA.

Karr, J.R. and Chu, E.W. 1995. Ecological integrity: Reclaiming lost connections. In L. Westra and J. Lemons, eds. *Perspectives on Ecological Integrity.* Kluwer Academic, Dordrecht. 34–48.

Karr, J.R. and Chu, E.W. 1999. *Restoring Life in Running Waters: Better Biological Monitoring.* Island Press, Covelo, CA.

Karr, J.R. and Dudley, D.R. 1981. Ecological perspective on water quality goals. *Environmental Management* 5:55–68.

Kavanagh, K. and Iacobelli, T. 1995. A protected areas gap analysis methodology: Planning for the conservation of biodiversity. World Wildlife Fund Canada, Toronto.

Kay, J.J. and Schneider, E. 1995. Embracing complexity: The challenge of the ecosystem approach. In L. Westra and J. Lemons, eds. *Perspectives on Ecological Integrity.* Kluwer Academic, Dordrecht. 49–59.

King, A.W. 1993. Considerations of scale and hierarchy. In S. Woodley, J. Kay, and G. Francis, eds. *Ecological Integrity and the Management of Ecosystems.* St. Lucie Press. 19–45.

KPMG Management Consulting. 1995. *Manitoba's Forest Plan . . . Towards Ecosystem Based Management.* Winnipeg.

MacLean, D.A., Woodley, S.J., Weber, M.G., and Wein, R.W. 1983. Fire and nutrient cycling. In R.W. Wein and D.A. MacLean, eds. *The Role of Fire in Northern Circumpolar Ecosystems.* SCOPE 18. John Wiley & Sons Ltd., New York. 111–132.

Miller, P. 1998. Entrenchment and vision in Canadian forest policy. *Business and Professional Ethics Journal* 17(1&2):29–45.

Moore, T.A. 1985. Seasonal fungal biomass dynamics in an interior Alaskan paper birch (*Betula papyrifera* Marsh) and quaking aspen (*Populus tremuloides* Michx.) stand and effects of long-term fertilization. Ph.D. thesis, Univ. Alaska.

Noss, R.F. 1992. The Wildlands Project: Land conservation strategy. *Wild Earth* (Special Issue):10–25.

Noss, R.F. 1995. *Maintaining Ecological Integrity in Representative Reserve Networks.* World Wildlife Fund Canada and World Wildlife Fund United States, Toronto and Washington, DC.

Payette, S. 1992. Fire as a controlling process in the North American boreal forest. In H.H. Shugart, R. Leemans, and G. Bonan, eds. *A Systems Analysis of the Global Boreal Forest.* Cambridge University Press, Cambridge. 144–169.

Plonski, W.L. 1981. *Normal Yield Tables (Metric) for Major Forest Species of Ontario.* Ontario Ministry of Natural Resources.

Rowe, J.S. 1983. Concepts of fire effects on plant individuals and species. In R.W. Wein and D.A. MacLean, eds. *The Role of Fire in Northern Circumpolar Ecosystems.* SCOPE 18. John Wiley & Sons Ltd. 135–154.

Saris, W.E. and Stronkhorst L.H. 1984. *Causal Modeling in Nonexperimental Research: An Introduction to the LISREL Approach*. Sociometric Research Foundation, Amsterdam.

Smyth, M. 1993. Grannies convicted in log war: B.C. court finds first 44 of Clayoquot 700 guilty. *Winnipeg Free Press*. October 7:A3.

(WCED) World Commission on Environment and Development. 1987. *Our Common Future*. Oxford University Press, New York.

Westra, L. 1998. *Living in Integrity: A Global Ethic to Restore a Fragmented Earth*. Rowman & Littlefield, Lanham, MD.

Pattern of Forest Integrity in the Eastern United States and Canada: Measuring Loss and Recovery

Orie Loucks

The prospect of implementing measures that set standards for areawide ecosystem integrity raises issues that are both moral and scientific. Indeed, the moral and value elements bear not only on how to define full or original integrity, but also on the troubling question of how much integrity is required to meet human (value) or ecological (scientific) system goals. Thus the objective of this chapter is to reason scientifically toward a means of measuring "how much" integrity is required to assure some stability in earth–human relationships, focused particularly on the forests of eastern North America. A related goal is to understand how science, in addition to philosophy, contributes to this reasoning, or to conclusions that may be drawn from it. In the belief that measurement and quantitation are fundamental to the contribution that science may make, this chapter seeks to advance the measurement of integrity in long-lived forest ecosystems.

The series of papers by Karr and coauthors (Karr 1981, Karr et al. 1986, Karr and Chu 1995) and others who have applied the index of biological integrity (IBI) in aquatic and other consumer systems has shown that the balance of living elements among biotic assemblages can be used to quantitate patterns in ecological integrity. However, forests are dominated by long-lived organisms that express change in relative abundances only slowly. In addition, forest ecosystems tend to be continuous over relatively large areas with an irregular overlay of locally intensive human use, alternating with relatively inaccessible tracts. Therefore, this chapter focuses also on making measurements of integrity over large areas of relatively unmanaged forest. While scholars often ask questions about the integrity of forests that are subject to harvests designed to imitate natural processes (such as periodic fire, as in central Canada), I will ask this further question: What reference context for the management of forest ecosystem integrity should we expect from large forest preserves, wild areas that are not subject to logging? In the eastern United States and Canada these remote areas are subject to long-distance transport and deposition of pollutants (ground-level ozone and acidic deposition), together with occasional introductions of exotic insects and diseases, all of which can impair ecological integrity.

Functions in Ecosystems: Toward Quantitation

Ecosystem functioning can be recognized at many levels of resolution, just as biological organization at many levels can be seen in ecosystem structure. However, ecosystems are commonly portrayed as having only a few dominant compartments of matter (the producers, consumers, decomposers, etc.), and for this chapter I focus on the major functions associated with the life-support processes for these compartments (Box 10.1).

However, many natural sources of fluctuation in ecosystem functioning occur in ecological systems as they respond to local perturbations (such as wind, drought, disease, or fire). The question to be addressed quantitatively, then, requires determining the magnitude of the naturally occurring departures from full function, phenomena that may take a year to a decade to pass. As long as the resilience of the system is capable of restoring full function, we may speak of perturbed systems as having full integrity, in spite of measurements indicating temporary departures therefrom.

Response Pattern of Net Primary Production as a Forest Ecosystem Function
In net primary production (NPP), as for other functions, one must be concerned with the natural fluctuations as well as the average level. Thus, following natural stressors such as large-area blowdown or fire, studies have shown at least a 50 percent reduction in NPP for up to 5 years (Heinselman 1973, Bormann and Likens 1979, Canham and Loucks 1984). Assuming such perturbations, in a reasonable worst case, cover 50 percent of a watershed, the result would be 25 percent reduction in growth for 5 years. For a 10-watershed local landscape, with no other fire or large-area blowdown, the result would be an average reduction in growth of 2.5 percent for 5 years.

Following industrial clear-cutting, however, studies show an average 75 percent reduction in growth (NPP) can occur on the clear-cut area for approximately 10 years (Likens et al. 1978). Assuming the overall timber removal is large-scale, then an average across multiple local clear-cuts in the watershed (covering 75 percent of the area over a decade) gives a 50 percent reduction in NPP on that watershed for those 10 years. Many fires, which

---

BOX 10.1

Ecosystem Functions for Health and Integrity

Net Primary Production
The process or amount of carbon fixing annually, after providing for respiration, expressed as biomass increment or woody forest growth.

Secondary Production
The process or amount of carbon fixed annually in consumer organisms such as insects, fish, mammals, birds; reflected also in invertebrate/biomass/diversity.

Hydrologic Pumping/Evapotranspiration
The process of mobilizing liquid water through plant tissues into water vapor (for photosynthesis) and to provide nutrient transport.

Biomass Decomposition
The process or quantities of organic carbon oxidized or decomposed annually, as expressed by CO_2 release or a decomposition rate constant.

Nutrient/Mineral Cycling
The process or amount of mobilizing of elemental nutrients—Ca, Mg, and others—from within organic matter onto soil exchange sites and into new plant or animal tissue.

---

burn erratically, would be in the same range, although some would be more severe (Heinselman 1973) and others less so. For a 10-watershed landscape with worst-case logging over a decade on 25 percent of all watersheds, the average would be a 12.5 percent reduction in growth for 10 years, followed by recovery.

Response Pattern of Secondary Production as an Ecosystem Function

For secondary production (SP) as an ecosystem function, stressors can be considered that are similar to those bringing about natural variation in NPP. For example, following large-area blowdown and fire, studies suggest that for a period of 20 or more years, responses can include a substantial increase in deer, bear, and small mammal populations, and increases in forest-edge and young-forest bird species. However, the same treatments can induce major decreases in interior forest bird species. Thus, for SP, there seems to be no clear dose–response relationship with natural stressors, except for quite specific species groups, as are used by Karr (1981, 1990). In the absence of clear, consistent, but also broad treatment–response relationships, secondary production, when treated as a general function in terrestrial ecosystems, appears unlikely to be feasible as an indicator of integrity.

Upland Hydrologic Flux Patterns as a Forest Ecosystem Function

Nearly all lists of major ecosystem functions include evaporation and transpiration, processes that are essential for much of the photosynthesis in an ecosystem, and for nutrient cycling. Weather fluctuations affect this function, giving it a natural source of variability in hydrologic flux (HF). The hydrogeochemical studies summarized by Likens and Bormann (1995) show that for temperate humid forest regions, reference streamflow (combining surface runoff and groundwater flow) is on the order of 62 percent of total precipitation input, and evapotranspiration is the remaining 38 percent. These are 80 cm and 50 cm, respectively, of a 130 cm annual input. Natural disturbances induce departures from these average flows, determined largely by the reduction in leaf area (or NPP) in a response pattern similar to that described above for NPP.

For anthropogenically stressed systems, hydrologic function can experience large increases in mean streamflow, up to 200 percent (Likens et al. 1978). Even larger increases in peak flow rates can occur. Clear-cutting reduces evaporation and increases runoff/streamflow generally in proportion to the NPP reduction. For the Hubbard Brook clear-cut, streamflow (and soil leaching potential) tripled due to the corresponding reduction in evaporation.

Response Pattern for Biomass Decomposition as a Forest Ecosystem Function

Extensive literature, beginning with Olson (1963), indicates that biomass decomposition (BD) is reasonably approximated by a rate constant (k) describing the negative exponential rate of breakdown of each annual pulse of litterfall, treated as organic matter. For example, Olson shows $k = 1/2$ (0.50) yields a steady-state surface organic (A_o) horizon biomass of 400 g per square meter; $k = 1/4$ (0.25) yields an A_o of 800 g; $k = 1/16$ (0.063) yields an A_o of 3,200 g, and the very slowly decomposing $k = 1/64$ (0.016) yields a steady-state A_o of 12,800 g/m^2. Studies show that for A_o accumulation, $k = 0.50$ (i.e., one-half of the litter decomposes in the first year) is an upper-bound rate of decomposition for a healthy, warm-temperature deciduous forest, with full integrity.[1] Specific sites may be lower for no recognizable reason. For a reference study site in Illinois, part of the Ohio Corridor Study (Loucks 1991), an observed rate, expressed with $|k = 64$,[2] indicates a "normal" departure from the maximum $|k = 0.70$ (for $k = 0.50$, noted above). This departure is 8.6 percent of the assumed maximum rate, an indication of natural variability.

For long-term, highly stressed environments, studies show that $k = 0.016$ (as has been seen around some smelters) is a devastating level of nonprocessing of annual litter inputs. This should be seen as a worst-case level of function degradation. To illustrate, data show $k = 0.042$ at an acid–altered site in Ohio, for $|k = 0.20$, an indicated impoverishment of 83 percent (17 percent short of the extreme degradation of smelter sites).

Response Pattern of Nutrient Cycling as an Ecosystem Function

Following experiments that reproduced many aspects of natural system processing and natural stressor events, studies at Hubbard Brook show the natural range of Ca leakage in broadleaf forests to be an annual leaching loss of 2 percent (11.5 kg/ha/yr) of the Ca available, and uptake by plants of 55 kg/ha/yr (Likens and Bormann 1995). Major blowdown and fire events would be expected to increase Ca export proportionally to the reduction in NPP or the change in biomass decomposition, as noted above.

Following industrial clear-cutting or long-term acid deposition, however, these studies (e.g., Likens et al. 1978 and 1996) show that anthropogenic stress on the nutrient cycling function would be undetectable if it were at an annual export rate of 10 to 15 kg/ha, while annual forest accretion of Ca is as high as $50-60$ kg/ha. At the same time, a maximum impairment of nutrient cycling (NC) can be seen in the clear-cut and treated watersheds at Hubbard Brook, where an annual export of 90 kg/ha/yr of Ca and ~0 net annual retention is observed (Likens et al. 1978; Likens and Bormann 1995). Thus the full gradient in nutrient cycling impairment can be represented minimally as the export of Ca at 15 kg/ha/yr, and maximally as an export of 90 kg/ha/yr. A number of other measures expressing the loss of Ca and other cations from the soil exchange pool can be seen as equivalent.

Mean Functional Integrity as a Measure for Large-Biomass Systems

If each of the above measures is normalized to a scale from 1 to 100, then several or all could be added, and divided by the number used, to obtain the mean across multiple functions. Thus mean functional integrity (MFI) is defined as the mean condition of two or more standard ecosystem functions scaled to a common range. When all are optimal, MFI corresponds to integrity (*sensu* Karr and Chu 1995), which is being complete or whole (all species, and fully functioning); when some functions are impaired beyond the natural range of variability for that function, MFI expresses whatever portion of full integrity is present.

The relationship of MFI to the potential range of natural and human impingements is shown schematically in Figure 10.1. Here "full" integrity is to be understood as a mean functioning that, although capable of being

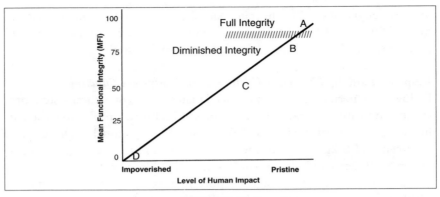

FIGURE 10.1

The simple relationship between the intensity of human intervention and ecological integrity (as expressed by MFI).

subtly altered, as with the introduction of an exotic species, is not measurably distinct from the unperturbed or "original" integrity. A goal for measurement, and for values assessment, would be to answer how much diminishment of integrity is consistent with long-term human and ecological sustainability. Figure 10.1 conveys an interesting dichotomy: Does integrity exist only for the clearly unaltered system? Or do we accept integrity as a continuum, as implied even within the uppermost levels of the figure?

Computing Mean Functional Integrity (MFI): Case Studies

Study Areas

To give examples and answer questions about levels of functional integrity, I will draw on data from six forest study areas under different levels of stressor input, and where long-term information is available. The spatial and temporal patterns of response among the six sites allow a test of epidemiological pattern for the resulting ecosystem integrity. Three of the sites represent a relatively high-dose treatment, while two represent only a moderate dose, and one is a light dose of pollutants (Figure 10.2). Historical up through recent data are available from all six sites, allowing comparison of system responses from as much as 20 to 30 years ago with recent system responses. Thus the study design allows consideration of the intensity of response over time for each treatment level, as well as the spatial treatment–response relationship itself.

The two northern study areas with moderate levels of pollutant deposition include:

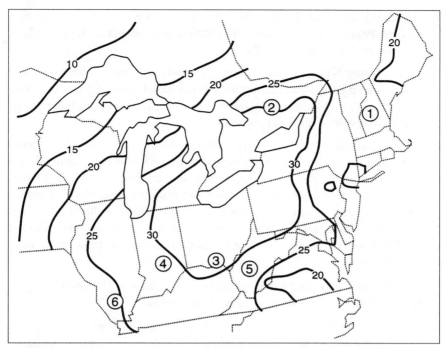

FIGURE 10.2

The pattern of wet sulfate deposition across six study sites: 1 and 2 are moderate dose, northeast; 3, 4, and 5 are high dose; and 6 is a light to moderate dose, west. (After Minns and Kelso 1985, in part.)

- *The Hubbard Brook Experimental Forest:* A protected part of the White Mountains National Forest, New Hampshire, this forest has been the site of long-term measurements of pollutant deposition, nutrient cycling, forest growth, and ecosystem change since the 1960s.

- *The Frost Center Forest, Haliburton Co., Ontario:* Located on the Canadian shield, the Center Forest is about 1300 sq. km in size. Logging has occurred recently in parts of the forest as a whole, but only light logging has occurred on the Clear Lake Preserve (of 2000 ha) and its surrounds, and for only one species, white pine, more than one hundred years ago. Pollution deposition has been significant, but only since the 1960s.

Three study areas with high deposition of strong acid ions and high ground-level ozone concentrations include:

- *The Edge-of-Appalachia Preserve, Adams Co., Ohio:* This preserve is 5000 ha, and is managed by The Nature Conservancy and Cincinnati Museum. It is situated nearly adjacent to the Shawnee State Forest, with a wilderness area of about 10,000 ha, and not far from the Wayne National Forest. All are in the Ohio Valley, and subject to high levels of pollutant deposition annually.

- *The Hoosier National Forest Deam Wilderness in Indiana:* This forest area was cleared partially in the nineteenth century, but has experienced one hundred years or more of recovery. However, it has been subject to significant levels of acidic deposition.

- *West Virginia Forest Inventory:* These forests experienced scattered clearing for settlement two hundred years ago, and more general logging beginning about one hundred years ago, but not in the steepest and highest terrain. Data on forest conditions are available from repeat measurements of the forest stock since the 1950s. Pollutant loadings have been very high, but the area has supported good populations of uncommon tree species such as birches, butternut, and magnolias until recent years.

A sixth study area on the western side of the eastern U.S. forest has been subjected to only a light to moderate pollutant load:

- *The Touch-of-Nature Preserve in Southern Illinois:* This preserve is operated by Southern Illinois University. The soils and forests are similar to those of the Indiana and Ohio study sites, but the pollutant loadings have been lower for most of the past 80 years (Loucks 1991).

Approach and Computations

Instead of casting biological integrity in terms of the relationships among the fully evolved complement of species present as an assemblage, expressing ecological integrity in terms of functions requires measurements of the full, evolved complement of ecosystem functions and services present. Having said that, let us look at the status of several functions for which we have data on forest ecosystem function along a gradient in a stressor complex, acidic deposition.

Of the five functions above, two or three have sufficient data at one or another of the study sites to implement a quantitation of MFI for eastern North American forests. In Table 10.1, measures of the nutrient cycling function, both as aspects of calcium supply, are shown for two sites characterizing ecosystems in areas of moderate pollution load. Together, they average to an MFI of 47, indicating an average loss of system function of about 50 percent, much more than the natural variation evaluated in the previous sections.

Table 10.2 presents data on two ecosystem functions, primary production and decomposition, for forests in a high-dose region in the Ohio Valley. The result is an average MFI of 18, indicating an average loss of

TABLE 10.1
Two Measures of Nutrient Function—Two Sites with
Moderate Pollution Load

	Reference Value	Recent Observed Value	Normalized Function Value[3] %
Mineralization and soil calcium supply			
Hubbard Brook, N.H.			
Ten-year mean, 1940–50	750[1]		
Five-year mean, 1987–92	450	60	
Retained calcium concentration, bolewood			
Frost Center, Ont.			
Heartwood, c. 1970s	410[2]		
Sapwood, 1981–85		140[2]	34
Mean functional integrity (MFI)			**47**
(mean of two measures)			(out of 100)

1. 10^6 kg/ha; see Likens et al. 1996.
2. Mean calcium concentration in the wood, ppm; see Pathak et al. 1985.
3. Observed, ratioed to mean reference value.

TABLE 10.2
Three Measures of Primary Production and Decomposition Function—
Two Sites under High Pollution Load

	Reference Value	Observed Value	Normalized Function Value (%)
Net woody biomass growth			
Edge-of-Appalachia, Ohio	42[1]	-33[1]	
(10-yr. mean '68–'77 vs. '78–'87)			
Deam Wilderness, Ind.	53	39	
Mean, Ohio and Ind.	50	6	12
Aggregate forest growth, West Virginia			
Net forest growth (bill. cu. ft.)	5.12	0.52[3]	
Growth rate (% per year)	2.64	0.33	13
Decomposer respiration by fauna			
Tennessee (two-year mean)	5.0[2]		
Illinois reference	3.3[2]		
(two-year average, 1988–90)			
Mean, Tenn. and Ill.	4.15		
Edge-of-Appalachia (obs.)		1.2[4]	29
Mean functional integrity (MFI)			**18**
(mean of four measures)			(out of 100)

1. 10^6 kg/ha (O. Loucks, file data).
2. billion cu. ft.; Tables 32 and 33 of DiGiovanni 1990.
3. billion cu. ft.; W. Va. Div. of Forestry (1996 press release).
4. Faunal carbon respiration as percentage of total carbon input (see Reichle 1977).

system function for the two measures (covering growth and soil faunal respiration) of 80 percent. Considerable consistency exists across these very different measures.

Each measure in Tables 10.1 and 10.2 represents a dual response pattern in an epidemiological design: change over time as well as change in relation to dose spatially, differences (in epidemiological terms) that can be evaluated independently of each other. The evidence indicates a consistent loss of integrity as pollutant dose increases, geographically and over time, as has been seen in other applications of integrity measures (Karr and Chu 1996).

The large-scale, state-wide decline in forest growth over nearly 20 years in West Virginia is explained in Tables 10.2 and 10.3. The decline in annual growth rate is from 2.64 percent/yr to 0.33 percent/yr, the latter 14 percent of the original, consistent with the general MFI estimate of 18 for this region. Some of the effects of recent clear-cutting and surface mining, through "mountaintop removal," are reflected in this statewide determination of growth, elements that were not present in the site-specific values shown in Tables 10.1 and 10.2.

These results are shown graphically in Figure 10.3, where we recognize that conditions such as have been seen around smelters, referred to as impoverished, lead to the nearly complete loss of ecosystem function. The average of the three measures of MFI (from Table 10.3) is plotted at the value of 18. These measures indicate that the high-dose sites documented here, functionally, are more to be compared with industrial brownfields or smelter sites than the fully functioning forests one might have expected. One aspect of this result seems to be that, because trees are large and experience only slow dieback, they leave a visual impression of a forest with full function, when it evidently has only minimal integrity.

HOW MUCH INTEGRITY, WHERE, AND WHEN?

The essential question being asked by the chapters in this volume, however, deals with how much integrity in the natural systems around us is needed, and in what spatial and temporal pattern is it needed? Given the pattern of MFI seen in Tables 10.1 and 10.2, one inevitably reflects on whether integrity is still being lost, and whether there may be other long-term negative outcomes that are not yet apparent. We must ask whether slipping to a level of 18 out of 100 is only inconvenient, or is there a high risk of serious consequences for neighboring ecosystems and for society?

We can explore answers to these questions by examining data from sites along a gradient in pollution loading and forest integrity extending from southern Illinois through Indiana to southern Ohio (Loucks 1991). The negative exponential relationship between the 30-year cumulative loading of acid ions (with associated changes in soil pH) and the number of soil

TABLE 10.3
West Virginia Forest Growth (USFS-Forest Inventory)

	1977–1989 (14 yrs)	1989–1995 (7 yrs)
Measured volumes	13.9–19.0[1] cu. ft	22.2–22.7[2] cu. ft
Net growth (by difference)	5.1[1] cu. ft	0.52 cu. ft
Growth as % change	37	2.3
Growth rate (% per year)	2.64/yr	0.33/yr

1. billion cu. ft.; Tables 32 and 33 of DiGiovanni 1990.

2. billion cu. ft.; W. Va. Div. of Forestry (1996 press release).

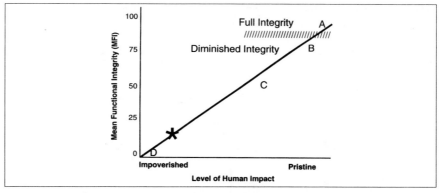

FIGURE 10.3

The continuum of biotic or ecological integrity, shown in relation to intensity of human impact, where A is pristine, B is slightly modified as in low-impact grazing or light-selection logging, C is seriously changed but healthy, as in sustainable agriculture, and D is devoid of health or integrity, as around former smelter sites or urban brownfield areas. The asterisk shows the current, measured level of integrity for the upper Ohio Valley, closer to a "brownfield" condition than to a heavily logged industrial forest.

macroinvertebrate species from four insect families (Sugg et al. in review) is shown in Figure 10.4. The loss of species shown here is, itself, an expression of progressive loss of integrity. But how much is needed?

Figure 10.5 shows some of the implications of species loss for the functional integrity of ecosystems, and begins to answer how much is needed. What is remarkable here is the very modest consequence for integrity across the initial range in species impoverishment. As more species are lost, however, the response in MFI is nonlinear, and at some point, possibly a threshold, system integrity falls sharply. Could ecological integrity approach zero at these sites, as it has in other industrial brownfields? Thus the

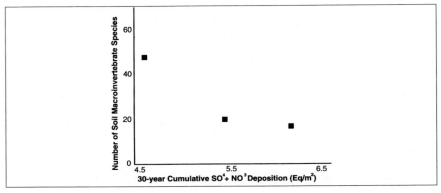

FIGURE 10.4

The pattern of loss of biological diversity in relation to cumulative acid ion loading and associated decreases in soil pH. (After Sugg et al., in review.)

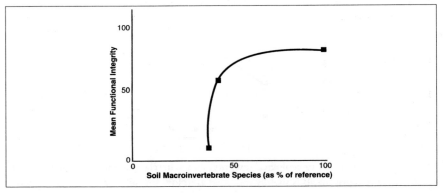

FIGURE 10.5

Mean functional integrity in relation to soil macroinvertebrate species for three forested sites
differing in acid dose from Illinois through Indiana to Ohio.

answer to the question, How much integrity? appears to lie in a sensitive, although not obviously impaired region where mean functional integrity
ranges from 60 to 80. When causal agents for the impairment of integrity
are present with a potential to induce still more loss, a pattern of ecosystem
destabilization can develop that leaves the system largely without useful
functions.

As with other kinds of values, society should consider conventions that
set standards of tolerable as opposed to intolerable levels of integrity loss.
"Implementation" of integrity guidelines would have to outline what these
values and thresholds are, and what societal risks follow from their being exceeded. In adopting such standards, however, society also has to be in-

formed by measurements and understanding of the long-term dynamics of both system impoverishment and potential for recovery. Functional measures of integrity provide these standards for long-lived, high-biomass ecosystems such as forests. Long-term and large-scale consequences are involved, both of which appear to be difficult for the human species to take seriously.

NOTES

1. k will normally range down to 0.25 in colder regions of the deciduous forests.
2. The square root of k is used to remove the nonlinearity, giving an upper bound of 0.7 and a minimum of 0.12, against which the 0.64 has been compared.

REFERENCES

Bormann, F. H. and G. E. Likens. 1979. *Pattern and Process in a Forested Ecosystem.* Springer-Verlag, New York.

Canham, C. D. and O. L. Loucks. 1984. Catastrophic windthrow in the presettlement forests of Wisconsin. *Ecology* 65(3):803–809.

DiGiovanni, D. M. 1990. *Forest Statistics for West Virginia—1975 and 1989.* USDA Forest Service Resource Bulletin NE-114. Radnor, PA.

Heinselman, M. L. 1973. Fire in the virgin forests of the Boundary Waters Canoe Area, Minnesota. *Quaternary Research* 3:329–382.

Karr, J. R. 1981. Assessment of biotic integrity using fish communities. *Fisheries* 6(6):21–27.

Karr, J. R. 1990. Biological integrity and the goal of environmental legislation: Lessons for conservation biology. *Conservation Biology* 4(3):244–250.

Karr, J. R. and E. W. Chu. 1995. Ecological integrity: Reclaiming lost connections. Pp. 34–48 in L. Westra and J. Lemons, eds. *Perspectives on Ecological Integrity.* Kluwer, Dordrecht, Netherlands.

Karr, J. R., K. D. Fausch, P. L. Angermeier, P. R. Yant, and I. J. Schlosser. 1986. *Assessing Biological Integrity in Running Waters: A Method and Its Rationale.* Illinois Natural History Survey, Special Publication 5.

Likens, G. E. and F. H. Bormann. 1995. *Biogeochemistry of a Forested Ecosystem.* 2nd ed. Springer-Verlag, New York.

Likens, G. E., F. H. Bormann, R. S. Pierce, and W. A. Reiners. 1978. Recovery of a deforested ecosystem. *Science* 199:492–496.

Likens, G. E., C. T. Driscoll, and D. C. Buso. 1996. Long-term effects of acid rain: response and recovery of a forest ecosystem. *Science* 272:244–246.

Loucks, O. L. (ed.). 1991. *Pattern of Air Pollutants and Response of Oak-Hickory Ecosystems in the Ohio Corridor.* Internal Report, Miami University, Oxford, OH.

Minns, C. K. and J. R. M. Kelso. 1985. Estimates of existing and potential impact of acidification on the freshwater fishery resources and their use in eastern Canada. In Hans C. Martin, ed., *Acidic Precipitation, Part 2.* D. Reidel Publishing Company, Boston.

Olson, J. S. 1963. Energy storage and the balance of producers and decomposers in ecological systems. *Ecology* 44(2):322–331.

Pathak, S. N., D. V. Love, and D. N. Roy. 1985. Determination of a chemical basis of air-pollution stress in wood of mature white pine trees in the susceptive forest ecosystems. In Hans C. Martin, ed., *Acidic Precipitation, Part 2*. D. Reidel Publishing Company, Boston.

Reichle, D. E. 1977. The role of soil invertebrates in nutrient cycling. In U. Lohm and T. Persson (eds.), Soil organisms as components of ecosystems. *Ecological Bulletins* 25:145–156.

Sugg, P. M., O. L. Loucks, and R. G. Kuperman. Soil biodiversity at risk: Apparent effect of acidic deposition. Manuscript in review.

Maintaining the Ecological Integrity of Landscapes and Ecoregions

Reed Noss

Biology—the science of life—and planning (for example, regional planning or land-use planning) have been considered totally separate disciplines, pursued by different people with different training and different interests. But, at a time when the ecological integrity of the Earth is declining rapidly and human land use is the major cause of this decline (Ehrlich and Ehrlich 1981, Wilson 1992, Noss and Cooperrider 1994), effective conservation requires that we bring biology and planning together. This convergence is necessary not just for planning networks of parks and other protected areas, but for planning and locating human activities generally. Where we put our developments and infrastructure on the landscape should follow from an awareness of nature's infrastructure. We have been ignoring biogeography and landscape ecology in going about our business for too long. The results— highways through precious wetlands, subdivisions in scrub rich in endemic species, tree farms replacing ancient forest—are painful to the biologist but go unnoticed by those unaware of natural patterns and processes.

I am a conservation biologist, trained as a scientist, but I work mostly in this new, hybrid area of conservation planning. In both conservation biology and conservation planning, what we are most interested in is maintaining or restoring biodiversity—the variety of life on Earth. Biodiversity and the related idea of ecological integrity—the healthy and complete condition of a natural landscape (Angermeier and Karr 1994, Westra 1994, Noss 1995)— provide a solid conceptual foundation for modern conservation.

Expanding Our Scale of Concern

But let's throw our lofty concepts aside for a moment. When most people think about nature, it is the big, charismatic wildlife and views of scenic

grandeur they are concerned about—not biodiversity or ecological integrity. It is well documented that most funding for wildlife has gone toward
a small set of attractive and usually huntable animals. Aldo Leopold, known
as the father of American wildlife management, defined it as "the art of
making land produce sustained annual crops of wild game for recreational
use" (Leopold 1933, p. 1). In practice, the species level of biodiversity is
where we have focused almost all of our attention, and to a very select group
of species, at that.

Recently there has been increasing concern about another kind of
species—endangered species (Kohm 1991). This concern is certainly war-
ranted. Endangered species, by definition, are in imminent danger of extinction. If we do not do something for them soon, they will be gone. But
the limitations of the endangered species approach are becoming obvious.
For many species, such as the California condor, many millions of dollars
have been spent without any assurance of recovery in the wild. In the
United States 50 percent of listed species occur only on private lands, where
regulatory authority is increasingly limited (Noss et al. 1997). Most actions
taken under the U.S. Endangered Species Act, and under similar laws and
policies in other countries, have taken place species by species, site by site,
and threat by threat. Conservation actions are not well coordinated and are
incapable of reconciling the sometimes conflicting needs of different
species.

Hence, for a variety of reasons, people from several camps have been
talking about the need to get beyond endangered species and try to do
something a bit more proactive. The increasing interest in conservation at
the ecosystem level is entirely consistent with the U.S. Endangered Species
Act of 1973, whose stated purpose is "to provide a means whereby the ecosystems upon which endangered species and threatened species depend may
be conserved" (Noss et al. 1997). Even in situations where no endangered
species are involved, it usually makes sense to manage at an ecosystem level,
that is, to maintain or restore ecological integrity as a whole. Conservation
biologists today are in general agreement with the idea that maintaining viable, intact ecosystems is likely to be more efficient, economical, and effective than a species-by-species approach.

What is the new approach people are advocating, which presumably
moves us beyond endangered species and into the realm of ecological integrity? It has been variously called an ecosystem approach, a greater ecosystem approach, ecosystem management (or ecosystem-based management), a coarse filter, a landscape approach, a bioregional or ecoregional
approach, or a "big picture" approach. I'm sure we could think of more descriptors. Different people, of course, interpret these approaches in different
ways. A developer or timber company executive is likely to have an idea of

ecosystem management different from that of an environmentalist. At least, however, the different camps are beginning to speak in a similar language about the same issues.

Might some of the confusion be eliminated if we had clear definitions of terms? It would seem that, if we are going to talk about managing and conserving ecosystems, we ought to have some general agreement on what an ecosystem is. In his influential third edition of *Fundamentals of Ecology*, Eugene Odum defined an ecosystem as "any unit that includes all of the organisms in a given area interacting with the physical environment so that a flow of energy leads to clearly defined trophic structure, biotic diversity and material cycles" (Odum 1971). This definition seems reasonable enough, but for practicing conservationists and land managers, we can see how it might seem a bit abstract and difficult to implement. Ecosystems are open systems, exchanging matter, energy, and organisms among them. Where we draw the lines between them appears largely arbitrary.

Although some people are troubled by the seemingly arbitrary boundaries of an ecosystem, I believe the flexibility of the ecosystem concept is one of its strengths. Depending on the problem or conservation objective at hand, we can be concerned with a particular plant community type or the whole mosaic of communities across a broad landscape, say, from the scale of a single stand of old-growth red pine in northern Minnesota to the huge Great Lakes basin ecosystem. What nature has provided us is a nested hierarchy of ecosystems within ecosystems. What level in this hierarchy we focus on depends on the problems we seek to address.

Increasingly, people are recognizing the need to conserve and manage ecosystems on a regional scale—so-called ecoregion-based conservation. Ecoregions are basically regional ecosystems: relatively large areas of land or water that harbor characteristic species, communities, ecological phenomena and processes, and environmental conditions. It is well recognized now that patterns of biodiversity are better reflected in ecoregional than political boundaries. World Wildlife Fund, The Nature Conservancy, the Sierra Club, and other conservation groups in North America and worldwide are now taking an ecoregional approach to conservation, or at least talking seriously about it.

The Status of Ecosystems

World Wildlife Fund (WWF) is in the process of conducting ecoregion-based conservation assessments worldwide; an assessment for the United States and Canada was recently completed. Among the goals of the WWF assessment were to (1) identify ecoregions that support globally outstanding biodiversity and emphasize the global responsibility to protect or restore them; (2) assess the types and immediacy of threats to North American ecoregions; and (3) identify appropriate conservation activities for each ecoregion based on its particular biological and ecological characteristics, conservation status, and threats (Ricketts et al. 1999). The 116 terrestrial ecoregions identified for the United States and Canada were divided into 10 Major Habitat Types to ensure good representation of terrestrial ecosystems and to compare only similar ecological systems. Regional and taxonomic experts assessed the biological distinctiveness and conservation status of each ecoregion at a workshop in August 1996. Biological distinctiveness was determined through an analysis of species richness, endemism, distinctiveness of higher taxa, unusual ecological or evolutionary phenomena, and global rarity of Major Habitat Types.

The conservation status of ecoregions was determined from an assessment of landscape-level features such as habitat loss, habitat fragmentation, the size and number of large blocks of habitat, the degree of protection, and current and potential threats. Different combinations of biological distinctiveness and conservation status were used to prioritize ecoregions for conservation action and identify the appropriate suite of conservation activities to be undertaken within them. A summary map (Figure 11.1) illustrates ecoregions of highest and most urgent conservation concern, and also suggests appropriate conservation actions for all ecoregions. No ecoregion is "written off" as a sacrifice zone (Ricketts et al. 1999), but it is implicitly recognized that when resources are limited, ecoregions that have the most to lose must receive priority attention. Admittedly, conservation prioritization carries certain dangers; effective conservation ultimately requires that each and every ecosystem be sensitively managed. But prioritization is consistent with the observation that biodiversity is not distributed randomly or uniformly; rather, at several spatial scales (i.e., both within and among ecoregions) biodiversity tends to be concentrated in certain areas—"hotspots" (Myers 1988). These hotspots are like vital organs—they must be protected for biodiversity as a whole to survive.

One of the more important questions for those engaged in conservation planning is how the region of concern has changed over time. Some of the changes in the North American landscape have been dramatic—for example, the 95–98 percent loss of old-growth forests in the lower 48 states (Noss et al. 1995). Changes in ecological processes—and therefore, ecological integrity—have also been severe. Among the best-documented changes have been related to fire suppression. In ponderosa pine (*Pinus ponderosa*) ecosystems of western North America, nearly a century of fire suppression has changed open, parklike forests maintained by frequent, low-intensity

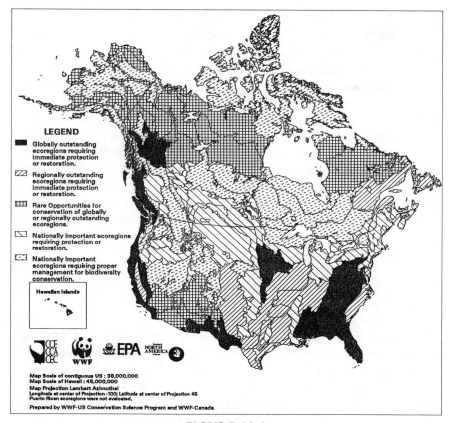

FIGURE 11.1

North American ecoregions of conservation concern, based on considerations of biological distinctiveness and conservation status. (From World Wildlife Fund.)

surface fires to dense, crowded forests containing many fire-sensitive species that invaded from off site when fire was eliminated. When fire now occurs in these forests, it is often catastrophic crown fire (Noss and Cooperrider 1994, Perry 1994).

The ecological analog of ponderosa pine in eastern North America is the longleaf pine (*Pinus palustris*) ecosystem of the southeastern coastal plain. This is one of the most endangered ecosystems in North America; it has declined by approximately 98 percent since European settlement (Ware et al. 1993). The early causes of decline were heavy logging and agriculture. Many sites logged in the nineteenth and early twentieth centuries recovered their longleaf pines over time because the logging was graciously sloppy and left a few live trees. Most of these recovered forests, however, have been hit by a second round of much more intensive forestry, where clear-cut sites are stripped to bare soil and planted with dense stands of faster-growing slash (*P. elliottii*) or loblolly (*P. taeda*) pines. Fire suppression, both active and passive (i.e., through habitat fragmentation, which prevents the natural spread of fires) has converted many longleaf pine forests to hardwoods. Some 27 federally listed species, plus, as of 1993, 99 species that were candidates for listing, are associated with longleaf pine and its dominant groundcover in most of the Southeast, wiregrass (*Aristida* sp.) (Noss et al. 1995). The best known of the listed species is the red-cockaded woodpecker (*Picoides borealis*), but most of the diversity and endangerment in this community is in the herbaceous layer, which is among the most species-rich in the world (Clewell 1989). The huge number of imperiled species associated with this and many other endangered ecosystems proves a point that should be obvious—as ecosystems decline in extent or quality, so do the species that compose them.

In most ecoregions of North America and other continents, we are forced to deal with landscapes that have been degraded to one degree or another, often to a very significant degree. Hence, the conservation paradigm for these degraded ecoregions must be one of ecological restoration. An essential first step in a restoration strategy is determining the changes that have occurred in the region or landscape of interest and have been associated with losses of biodiversity and other values. Such trends for forests, for example, include a shift from old to young forests, from structurally rich to simplified stands, from large and connected patches to smaller and more isolated patches, from no roads to high road density, and so on (Noss and Cooperrider 1994, Noss 1999). Knowing what these trends are, we can set out to reverse them. Where we stop in such a process of restoring an ecosystem to natural or historic condition depends on many factors, socioeconomic and cultural as well as biological.

Developing Conservation Plans

Knowing the present status of an ecosystem and how it has changed over time, how can science be applied to the design and management of regional landscapes for maintenance of ecological integrity? We must begin by recognizing that conservation is a value-laden exercise. These values should not be hidden. A conservation plan should be founded on a set of explicit goals, determined by the shared values of those engaged in the planning exercise. Not everyone will accept these goals, and a conservation plan that seeks to achieve complete consensus among all stakeholders will inevitably flounder. It is often difficult enough just to find consensus among people sincerely interested in biological conservation. Yet these are the people, local and otherwise, who care about the nonhuman life of a region and have a legitimate say about what becomes of it. Essentially, these people speak for the voiceless.

Commonly accepted goals of conservation include (1) representing all kinds of ecosystems, across their natural range of variation, in protected areas; (2) maintaining viable populations of all native species in natural patterns of abundance and distribution; (3) sustaining ecological and evolutionary processes within their natural ranges of variability; and (4) building a conservation network that is adaptable to environmental change (Noss 1992). These goals are ambitious and inclusive. Hence, any strategy for attaining these goals must be similarly broad and pluralistic. Yet a strategy that seeks to protect absolutely everything is not practical; some species and habitats are common, well represented in existing reserves, adaptable to human disturbances, or otherwise at low risk of loss. Or perhaps they are being addressed adequately by existing conservation initiatives. Thus the challenge is to design a nonredundant strategy that has a high probability of protecting those species and habitats that might otherwise disappear within the foreseeable future.

Traditionally, protected areas have been the cornerstone of conservation. I believe they remain an essential element, but we need to look beyond core reserves themselves in landscape design and consider other components such as buffer zones, corridors, and the surrounding matrix (Noss and Cooperrider 1994). Most core reserves are too small to remain viable in the long term unless they are connected and buffered. Most species are distributed largely outside reserves. We may never have enough area in reserves to meet conservation goals, though it is not unreasonable to strive for an order-of-magnitude increase over our present 5 percent or so worldwide.

Although some modern proponents of ecosystem management have questioned the need for protected areas (e.g., Everett and Lehmkuhl 1997), most conservation biologists agree that they are fundamental (Noss et al. 1999a). Among those who accept the need for protected areas, the most commonly asked question is, How much is enough? (Noss 1996). This is an unfortunate question. We cannot answer this question in the abstract or come up with a precise percentage that applies across ecoregions. Rather, we must approach the question empirically, case by case, while relying for a foundation on a series of empirical generalizations that serve as guiding principles. Nevertheless, most estimates of the area needed in reserves in order to attain well-accepted conservation goals range from 25 to 75 percent of a region (Noss 1996).

Three Tracks of Science-Based Conservation Planning

Since scientists became involved in conservation planning, many different methods have been used to identify areas for protection, but most are variants of three basic approaches that, in turn, reflect different areas of emphasis: (1) protection of special elements, such as rare species hotspots, old growth, critical watersheds, and roadless areas; (2) representation of all habitats, vegetation types, or species within certain "indicator" or "surrogate" taxa, within a network of reserves; and (3) meeting the needs of particular focal species, especially those that are area-dependent and sensitive to human activities (Vance-Borland et al. 1995/96, Noss 1996, Noss et al. 1999a, 1999b).

Some colleagues and I have united these three streams in a conservation research and planning project in the Klamath-Siskiyou ecoregion (Noss et al. 1999b). This ecoregion, comprising nearly 10.8 million acres in northwestern California and southwestern Oregon, is one of the biologically richest temperate coniferous forests in the world. Considered an Area of Global Botanical Significance by the World Conservation Union (IUCN), the region holds some 3,500 plant species, 281 endemic plant taxa (at the subspecies level), and the highest number of temperate conifer species in North America (30 species, including six endemic to the region) (Smith and Sawyer 1988, DellaSala et al. 1999). World Wildlife Fund, in the study mentioned earlier, rated the Klamath-Siskiyou ecoregion one of its five highest priorities in North America (Ricketts et al. 1999).

Despite its superlative biological values, few people other than scientists and activists on the West Coast have heard of the Klamath-Siskiyou region; fewer still are aware of its global conservation significance. With a national public largely ignorant of the Klamath-Siskiyou, threats such as mining, logging, road-building, livestock grazing, fire suppression, and other activities proceed with little notice.

In our conservation plan for the Klamath-Siskiyou, we treated the three major approaches to conservation planning as three tracks or streams of a comprehensive strategy for identifying and protecting areas of high biological value and for assuring the ecological integrity of the region as a whole (Figure 11.2). We believe such an approach can—and should—be pursued in every ecoregion, regardless of its conservation status.

The first track, special elements, seeks to identify areas of concentrated conservation value. Perhaps the best-known special elements in the United States are the "elements of diversity" ranked and tracked by the natural heritage programs established by The Nature Conservancy. The elements of greatest concern are those species and plant communities ranked as "critically imperiled globally" (G1) and "imperiled globally" (G2) based on their

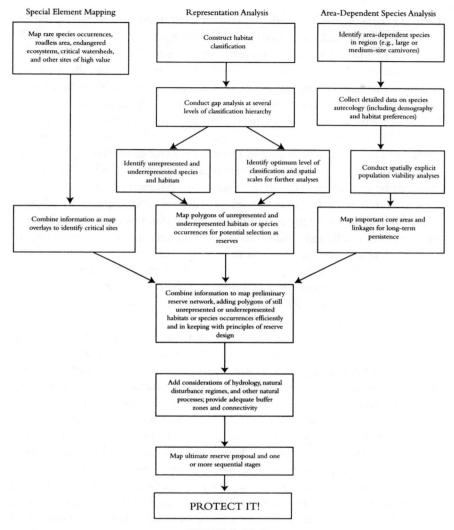

FIGURE 11.2

Three tracks of reserve selection and design, which converge in a defensible reserve system. These three tracks have rarely been combined in practice, as researchers usually pursue their specialized interests independently. (Adapted from Noss 1996.)

rarity and threats (see Noss and Cooperrider 1994). "Element occurrences" are mapped locations of these elements. At the scale of the Klamath-Siskiyou ecoregion, we looked not for individual occurrences but for geographic clusters of occurrences (hotspots). Besides hotspots, other special elements we mapped included old-growth forests; serpentine areas (which are rich in endemics and rare plant communities); watersheds with Port

Orford cedars (one of the endemic conifers) relatively uninfected by the exotic root disease; and watersheds of high value for native fisheries (especially imperiled salmonid stocks) and aquatic biodiversity (Noss et al. 1999b).

Protection of special elements—which often comprise the rare and unique in nature—does not assure that all species and habitats in a region will be adequately protected. In particular, species groups that are poorly known or inventoried (for example, soil invertebrates and fungi) may be missed. Hence, our second track of planning was a "coarse filter" or representation approach, which sought to protect intact examples of each vegetation and physical habitat type in the region (see Noss 1987). Representation can be considered complementary to special element protection. The assumption is that, because species distributions correspond to physical habitat gradients, protecting examples of all habitat types (i.e., complete environmental gradients) will capture occurrences of a vast majority of species. The gap analysis projects in several countries are examples of this approach (Scott et al. 1993), and many scientists are carrying out quantitative analyses of representation and how to achieve it most efficiently (e.g., Pressey and Nicholls 1989, Bedward et al. 1992, Pressey et al. 1993, 1996, Church et al. 1996, Csuti et al. 1997).

In the Klamath-Siskiyou we conducted gap analyses of both physical habitats and vegetation (Noss et al. 1999b). Our classification of physical habitats is based on climate and soil variables, which are known to be important for determining the distributions of organisms. Physical habitat gradients are hypothesized to represent the range of biotic variation within vegetation types, which are classified according to remotely sensed overstory vegetation. A combination of 26 vegetation types and 19 physical habitats yielded 215 "repclasses." Approximately one-third of these habitats had less than 10 percent of their area currently represented in reserves. These underrepresented types were generally lowlands with the most fertile soils, whereas the best represented types were high-elevation habitats with poor soils. Hence, existing protected areas fail to include the landscapes that naturally would be richest in biodiversity. These results are similar to findings in other regions, where protected areas tend to be concentrated in extreme, low-biodiversity sites that are not useful for timber or other resource production (Noss and Cooperrider 1994).

Focal species analysis was the third track in our research. Again, we found it complementary to the other two tracks. Whereas the locations of special elements and underrepresented habitats point to particular sites and landscapes that require protection, focal species analysis identifies additional high-value habitats and addresses questions concerning the configuration of habitat areas required to maintain viable populations. These questions form the linkage from reserve selection to reserve design. For example, one cannot design meaningful habitat corridors between reserves without knowledge of the species expected to use the corridors, what kinds of habitats the animals will and will not travel through, how far individuals will disperse, and so on.

The Klamath-Siskiyou region, together with the adjacent California northcoast or redwoods region, is one of the last refuges of the Pacific fisher (*Martes pennanti pacifica*), a threatened forest carnivore. Based on the presumed importance of the Klamath-Siskiyou region for the fisher and preliminary information linking it to older forest and suggesting sensitivity to fragmentation, we selected the fisher as a potential focal species. By combining data from regional forest carnivore surveys with habitat data derived from satellite imagery, we were able to predict with great accuracy the distribution of the fisher in the large portions of the region that have not been surveyed (Carroll et al. 1999). Critical core areas and landscape linkages were identified and incorporated into the conservation plan.

Among the general conclusions that emerged from this analysis was that the most important fisher habitat lies outside existing protected areas, primarily in low to mid-elevation, biologically productive forests with a significant hardwood component (Carroll et al. 1999). Many of these areas have been degraded to some extent by logging and roading. Although they previously attracted scant conservation interest for this reason—that is, they generally are not potential wilderness areas—our research found they represent critical habitat for mesocarnivores. Another important conclusion was that the presence of fishers in any particular watershed is determined by regional population processes operating at scales larger than those usually considered by land-managing agencies. Hence, a successful conservation plan for the fisher will require a multiownership, regional strategy that insures that habitat areas are large and well connected.

Although the fisher study provided important insights for our conservation plan, we determined that studies of other focal species are also needed. For example, the fisher is a habitat specialist on older forest but appears relatively tolerant of roads. Therefore, it would not make a good umbrella for wilderness-dependent species. In order to incorporate the needs of species with the greatest sensitivity to human activities, we initiated a second phase of our focal species analysis: evaluating the feasibility of reintroducing large carnivores to the region. The potential focal species are the gray wolf (*Canis lupus*), grizzly bear (*Ursus arctos*), and wolverine (*Gulo gulo*). These species are either extirpated (wolf and grizzly) or believed extirpated or present at very low densities (wolverine). The grizzly's sensitivity to roads and human disturbance makes it a valuable umbrella species for defining core reserves. The gray wolf is a habitat generalist with relatively high fecundity whose survival also is mainly limited by human persecution, often associated with roads. The wolf may prove useful to help define buffer zones and corridors, as it is more tolerant of human presence than is the grizzly. The wolverine has an extremely large home range size (an average of 1,500 km² for males in Idaho). In the long term, all of these carnivore species will require inter-regional habitat linkages (for example, to the California and Oregon coastal ranges, Cascade Mountains, and Sierra Nevada) in order to maintain viable populations. Evaluation of these species will help initiate a campaign to re-store the ecological integrity of the Pacific Northwest by restoration of the full complement of native predators. Our strategy for all these species is to assess biological feasibility first. If reintroduction is biologically feasible in the near or medium term, we will then proceed to investigate socioeco-nomic feasibility.

Because species biology is more advanced than most areas of conserva-tion biology, many principles are available to guide reserve design based on the needs of focal species. They include such well-accepted empirical gen-eralizations as: (1) species well distributed across their native range are less susceptible to extinction than species confined to small portions of their range; (2) large blocks of habitat, containing large populations, are better than small blocks with small populations; (3) blocks of habitat close together are better than blocks far apart; (4) habitat in contiguous blocks is better than fragmented habitat; (5) interconnected blocks of habitat are better than isolated blocks; and (6) blocks of habitat that are roadless or otherwise inac-cessible to humans are better than roaded and accessible habitat blocks (Wilcove and Murphy 1991, Noss 1992, Noss et al. 1997).

Although these principles are well supported by empirical data, they have exceptions; their application to specific cases is not usually straightforward. Proper interpretation of these principles can be made only by competent biologists familiar with the organisms and landscapes in question. Simplistic and uncritical application of general principles is distressingly common and threatens to undermine the contributions science might make to real-world conservation. For example, corridors have become somewhat of a fad in conservation, to the point that well-meaning conservationists often draw corridors into their proposals without doing the necessary work to deter-mine which species in their region might benefit from corridors and what design of corridors will work best for these species. In some cases corri-dors—especially narrow ones that favor weedy, edge-adapted species—may do more harm than good. Unfortunately, we know little about what deter-mines functional connectivity for most species sensitive to fragmentation. In the absence of case-specific information, it is virtually always a good idea to maintain natural connectivity in a landscape and restore it where we can (Noss and Cooperrider 1994, Beier and Noss 1998).

Joining the three tracks—special elements, representation, and focal species—together into a comprehensive assessment and plan for the Klamath-Siskiyou ecoregion was challenging. Somewhat to our surprise, we found that roadless areas on public lands could serve as the basic "building blocks" of our reserve design. Roadless areas of 1,000 acres or more (or smaller, if they adjoined existing protected areas) that scored highest in terms of their contributions to protecting special elements, representing habitats, and serving focal species, were incorporated into our proposed reserve design. These areas, supplemented by some additional public lands and small areas of private land, form our Phase I proposal (Noss et al. 1999b). If we liberally include the late successional reserves established under President Clinton's Northwest Forest Plan as protected areas, some 32 percent of the Klamath-Siskiyou ecoregion currently is protected. Our proposal would increase the protected acreage by 21 percent, placing some 53 percent of the region in reserves with moderate to strict protection. This increase in protected land would provide major gains toward meeting conservation goals in the region (Table 11.1).

TABLE 11.1
Comparison between the Current Reserve Network and Our Proposed Reserve Design (Phase I) for the Klamath-Siskiyou Ecoregion

	Current Condition			Proposed Phase I			
Criterion	GAP 1	GAP 2	GAP 1+2	GAP 1	GAP 2	GAP 1+2	–
G1/G2 species occurrences	11.0	25.0	36.0	68.0	14.0	82.0	+46.0
All heritage elements	8.0	30.0	38.0	45.0	21.0	66.0	+28.0
Late-seral forest	16.5	27.0	43.5	50.0	18.0	68.0	+24.5
Serpentine	18.0	25.0	43.0	50.5	11.0	61.5	+18.5
Port Orford cedar							
(high presence, low disease)	36.0	46.5	82.5	88.0	8.0	96.0	+13.5
(moderate presence, low disease)	31.0	42.0	73.0	73.0	12.0	85.0	+12.0
Key watersheds	27.0	32.0	59.0	62.0	16.0	78.0	+18.0
Roadless areas (designated wilderness excluded)	1.0	48.0	49.0	83.0	9.0	92.0	+43.0
Representation (>10%)	na	na	72.5	na	na	86.0	+13.5
(>25%)	na	na	59.5	na	na	77.0	+17.5
(≥50%)	na	na	39.0	na	na	59.0	+20.0
High-quality fisher habitat	na	na	36.0	na	na	50.0	+14.0

Note: The current reserve network includes the Northwest Forest Plan, with late successional reserves as GAP Status 2. Values are in percent area and include combined GAP Status 1 and 2 (strict and moderate protection, respectively) for both alternatives. GAP distinctions are not available (na) for representation and fisher components. The column on the far right (–) indicates the difference or change in percent coverage from the current condition to the proposed Phase I design. These gains would be realized by increasing protected acreage in the region by 21 percent.

Source: From Noss et al. 1999b.

A second proposed phase of research would assess, in more detail, private lands and additional public lands for their potential contributions to meeting habitat representation goals. We also will integrate the results of our wolf–grizzly bear–wolverine habitat analysis into designs for connectivity within the region and for linkages of the Klamath-Siskiyou to surrounding regions. Also needed is more attention to management issues, especially regarding the role of fire, which appears necessary for restoring and maintaining the ecological integrity of such plant communities as oak woodlands and savannas.

Ecosystem Management

A lingering question is how the conservation networks that emerge from science-based conservation planning will be managed. The prevailing model for public lands management today is ecosystem management (Grumbine 1994). But how ecosystem management is interpreted is a matter of philosophy and values. Values determine the fundamental insights and goals of managers.

The dominant paradigm of ecosystem management is one where human interests are paramount. This model (Figure 11.3), which I call the Forest Service version because it has been endorsed in many Forest Service publications, carries the implicit, anthropocentric assumption that human needs and desires—and the needs of an expanding economy and technology—

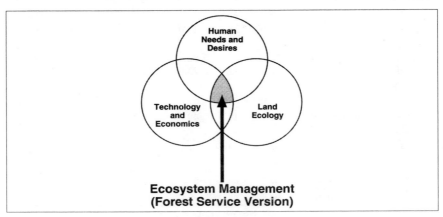

FIGURE 11.3

An anthropocentric model of ecosystem management, as endorsed by the U.S. Forest Service, which carries the assumption that human society is largely independent from natural ecosystems. (Adapted from U.S. Forest Service publications [e.g., Eastside Forest Health Assessment Team 1993].)

can be met mostly independently from the land. This assumption—almost certainly false—is indicative of what Ehrenfeld (1978) called "the arrogance of humanism." Any ecosystem management project that operates under this assumption will ultimately fail, as it will not maintain ecological integrity.

An alternative paradigm of ecosystem management (Figure 11.4) would be an ecocentric one, where human needs and desires, as well as the realities of economics and technology, are acknowledged, but along with the needs of nonhuman species. Furthermore, this new paradigm would recognize that none of these needs can be met independently from the land. This paradigm places us, in Aldo Leopold's words, as plain members and citizens of the biotic community (Leopold 1949).

Top-Down or Bottom-Up?

The conservation strategy I have endorsed here is what many would call "top-down." It determines conservation priorities from a broad (ultimately global) context, designs and implements conservation plans on a landscape or regional scale, and generally considers the "big picture" over purely local concerns. A top-down approach is eminently reasonable in a world where funding for conservation is limited. Those areas on each continent that have the most to lose—those that possess high biological richness and endemism coupled with immediate threat—arguably must be priorities for action.

The top-down approach has its limitations, however. Taken to an ex-

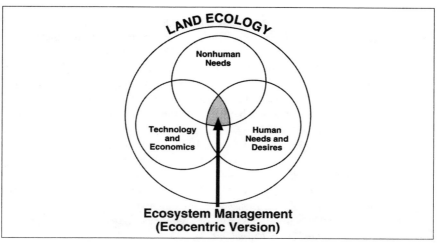

FIGURE 11.4

An alternative model of ecosystem management, based on biocentric values and recognizing the dependence of human society on land ecology.

treme, it may lead to neglect of ecoregions that do not score high from the standpoint of global or continental biodiversity, to undue emphasis on high-tech geographic information system mapping at the expense of ground-based field surveys, and to a detachment of people from the land. Global ecological integrity demands that each and every region maintain its native biotas and natural functioning. It requires the "hands-on" participation of local people who have considerable knowledge about their home land-scapes and a passionate attachment to those areas. That most local people do not possess this knowledge and sense of attachment is only a symptom of the cultural degeneration of our time.

On the other hand, the bottom-up approach that many grassroots ac-tivists and bioregionalists champion also has its drawbacks. It often fails to consider local issues from a broader spatial or historical perspective. It is often highly parochial and prejudiced. And it may be incapable of learning from lessons gained elsewhere.

Top-down and bottom-up approaches, however, are not mutually exclu-sive—they can be pursued in combination, achieving the advantages of each without the limitations. If we can combine local knowledge and ap-preciation of nature in our own backyards with the contextual, farsighted thinking enabled by a broad, biogeographic perspective, we have a basis for fully informed conservation planning. Think globally, act locally? No— think *and* act locally, regionally, and globally.

REFERENCES

Angermeier, P.L., and J.R. Karr. 1994. Biological integrity versus biological diver-sity as policy directives. *BioScience* 44:690–697.

Bedward, M., R.L. Pressey, and D.A. Keith. 1992. A new approach for selecting fully representative reserve networks: Addressing efficiency, reserve design, and land suitability with an iterative analysis. *Biological Conservation* 62:115–125.

Beier, P., and R.F. Noss. 1998. Do habitat corridors provide connectivity? *Conser-vation Biology* 12:1241–1252.

Carroll, C., W.J. Zielinski, and R.F. Noss. 1999. Using presence-absence data to build and test spatial habitat models for the fisher in the Klamath region, U.S.A. *Conservation Biology* 13:1344–1359.

Church, R.L., D.M. Stoms, and F.W. Davis. 1996. Reserve selection as a maximal covering location problem. *Biological Conservation* 76:105–112.

Clewell, A.F. 1989. Natural history of wiregrass (*Aristida stricta* Michx., Gramineae). *Natural Areas Journal* 9:223–233.

Csuti, B., S. Polasky, P.H. Williams, R.L. Pressey, J.D. Camm, M. Kershaw, A.R. Kiester, B. Downs, R. Hamilton, M. Huso, and K. Sahr. 1997. A comparison of reserve selection algorithms using data on terrestrial vertebrates in Oregon. *Biological Conservation* 80:83–97.

DellaSala, D.A., S.B. Reid, T.J. Frest, J.R. Strittholt, and D.M. Olson. 1999. A global perspective on the biodiversity of the Klamath-Siskiyou ecoregion. *Natural Areas Journal* 19:300–319.

Eastside Forest Health Assessment Team. 1993. *Eastside Forest Health Assessment.* Volume 1, *Executive Summary.* Washington, DC: USDA Forest Service.

Ehrenfeld, D. 1978. *The Arrogance of Humanism.* New York: Oxford University Press.

Ehrlich, P.R., and A.H. Ehrlich. 1981. *Extinction: The Causes and Consequences of the Disappearance of Species.* New York: Random House.

Everett, R.L., and J.F. Lehmkuhl. 1997. A forum for presenting alternative viewpoints on the role of reserves in conservation biology? A reply to Noss (1996). *Wildlife Society Bulletin* 97:575–577.

Grumbine, R.E. 1994. What is ecosystem management? *Conservation Biology* 8:27–38.

Kohm, K.A., editor. 1991. *Balancing on the Brink of Extinction: The Endangered Species Act and Lessons for the Future.* Washington, DC: Island Press.

Leopold, A. 1933. *Game Management.* New York: Charles Scribner's Sons.

Leopold, A. 1949. *A Sand County Almanac.* New York: Oxford University Press.

Myers, N. 1988. Threatened biotas: "Hot spots" in tropical forests. *Environmentalist* 8:187–208.

Noss, R.F. 1987. From plant communities to landscapes in conservation inventories: A look at The Nature Conservancy (USA). *Biological Conservation* 41:11–37.

Noss, R.F. 1992. The Wildlands Project: Land conservation strategy. *Wild Earth* (Special Issue):10–25.

Noss, R.F. 1995. *Maintaining Ecological Integrity in Representative Reserve Networks.* Toronto, Ontario: World Wildlife Fund Canada.

Noss, R.F. 1996. Protected areas: How much is enough? Pages 91–120 in R.G. Wright, ed. *National Parks and Protected Areas.* Cambridge, MA: Blackwell Science.

Noss, R.F. 1999. Assessing and monitoring forest biodiversity: A suggested framework and indicators. *Forest Ecology and Management* 115:135–146.

Noss, R.F., and A.Y. Cooperrider. 1994. *Saving Nature's Legacy: Protecting and Restoring Biodiversity.* Washington, DC: Island Press.

Noss, R.F., E.T. LaRoe, and J.M. Scott. 1995. *Endangered Ecosystems of the United States: A Preliminary Assessment of Loss and Degradation.* Biological Report 28. Washington, DC: USDI National Biological Service.

Noss, R.F., M.A. O'Connell, and D.D. Murphy. 1997. *The Science of Conservation Planning: Habitat Conservation under the Endangered Species Act.* Washington, DC: Island Press.

Noss, R., E. Dinerstein, B. Gilbert, M. Gilpin, B. Miller, J. Terborgh, and S. Trombulak. 1999a. Core areas: Where nature reigns. Pages 99–128 in M.E. Soulé and J. Terborgh, eds. *Continental Conservation: Scientific Foundations of Regional Reserve Networks.* Washington, DC: Island Press.

Noss, R.F., J.R. Strittholt, K. Vance-Borland, C. Carroll, and P. Frost. 1999b. A conservation plan for the Klamath-Siskiyou ecoregion. *Natural Areas Journal* 19:392–411.

Odum, E.P. 1971. *Fundamentals of Ecology.* Third edition. Philadelphia: W.B. Saunders.

Perry, D.A. 1994. *Forest Ecosystems.* Baltimore: Johns Hopkins University Press.

Pressey, R.L., and A.O. Nicholls. 1989. Application of a numerical algorithm to the selection of reserves in semi-arid New South Wales. *Biological Conservation* 50:263–278.

Pressey, R.L., C.J. Humphries, C.R. Margules, R.I. Vane-Wright, and P.H. Williams. 1993. Beyond opportunism: Key principles for systematic reserve selection. *Trends in Ecology and Evolution* 8:124–128.

Pressey, R.L., H.P. Possingham, and C.R. Margules. 1996. Optimality in reserve selection algorithms: When does it matter and how much? *Biological Conservation* 76:259–267.

Ricketts, T.H., E. Dinerstein, D.M. Olson, C.J. Loucks, W.M. Eichbaum, D.A. DellaSala, K.C. Kavanagh, P. Hedao, P.T. Hurley, K.M. Carney, R.A. Abell, and S. Walters. 1999. *A Conservation Assessment of the Terrestrial Ecoregions of North America.* Volume 1, *The United States and Canada.* Washington, DC: Island Press.

Scott, J.M., F. Davis, B. Csuti, R. Noss, B. Butterfield, C. Groves, J. Anderson, S. Caicco, F. D'Erchia, T.C. Edwards, J. Ulliman, and R.G. Wright. 1993. Gap analysis: A geographical approach to protection of biological diversity. *Wildlife Monographs* 123:1–41.

Smith, J.P., and J.O. Sawyer. 1988. Endemic vascular plants of northwestern California and southwestern Oregon. *Madroño* 35(1):54–69.

Vance-Borland, K., R. Noss, J. Strittholt, P. Frost, C. Carroll, and R. Nawa. 1995/96. A biodiversity conservation plan for the Klamath/Siskiyou region: A progress report on a case study for bioregional conservation. *Wild Earth* 5(4):52–59.

Ware, S., C.C. Frost, and P. Doerr. 1993. Southern mixed hardwood forest: The former longleaf pine forest. Pages 447–493 in W.H. Martin, S.G. Boyce, and A.C. Echternacht, eds. *Biodiversity of the Southeastern United States: Lowland Terrestrial Communities.* New York: Wiley.

Westra, L. 1994. *An Environmental Proposal for Ethics: The Principle of Integrity.* Lanham, MD: Rowman & Littlefield.

Wilcove, D.S., and D.D. Murphy. 1991. The spotted owl controversy and conservation biology. *Conservation Biology* 5:261–262.

Wilson, E.O. 1992. *The Diversity of Life.* Cambridge, MA: Belknap Press of Harvard University Press.

Health, Integrity, and Biological Assessment: The Importance of Measuring Whole Things

James R. Karr

For millennia, nature—specifically living systems—provided food and fiber to nourish and clothe us and materials to build us homes and transport. Living systems conditioned the air we breathe, regulated the global water cycle, and created the soil that sustained our developing agriculture. They decomposed and absorbed our wastes. Beyond practicality, nature fed the human spirit.

But pressure on nature from the impact of 6 billion humans is taking its toll. Living systems worldwide are collapsing (Woodwell 1990, Karr 1993, Karr and Chu 1995, Vitousek et al. 1997, Lubchenco 1998). Changes in Earth's biota caused by human actions range from indirect depletion caused by altering Earth's physical and chemical environment to direct depletion of human and nonhuman life (Karr and Chu 1995).

We have not always had such devastating effects. When modern humans emerged some 200,000 years ago, changes we caused happened slowly, and over relatively small geographic scales. But now change is fast, fueled by unconstrained population growth and advancing technologies. "Human-dominated ecosystems" are not simply farm fields but the entire planet (Vitousek et al. 1997). The ecological footprint of modern human society is huge (Rees, chapter 8, this volume). The result is global ecological disruption and biotic impoverishment. Yet modern society continues to behave as if there were no long-term consequences of transforming the biosphere, as if we were not connected to nature's life-support systems.

Current environmental challenges come straight from our failure to understand the risks associated with sickening and ultimately killing life on Earth. The lens through which we have seen challenges to human health has been too narrow. Despite dramatic medical improvements, our approach to human health and health care has not kept pace with changing threats to individuals or the well-being of society.

Tracking Well-Being

For thousands of years, people worried most about the health of individuals, including injuries in fights or wars, periodic famine, vector-borne diseases, and accidents (McMichael 1993). Modern agriculture and the domestication of animals created new health challenges by transferring a vast array of new contagious diseases to humans (Diamond 1997). The industrial revolution brought some relief; wastewater treatment, for example, reduced the incidence of waterborne diseases. But new technologies generated new threats, ranging from toxic industrial chemicals to global transportation systems that spread infectious diseases and exposed individuals to a greater variety of diseases. Modern environmental regulation and medicine have attacked these problems, but they struggle to stay ahead of evolving, unforeseen consequences, such as the resistance of many disease organisms to antibiotics.

The human condition has, of course, been the subject of intellectual and practical concern since civilization began. But economic and political changes during the industrial revolution moved humans away from their ties to the land. Technology and trade liberated people from concerns about life-support systems, or so it seemed. Lessons of the past—especially accumulated knowledge about connections to living systems—seemed increasingly irrelevant (Schorske 1998). Emerging economic theories suggested that "the market" would, if allowed to operate freely, provide for humankind. So-called neoclassical economics argued (incorrectly) that economic growth and the forces that promote it are good for the environment and for the poor. The attainment of societal well-being was assumed to be an inevitable by-product of a market economy. Present environmental trends and the growing gap between rich and poor demonstrate that this assumption is flawed (Homer-Dixon 1999).

A still greater flaw in how we track societal well-being is our failure to recognize the importance of health beyond bodily and economic health, our failure to recognize the importance of ecological health. Whereas bodily health threats used to come *from* the surrounding environment, modern affluence (aptly named "affluenza") has brought threats *to* the wider environment, especially to the life-supporting systems that nurture humans and all other species. In the long term, and the broadest view, a critical frontier of health care should be the protection of clean air, pure water, fertile soils, and above all else our home planet's mantle of life.

Ignoring ecological health goes back at least two centuries, during which secular society turned away from a view of whole things that was once commonplace. In the eighteenth century, a biogeographer named Baron Alexander von Humboldt wanted to catalog the natural world in detail and to formulate a grand theory that would unify and link natural phenomena, including humanity's place within nature's interdependent relationships (Sachs 1995). But von Humboldt's whole-systems view was soon supplanted by views of fragments, of phenomena broken down into their supposed component parts; this view has dominated science and characterized most scientists ever since. Science was taken over by narrow specializations, and, in the rush to gain in-depth knowledge, science and society lost sight of the need to tie the knowledge together. Generalists like von Humboldt—which David Orr (1999) has defined as specialists in whole things—disappeared. As a result, all of society began to deny the reality that humans are tied to the complex interrelationships that constitute life on Earth, the ecological health that holds together the biosphere.

What Is *Health*?

Webster's dictionaries define *health* as a flourishing condition, well-being, vitality, or prosperity. A healthy person is free from physical disease or pain; a healthy person is sound in mind, body, and spirit. An organism is healthy when it performs all its vital functions normally and properly, when it is able to recover from normal stresses, when it requires minimal outside care. A country is healthy when a flourishing economy provides for the well-being of its citizens. An environment is healthy when the supply of goods and services required by both human and nonhuman residents is sustained. *Health* is short for "good condition."

Despite—or perhaps because of—the simplicity and the breadth of this concept, the intellectual literature is rife with arguments over whether it is appropriate to speak of "ecological health" (Meyer 1997, Rapport et al. 1998a, Callicott et al. 1999, Goldstein 1999, Karr 1999).

These arguments—with refinements based on theoretical, philosophical, scientific, ethical, and moral foundations—will likely continue forever. Regardless of the conclusions, the plain fact is that humans must grapple with the reality of environmental deterioration. At its core, this deterioration means a loss of life, the removal of *bio-* from the *biosphere*. It means the loss of the whole things that have nurtured all life, including humans.

In my view, *health* as a word and concept in ecology is useful precisely because it is a familiar concept. It is an effortless intuitive step from "my health" to "ecological health." Granted that we must operationalize the term—define it and find ways to measure it. But as a policy goal, protecting health—whether of landscapes, rivers, children, or wildlife—has a fighting chance of engaging public interest and support.

What Is *Integrity?*

Protecting biological or ecological integrity is the core principle of national laws and international agreements in North America, Europe, and elsewhere (e.g., the U.S. Clean Water Act, Canada's National Park Act, the Great Lakes Water Quality Agreement between the United States and Canada, and water policy directives being developed by the European Community). Like health, this term too needs to be operationalized. And it can be. When properly defined, *integrity* can serve as a benchmark of biological condition to clarify and understand humans' relationship with their surroundings.

Biological integrity refers to the condition of places at one end of a continuum of human influence, places that support a biota that is the product of evolutionary and biogeographic processes with little or no influence from industrial society (Figure 12.1). This biota is a balanced, integrated, adaptive system having its full range of elements (genes, species, assemblages) and processes (mutation, demography, biotic interactions, nutrient and energy dynamics, and metapopulation processes) expected in areas with minimal human influence (Karr 1991, Angermeier and Karr 1994). Human society depends on both elements and processes of living systems.

As human activity alters biological systems, they—and we along with them—move along a gradient, ultimately to a state where little or nothing is left alive (see Figure 12.1). Once human actions alter a place so that it no longer possesses biological integrity as just defined, then the question arises whether the place is ecologically healthy. That decision will often be based on a judgment tied to societal values. Does the society value the new biological condition that results? Are there shifts in the parts and processes of living systems (e.g., loss of salmonids as stream temperature increases or area-sensitive birds as forests are fragmented)? But these decisions cannot be only value based. Degradation may proceed to the point where value-based land uses that are acceptable may not be sustainable. When that threshold is crossed (Figure 12.1), the situation shifts from healthy to unhealthy, sustainable to unsustainable.

Two factors are important in helping to set standards that will avoid depletion of living systems. Environmental policies from land use to setting of

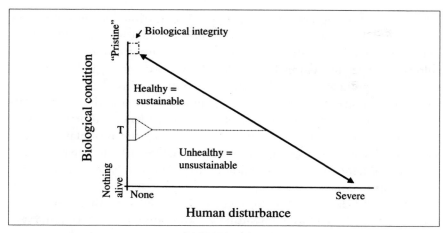

FIGURE 12.1

Biological condition declines away from biological integrity as human disturbance increases. Biological integrity is the condition of a place that has its evolutionary legacy—parts (e.g., species) and processes (e.g., nutrient cycles)— intact. On the basis of contemporary societal values, a site or region may still be considered healthy despite some decline below integrity. Biological condition can, however, degrade beyond a threshold (in the vicinity of T) where the situation becomes unhealthy because it is unsustainable. T is not necessarily an easily measured threshold, especially over short time scales. Rather it is a biological tipping point beyond which neither the natural biota nor human activity can be sustained in that place.

fish harvest quotas should not be justified by invoking values when human activity alters the long-term ability of places to supply critical goods and services. For example, healthy agriculture should not deplete soil or water so that agricultural activity cannot be sustained; industrial sites should not become so polluted that people cannot work at those sites. Moreover, human uses should not degrade other areas (e.g., downstream or downwind).

Two examples illustrate what can happen if society makes decisions based on values not leavened by understanding of environmental consequences. Flood-control efforts on Florida's Kissimmee River created a canal that compromised local and regional natural resources. In this case, pursuit of narrow flood-control values trumped concerns about other environmental degradation. Calls for restoration arose soon after the project was completed. Twenty-eight years later a project to reverse the original channelization is under way. The explicit goal is to restore the river and its connections with its floodplain—to restore the biological integrity of the Kissimmee River landscape (Toth 1993, Karr 1994).

Agriculture in much of eastern Colorado depends on irrigation. But in addition to allowing crops to be produced, irrigation adds moisture and energy to the atmosphere. This process, in turn, increases humidity, moderates temperature extremes, and increases convective storm activity. The resulting change in regional heat flux transports more industrial and agricultural pollutants from the plains to the mountains, depositing excess nitrogen and stressing alpine and subalpine ecosystems (Rapport et al. 1998b). Those ecosystems are the foundation of a lucrative tourist industry and the source of water for cities at the base of the mountains. What Coloradans may gain in agricultural production, they stand to lose in biology of the Continental Divide, including perhaps the already dwindling water supplies for Colorado's cities.

In both Florida and Colorado, decisions based on values that later turned out to be inappropriate have unwittingly compromised regional natural systems. At the very least, appeal to the preeminence of societal values to justify human activities should include a careful evaluation of the likely unintended biological consequences of those actions.

Benchmark, Guide, and Goal

Aided by the language of health and integrity, environmental decision-makers can and should use the condition of living systems as benchmark, guide, and goal for their work. The biota of minimally disturbed sites—those with integrity—provides a benchmark, a standard by which others are measured. The protection of that standard, or something very close to it, is likely to be the goal—the end toward which effort is directed—in relatively few places (e.g., national parks). The modern reality is that we are not able to preserve all areas in this benchmark condition. For example, restoring salmon to every Pacific Northwest stream is not realistic, yet a restoration goal that includes viable populations of cutthroat trout may be reasonable even in many urban or suburban streams.

Finally, using the condition of living systems as a guide—something to steady or direct what we do—is vital when it comes to protecting the biosphere. Because it took a century or more to produce present conditions, recovery will not be immediate. Routine evaluation of biological condition can guide us by telling us whether we are going in the right direction and at what rate.

In the past, attainment of policy goals and enforcement of environmental regulations were too often assessed in terms of bureaucratic endpoints (number of permits issued, reduction in contaminated effluent; Yoder and Rankin 1998). Even when assessment criteria pretended to measure "ambient condition," they really counted agency or institutional activity (number of trees planted or effluent not released) rather than tracking the condition of the system we sought to protect or restore.

The Clean Water Act in the United States illustrates this problem. Section 101(a) provides a mandate to "restore and maintain the chemical, physical, and biological integrity of the Nation's waters." By integrity, Congress intended to "convey a concept that refers to a condition in which the natural structure and function of ecosystems is maintained," a benchmark concept that is explicit in Figure 12.1. Too many water managers in the United States have failed to use living systems as benchmark, guide, or goal.

Understanding this baseline, or benchmark condition, must be the foundation for assessing change caused by humans. Only then can we make informed decisions in response to the question, Is this level of change acceptable? Are the landscape and its component ecosystems healthy?

Goals, Models, and Actions

As humans continued to conquer new frontiers, concepts such as ecological health or biological integrity were rarely used to evaluate the consequences of development. Land and water were there to be farmed or allocated, developed or consumed; more was always available. Voices who spoke up for land health and a civil relationship between people and their landscapes were heard but rarely heeded (Leopold 1949, Carson 1962, Freyfogle 1998, Lear 1998, Callicott and Freyfogle 1999). Conversion of lands and waters to some "productive" purpose was the only reasonable use, even though liquidation of natural capital was the result. Lack of civility toward landscapes was mirrored by "man's inhumanity to man," as powerful cultures dominated and decimated other, usually economically powerless, cultures or communities (Donahue and Johnston 1998).

Society—oblivious to either human or ecological health risks of radically altering landscapes—has chronically undervalued their biological components. We have behaved as if we could repair or replace any lost or broken parts of living systems, much as we replace appliances and even living hearts or livers. We are rapidly converting the world to corn, cows, cars, cancer, carbon dioxide, and computers (virtual reality). This disregard for living systems has only worsened the lack of coherence in environmental laws and regulations. The result in the United States is a body of federal, state, and local law that fails to make the connections between human actions and the quality of life. This disconnectedness was one thing when few people lived on a vast landscape; with 6 billion people in the world, it is quite another.

We need a new approach, one based in new conceptual models of how landscapes, living systems, and human society interact. In the United

States, for example, conceptual models guiding water law went from "We must not dump raw sewage and oil into our waterways" to "We must not dump dangerous chemicals into our waterways" to "We must 'restore and maintain the chemical, physical, and biological integrity of the Nation's waters'" (1972 Water Pollution Control Act Amendments, sec. 101[a]). Yet any model we use is only as good as its ability to evaluate the consequences of actions that influence land and water health. One challenge is to develop models that can make real progress toward this goal. Another is to staff agencies and give them the will and power to enforce laws based on those models.

New Approaches

Several advances have been made in the past decade to spread recognition of the fractured connection between humans and other living systems. All strive to take into account the whole things that have been left out for nearly two centuries.

Recognizing that conventional neoclassical economics ignores the ecological costs of human activities as well as the value of ecological goods and services, a group of ecologists and economists developed the field of ecological economics. This approach uses many of the concepts and much of the language of neoclassical economics and tries to put monetary values on the goods and services supplied by ecological systems (e.g., Prugh et al. 1995).

Monetary Valuation

Costanza et al. (1997), for example, estimated the total monetary value to human society of natural capital flows. The researchers estimated that the current economic value of 17 ecosystem services for 16 biomes averages U.S.$33,000 billion per year, an amount about twice the global gross national product. Pimentel et al. (1997), focusing on vital services the biota provides (e.g., soil formation, crop breeding, pollination), estimated the total economic benefits of biodiversity for the United States ($319 billion) and the world ($2,928 billion)—5 percent and 11 percent of their respective gross domestic products. Both these studies attempt to engage those who think almost exclusively in economic terms, by putting a monetary value on (often declining) natural capital that supports human society. The primary message is that those long-ignored values are very high, even if the figures are not definitive. The studies are instructive because they stimulate discussion; they work less well for defining actions, identifying ecological limits, or describing competing uses of nature (Wackernagel et al. 1999).

Ecological Footprints

Another approach examines the extent to which human activities usurp or appropriate the products of Earth's systems. An early effort (Vitousek et al. 1986) examined human appropriation of the products of photosynthesis. Vitousek and colleagues calculated the global energy consumption of human society and compared it with the Earth's cumulative primary production. Humans in 1986 consumed the equivalent of nearly 40 percent of the net annual production of the Earth's terrestrial ecosystems (25 percent of marine and terrestrial systems combined). Perennial optimists might assume that we therefore still have 60 percent of net annual production at our disposal, but most of that 60 percent is not available for human use (e.g., located in widely dispersed, inaccessible areas). Rather, 40 percent of the Earth's plant productivity goes to support only one of the biosphere's tens of millions of living species.

Vitousek's study was an antecedent of ecological footprint analysis (Folke et al. 1997, Wackernagel et al. 1999, Rees, chapter 8 this volume). Footprint analysis improves on the appropriation calculus by expanding from primary production to a broad range of resources (e.g., various forms of energy, food consumption, arable land, carbon sequestering). A powerful accounting tool, footprint analysis estimates the area of land and water required to produce consumed resources and to absorb the wastes generated by a human community (Rees 1996, chapter 8 this volume). Demand and supply (based on the productive or absorptive capacity of natural systems) are combined to yield an estimate of the area "occupied"—in other words, taken over or appropriated by the population.

Footprint analyses have been completed at scales ranging from cities to nations. The 29 largest cities of Baltic Europe, for example, appropriate areas of forest, agricultural, marine, and wetland ecosystems that are at least 565 to 1,130 times larger than the areas of the cities themselves (Folke et al. 1997). The 1.1 billion people living in the world's 744 largest cities appropriate a forest area for assimilating CO_2 emissions that exceeds the full sink capacity of global forests by 10 percent.

Nations' ecological footprints in hectares per capita (1997) range from a high of 10.3 for the United States to 0.5 for Bangladesh. Both exceed each nation's own available biocapacity in the same units. The average per capita footprint for 52 nations in 1997 was 2.8 ha per capita, yet average available biocapacity was 2.0 ha per capita. Thirty-four of 52 nations are currently operating with such ecological deficits; their material standards are subsidized by exploiting other nations' capital.

As of autumn 1999, the human population of Earth stands at 6 billion. Raising all those people to living standards, and thus ecological footprints, equal to that of a U.S. citizen would require an additional two planets.

These analyses show that sustainable city or sustainable nation initiatives must understand the demands placed on a geographically wider ecological resource base. It also seems obvious that life for the inhabitants of modern cities will soon become intolerable if actions are not taken to protect the supply of goods and services that derive from living systems outside the boundaries of those cities. Cities too must do more to reflect on the ethical and moral responsibilities involved when they usurp the resources of people and cultures in regions occupied by their footprint.

By aggregating consumption in an ecologically meaningful way, and thus supplementing conventional measures of gross domestic product, ecological footprint analysis offers us something never before available to human society. It shows us the ecological deficits we are accumulating and clearly outlines the global sustainability gap we face (Rees 1996).

Both monetary evaluation and ecological footprint analysis provide valuable insight into the dangers of industrial consumerism on local and global scales. Each offers a clearer view than ever before of humans' dominion over Earth and the biosphere. The insights can be easily communicated in decisionmaking circles. But both approaches still use a human-centered accounting system. Both still consider living systems as providers of so many commodities. Neither starts from the premise that the world is a whole thing, not just a collection of parts. Neither directly measures the condition of the biosphere itself.

Biological Assessment

Direct assessment of living systems has come into its own only within the last two decades or so, ever since, in the United States, the National Environmental Policy Act of 1969 began requiring environmental impact statements prior to development. Counts of species recognized as threatened or endangered under the Endangered Species Act became a primary currency for these assessments. This focus altered the harvest of commodities when harvest was likely to affect populations of an imperiled species (e.g., spotted owl in the Pacific Northwest).

The important but narrow context of the imperiled-species perspective stimulated many in and out of government to focus on endangered ecosystems (Abell et al. 1999, Ricketts et al. 1999). Governmental agencies and nongovernmental organizations are using these compilations to identify the least disturbed places especially deserving of park or reserve status.

The central problem with counting imperiled species is that, though effective in communicating losses, species counts still focus on ecological parts, not ecological wholes—as if imperiled species were another commodity that humans are losing from our storehouse of natural capital. Even cataloging ecoregions still emphasizes the parts, not an integrated view of the condition of whole landscapes. It is true that species-rich places are likely to be more healthy than species-poor places, most deserving of conservation. But it is not enough to protect only the highest-biodiversity places. Places with naturally low biodiversity that still have their full complement of parts and processes (e.g., desert ponds, small wetlands, rocky outcrops, temperate as opposed to tropical forest) deserve protection as well. Good places near people deserve protection or restoration to connect local people to living systems.

For these and other reasons, society needs an objective measure of the condition of all places, so we can judge whether our actions are compromising the health and integrity of those places. We need a measure of biological condition other than dollars, other than units of energy; we need a broader yardstick for the health of living systems.

Ambient biological assessment tells us about the condition of landscapes, and about the needs of the people living in those landscapes. Such assessment focuses on biological endpoints as the most integrative measures of biological integrity or ecological health. Biological assessments provide ground truth to evaluate the connections between monetary valuation and ecological footprints and actual conditions in living systems. Biological assessments permit a new level of integration because living systems register the accumulated effects of all forms of degradation caused by human actions.

Efforts to assess the condition of aquatic systems in biological terms have been much stronger than those in terrestrial environments. At least two major aquatic approaches have been developed independently over the past 25 years. The underlying principle of both approaches is that the biota is the ultimate integrator of all human actions. Both attempt to look at whole things, not just the component parts.

One approach, the multimetric index of biological integrity (IBI), arose as an offshoot of basic research in aquatic ecology (Box 12.1; Karr 1981, Karr et al. 1986, Karr 1991). The concept was adopted quickly by a variety of state (Ohio EPA, 1988) and federal (Plafkin et al. 1989) agencies and in geographic regions throughout the world (Oberdorff and Hughes 1992, Davis and Simon 1995, Rossano 1996, Thorne and Williams 1997, Deegan et al. 1997). IBI has helped scientists, resource managers, and citizen volunteers to understand, protect, and restore rivers worldwide.

Effective multimetric biological indexes avoid indicators that are either theoretically or empirically flawed (see Karr and Chu [1999] for a review). They incorporate components of biology that are sensitive to a broad range of human actions (sedimentation, organic enrichment, toxic chemicals, flow alteration). Common metrics include those that illustrate changes in taxa richness (biodiversity), shifts in species composition reflecting human

BOX 12.1

Summary of Contexts and Use of the Multimetric IBI

- Tells us whether we are maintaining water bodies, water supply, and flow through the water cycle, along with the vital resources the water cycle supports.
- Works in streams, rivers, lakes, wetlands, estuaries, and coastal marine and terrestrial systems.
- Integrates elements that conventionally have been fragmented in water policy and decisionmaking, such as water quality and water quantity, surface water, and groundwater.
- Stands up to scientific and legal scrutiny and is actually improving the legal and regulatory approaches used by governments to protect the public's interest in water resources.
- Directly addresses the central call of the U.S. Clean Water Act and the European Union's Water Framework to protect the integrity of water.
- Is simple to develop and use, demanding no advanced technologies beyond the reach of developing countries with limited financial means or of citizen groups seeking to understand the condition of their local and regional watersheds.
- Defines the health of a water resource system and aids in diagnosing and identifying causes of any detected degradation.
- Enables us to identify and protect the places most deserving of conservation, defines places where restoration is possible and practical, and guides development activities to prevent or minimize damage to water resources.
- Provides results that can be used to assess the effectiveness of particular resource management decisions and to set funding priorities.
- Extends the concept of taking multiple measures to assess health—long central in economics and medicine—to environmental assessments.
- Integrates precise biological measurements of the condition of waters and their associated resources into numbers and words that are easily understood by diverse audiences.
- Allows us to compare the effects of single acts with the cumulative effects of many activities.
- Permits comparisons across time and space: of the effects of different human activities through time at the same site or of landscape condition in different geographic regions.
- Allows us to measure and compare the relative impacts of different human land uses, including recreation, farming, logging, and urbanization, and to compare such impacts with those affecting water bodies directly, such as pollution, channelization, or dam building.
- Can be applied with a broad range of taxa, from algae and vascular plants to invertebrates and fishes.

Source: After Karr and Chu 2000.

effects (sedimentation or nutrient enrichment), individual health, food web organization, and other biological attributes that respond to human influence. Multimetric indexes thus integrate multiple dimensions of complex systems. In this respect, they are similar to the indexes used to measure the health of regional and national economies (e.g., index of leading economic indicators or consumer price index in the United States). The result is an index that integrates the responses of the parts and processes of biological systems to human actions.

The other approach relies on multivariate statistical methods to discern patterns in taxonomic composition, often but not always at the family level. Examples include RIVPACS (Wright 1995), AUSRIVAS (Parsons and Norris 1996), BEAST (Reynoldson et al. 1995), and the aquatic life classification models used in Maine (Davies et al. 1995).

The two approaches overlap in many important ways (Karr and Chu 2000). Both, for example, (1) focus on biological endpoints to define river condition; (2) use a concept of reference condition as a benchmark; (3) organize sites into classes with a select set of environmental characteristics; (4) assess changes that result from human actions; (5) require standardized sampling, laboratory, and analytical methods; (6) score sites numerically to reflect their condition; (7) define "bands," or condition classes, representing degrees of degradation; and (8) furnish needed analyses for selecting high-quality areas as acquisition and conservation priorities. Despite these shared properties, the details of RIVPACS and IBI also differ in important ways (Table 12.1).

Perhaps the most important difference between RIVPACS and IBI is the biological information used to frame the assessment process. The early goal of RIVPACS was to select better sites for conservation (Wright et al. 1984). As a result, recognizing patterns of species composition was and continues to be the core of RIVPACS analyses. In contrast, IBI was developed to measure river condition across a gradient like that illustrated in Figure 12.1. In addition, a goal of multimetric assessments is to diagnose causes of degradation. As a result, the biological signals that make up IBI analyses are broader, including taxa richness and composition, trophic or other aspects of ecological organization, presence and relative abundance of tolerant and intolerant taxa, and presence of diseased individuals or individuals with other anomalies (Karr 1991, Karr and Chu 1999). A primary goal of IBI is to define the attributes of living systems that change systematically in diverse situations when exposed to the activity of humans.

These and other differences notwithstanding, both RIVPACS and IBI have changed the way many scientists and water managers think. Developing and testing these integrative approaches to water resource assessment

TABLE 12.1

Comparative Analysis of the Conceptual, Sampling, and Analytical Characteristics of Multivariate and Multimetric Approaches to River Monitoring and Assessment (based on the most common current applications)

	RIVPACS[1] (multivariate)	IBI[2] (multimetric)
Site classification or characterization	Stream size, geography, substrate particle size, water chemistry	Geology, stream size and temperature, altitude
Reference standard	Sites without serious pollution (RP); other human influences not considered. Broader in recent applications (AR)	Sites with little or no human influence
Model foundations	Multivariate associations between environmental variables and species present	Empirically defined measures; dose-response graphs plotting human influence against biological response
Decision criteria	Species presence or absence (observed vs. expected ratios) from probabilistic models; sometimes tolerance measures	Biological attributes such as taxa richness, relative abundance, taxa composition, tolerance and intolerance
Microhabitat sampled	Multiple (e.g., riffle, edge, pool-rock: RP); riffles (AR)	Riffles
Subsampling	Varies regionally and with application	Full samples counted
Stream applications available	Benthic invertebrates	Benthic invertebrates, fish, algae
Data set required	Extensive, hundreds of sites; regional foundation; some smaller scale applications being developed	Fifteen to 20 sites representing a broad gradient of human disturbance; can be developed locally or over larger areas
Transferability	Extensive data sets and new species-specific models needed for each region	Consistency in selected measures and biological responses across regions
Treatment of rare species	Often excluded from analyses	Included in analyses
Sampling period	RP: combined three-season model; AR: model for each season	Defined period for sampling
Analytical basis	Species presence-absence	Diverse dimensions of biological and natural history patterns
Human influence	Largely chemical contamination	Full spectrum of human influences
Diagnostic capability	Not explored	Moderately well developed
Communication	Statistical foundations difficult; signal narrow (O/E [observed/expected species] ratio); pollution tolerance	Simple dose-response curves similar to toxicology; broad range of biological signal

1. RIVPACS (RP) developed in England and cloned as AUSRIVAS (AR) in Australia for rivers and streams; being applied in rivers in other regions.

2. IBI developed in midwestern United States for rivers and streams; now used internationally. Applications for other habitats available and in development.

Source: After Karr and Chu 1999b.

have provided a long-needed counterpoint to the history of monitoring chemical water quality and simple water quantity. Such shifts in thinking—from regarding the parts and processes of living systems as so many commodities and coins in our natural savings accounts to seeing them as the whole, independent living systems they are—are vital to protecting the interests of all life as we enter the twenty-first century.

ACKNOWLEDGMENTS

This chapter was prepared with support from the Consortium for Risk Evaluation with Stakeholder Participation (CRESP) by Department of Energy Cooperative Agreement #DE-FC01-95EW55084.S and was aided by numerous grants from the U.S. Environmental Protection Agency. Ellen W. Chu and Elena S. Karr provided invaluable advice that substantially improved the chapter.

REFERENCES

Abell, R. A., D. M. Olson, E. Dinerstein, P. T. Hurley, J. T. Diggs, W. Eichbaum, S. Walters, W. Wettengel, T. Allnutt, C. J. Loucks, and P. Hedao. 1999. *Freshwater Ecoregions of North America: A Conservation Assessment.* Washington, DC: Island Press.

Angermeier, P. L. and J. R. Karr. 1994. Biological integrity versus biological diversity as policy directives. *BioScience* 44:690–697.

Callicott, J. B. and E. T. Freyfogle, editors. 1999. *Aldo Leopold: For the Health of the Land.* Washington, DC: Island Press.

Callicott, J. B., L. B. Crowder, and K. Mumford. 1999. Current normative concepts in conservation. *Conservation Biology* 13:22–35.

Carson, R. 1962. *Silent Spring.* Boston: Houghton Mifflin.

Costanza, R., R. dArge, R. deGroot, S. Farber, M. Grasso, B. Hannon, K. Limburg, S. Naeem, R. V. O'Neill, J. Paruelo, R. G. Raskin, P. Sutton, and M. vanden-Belt. 1997. The value of the world's ecosystem services and natural capital. *Nature* 387:253–260.

Davies, S. P., L. Tsomides, D. L. Courtemanch, and F. Drummond. 1995. *Maine Biological Monitoring and Biocriteria Development Program.* Maine Department of Environmental Protection, Bureau of Land and Water Quality, Division of Environmental Assessment, Augusta.

Davis, W. S. and T. P. Simon, editors. 1995. *Biological Assessment and Criteria: Tools for Water Resource Planning and Decision Making.* Boca Raton: Lewis Publishers.

Deegan, L. A., J. T. Finn, S. G. Ayvazian, C. A. Ryder-Kieffer, and J. Buonaccorsi. 1997. Development and validation of an estuarine biotic integrity index. *Estuaries* 20:601–617.

Diamond, J. 1997. *Guns, Germs, and Steel: The Fates of Human Societies.* New York: Norton.

Donahue, J. M. and B. R. Johnston, editors. 1998. *Water, Culture, and Power: Local Struggles in a Global Context.* Washington, DC: Island Press.

Folke, C., A. Jansson, J. Larsson, and R. Costanza. 1997. Ecosystem appropriation by cities. *Ambio* 26:167–172.

Freyfogle, E. T. 1998. *Bounded People, Boundless Lands: Envisioning a New Land Ethic.* Washington, DC: Island Press.

Goldstein, P. Z. 1999. Functional ecosystems and biodiversity buzzwords. *Conservation Biology* 13:247–255.

Homer-Dixon, T. F. 1999. *Environment, Scarcity, and Violence.* Princeton: Princeton University Press.

Karr, J. R. 1981. Assessment of biotic integrity using fish communities. *Fisheries* 6(6):21–27.

Karr, J. R. 1991. Biological integrity: A long-neglected aspect of water resource management. *Ecological Applications* 1:66–84.

Karr, J. R. 1993. Protecting ecological integrity: An urgent societal goal. *Yale Journal of International Law* 18:297–306.

Karr, J. R. 1994. Landscapes and management for ecological integrity. In *Biodiversity and Landscapes: A Paradox of Humanity,* edited by K. C. Kim and R. D. Weaver, 229–251. Cambridge: Cambridge University Press.

Karr, J. R. 1999. Defining and measuring river health. *Freshwater Biology* 41:221–234.

Karr, J. R. and E. W. Chu. 1995. Ecological integrity: Reclaiming lost connections. In *Perspectives on Ecological Integrity,* edited by L. Westra and J. Lemons. Dordrecht, Netherlands: Kluwer Academic.

Karr, J. R. and E. W. Chu. 1999. *Restoring Life in Running Waters: Better Biological Monitoring.* Washington, DC: Island Press.

Karr, J. R. and E. W. Chu. 2000. Sustaining living rivers. *Hydrobiologia.*

Karr, J. R., K. D. Fausch, P. L. Angermeier, P. R. Yant, and I. J. Schlosser. 1986. *Assessing Biological Integrity in Running Waters: A Method and Its Rationale.* Special Publication No. 5. Champaign: Illinois Natural History Survey.

Lear, L. 1998. *Lost Woods: The Discovered Writing of Rachel Carson.* Boston: Beacon Press.

Leopold, A. S. 1949. *A Sand County Almanac.* New York: Oxford University Press.

Lubchenco, J. 1998. Entering the century of the environment: A new social contract for science. *Science* 279:491–497.

McMichael, A. J. 1993. *Planetary Overload: Global Environmental Change and the Health of the Human Species.* New York: Cambridge University Press.

Meyer, J. L. 1997. Stream health: Incorporating the human dimension to advance stream ecology. *Journal of the North American Benthological Society* 16:439–447.

Oberdorff, T. and R. M. Hughes. 1992. Modification of an index of biotic integrity based on fish assemblages to characterize rivers of the Seine-Normandie basin, France. *Hydrobiologia* 228:117–130.

Ohio EPA (Environmental Protection Agency). 1988. *Biological Criteria for the Protection of Aquatic Life,* vol. 1–3. Columbus, Ecological Assessment Section, Division of Water Quality Monitoring and Assessment, Ohio EPA.

Orr, D. W. 1999. Verbicide. *Conservation Biology* 13:696–699.

Parsons, M. and R. H. Norris. 1996. The effect of habitat-specific sampling on biological assessment of water quality using a predictive model. *Freshwater Biology* 36:419–434.

Pimentel, D., C. Wilson, C. McCullum, R. Huang, P. Dwen, J. Flack, Q. Tran, T. Saltman, and B. Cliff. 1997. Economic and environmental benefits of biodiversity. *BioScience* 47:747–757.

Plafkin, J. L., M. T. Barbour, K. D. Porter, S. K. Gross, and R. M. Hughes. 1989. *Rapid Bioassessment Protocols for Use in Streams and Rivers: Benthic Macroinvertebrates and Fish.* EPA/440/4-89-001. Washington, DC: Assessment and Water Protection Division, U.S. Environmental Protection Agency.

Prugh, T., R. Costanza, J. H. Cumberland, H. Daly, R. Goodland, and R. Norgaard. 1995. *Natural Capital and Human Economic Survival.* Solomons, MD: International Society for Ecological Economics Press.

Rapport, D., R. Costanza, P. R. Epstein, C. Gaudet, and R. Levins. 1998a. *Ecosystem Health.* Malden, MA: Blackwell Science.

Rapport, D. J., C. Gaudet, J. R. Karr, J. S. Baron, C. Bohlen, W. Jackson, B. Jones, R. J. Naiman, B. Norton, and M. M. Pollock. 1998b. Evaluating landscape health: Integrating societal goals and biophysical processes. *Journal of Environmental Management* 53:1–15.

Rees, W. E. 1996. Revisiting carrying capacity: Area-based indicators of sustainability. *Population and Environment* 17:195–215.

Reynoldson, T. B., R. C. Bailey, K. E. Day, and R. H. Norris. 1995. Biological guidelines for freshwater sediment based on Benthic Assessment of Sediment (the BEAST) using a multivariate approach for predicting biological state. *Australian Journal of Ecology* 20:198–219.

Ricketts, T. H., E. Dinerstein, D. M. Olson, and C. Loucks. 1999. Who's where in North America? Patterns of species richness and the utility of indicator taxa for conservation. *BioScience* 49:369–382.

Rossano, E. M. 1996. *Diagnosis of Stream Environments with Index of Biological Integrity.* (In Japanese and English.) Tokyo, Japan: Museum of Streams and Lakes, Sankaido Publishers.

Sachs, A. 1995. Humboldt's legacy and the restoration of science. *World Watch* 8(2):28–38.

Schorske, C. E. 1998. *Thinking with History: Explorations in the Passage of Modernism.* Princeton: Princeton University Press.

Thorne, R. St. J. and W. P. Williams. 1997. The response of benthic invertebrates to pollution in developing countries: A multimetric system of bioassessment. *Freshwater Biology* 37:671–686.

Toth, L. A. 1993. The ecological basis of the Kissimmee River restoration plan. *Florida Scientist* 56:25–51.

Vitousek, P. M., P. R. Ehrlich, A. H. Ehrlich, and P. A. Matson. 1986. Human appropriation of the products of photosynthesis. *BioScience* 36:368–373.

Vitousek, P. M., H. A. Mooney, J. Lubchenco, and J. M. Mellilo. 1997. Human domination of Earth's ecosystems. *Science* 277:494–499.

Wackernagel, M., L. Onisto, P. Bello, A. C. Linares, I. S. L. Falfan, J. M. Garcia, A. I. S. Guerrero, and C. S. Guerrero. 1999. Natural capital accounting with the ecological footprint concept. *Ecological Economics* 29:375–390.

Woodwell, G. M. 1990. *The Earth in Transition: Patterns and Processes of Biotic Impoverishment.* New York: Cambridge University Press.

Wright, J. F. 1995. Development and use of a system for predicting the macroinvertebrate fauna in flowing waters. *Australian Journal of Ecology* 20:181–197.

Wright, J. F., D. Moss, P. D. Armitage, and M. T. Furse. 1984. A preliminary classification of running-water sites in Great Britain based on macro-invertebrate species and the prediction of community type using environmental data. *Freshwater Biology* 14:221–256.

Yoder, C. O. and E. T. Rankin. 1998. The role of biological indicators in a state water quality management process. *Environmental Monitoring and Assessment* 51:61–88.

Global Change, Fisheries, and the Integrity of Marine Ecosystems: The Future Has Already Begun

Daniel Pauly

Given that the sun continues to shine as it does now, the physicists can tell us that further increases of greenhouse gases will cause the Earth's atmosphere to become warmer, a strong and most probably correct prediction. Meteorologists and other atmospheric scientists—especially those with access to global climate models—can predict the regional structure of the climate that should result, in two to five decades, from a generally warmer atmosphere (see e.g., contributions in MacCracken et al. 1990). I am not aware of substantial agricultural or agroforestry programs being implemented on the basis of these predictions, but at least they exist and are being refined, i.e., the science is being done.

Oceanographers, given these anticipated developments, are being asked to predict changes in regional oceanographic features. However, the prospects for these predictions to be precise enough for international organizations or countries to take preventive measures appear bleak, except perhaps for sea-level changes, which, although global, would have strongly differing impacts from region to region.

Where does this leave marine ecosystems and the fisheries they support, given the meteorologists' and the oceanographers' uncertainties? Put simply, I believe that fisheries scientists cannot predict what global changes will do regionally to marine fish stocks, and that if they could, it wouldn't matter, given the other forces at work, here illustrated by the case of Northern cod (Figure 13.1; Box 13.1).

Indeed, we often do not know accurately how large the existing fisheries are, and where they operate, because of widespread cheating and budget constraints for the national and international agencies mandated with monitoring fisheries. Thus it was only recently realized that over 25 percent of

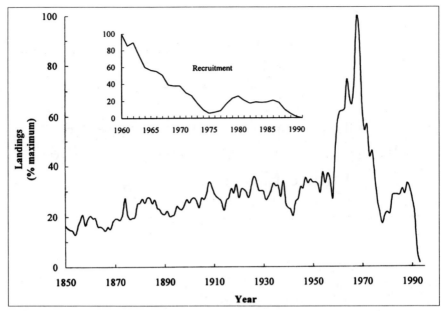

FIGURE 13.1

Time series of landings of Northern cod around Newfoundland, Canada, documenting the sustainable, inshore, small-scale fishery that caught 150–250,000 t per year for over one hundred years, until foreign deep-sea trawlers (1960s to mid-1970s) and the local trawl fleet that succeeded them (1980s) drove catches up, recruitment down, and the fishery into collapse (see insert; data from Myers et al. 1995).

the world catch of marine fish is discarded at sea (Alverson et al. 1994) and that globally, fisheries earn 50×10^6 U.S. dollars per year less than their cost, the rest being covered by government subsidies (see Beddington 1995, Christy 1997). Moreover, topping all this waste, fisheries destroy the structural integrity of marine food webs (Pauly et al. 1998). It is for these and a number of related reasons that marine fisheries resources and the ecosystems supporting them are now endangered, even before the global changes that will be induced by increased emission of greenhouse gases have begun to take hold (hence the second part of this chapter's title).

What scientists can do, on the other hand, is to try to identify key processes impacting marine fisheries and ecosystems, with a comparable scientific basis to, for example, the physical laws behind the prediction of the greenhouse effect. One could then infer some trends that might prevail, given the social and ecological conditions that might obtain two to five

---

BOX 13.1

A Lesson: The Collapse of Northern Cod

Northern cod (*Gadus morhua*) sustained vibrant fisheries for centuries and is indeed one of the key factors behind the colonization of Newfoundland, now a province of Canada. These fisheries, which used handlines or traps, left refuges—in deeper waters—for the large adults producing the recruits that sustained the fisheries.

In the 1970s, European trawler fleets started exploiting this resource, concentrating on the deeper waters. Catches shot up, and predictably, the spawning stock declined. In the 1980s, with the advent of the new Law of the Sea, the foreign fleet lost access to the cod stocks, now within the Canadian Exclusive Economic Zone, and was replaced by a new national fleet. In the early 1990s, the stock was completely devastated, and the century-old fishery for Northern cod was closed.

While the overwhelming preponderance of scientific evidence points at overfishing as the *sole* cause for the debacle (Hutchings and Myers 1994), there is evident support within the agency that managed the fishery for an account in which "environmental effects" conspired to destroy Northern cod, low temperatures and seals being most frequently blamed. However, the available time series of catches, dating back to 1850 and spanning several periods of intense cold, do not provide any support for low temperatures being a cause for the demise of Northern cod (Figure 13.1). And if seal predation has become relatively more important than it was before, it is because the cod biomass was reduced by fishing.

Following the collapse of Northern cod, a trawl fishery on bottom invertebrates developed around Newfoundland, targeting organisms that were low in the food web and that were earlier spurned by fishers. There is little need here to emphasize that catching these organisms is not going to help toward rebuilding, around Newfoundland, the population of this bottom-feeding fish.

I believe that these events reflect a generic feature of marine fisheries: our technical ability to catch fishes and their prey, left unchecked, will destroy all marine fisheries resources and ecosystems of the world, one after the other, and we will blame the "environment," or El Niño. In a few years, we will blame "global change."

---

decades hence (as represented by "scenarios" *sensu* Jamieson 1988). Examples of four such processes follow.

The first process is demographic: the same one that drives the production of greenhouse gases, i.e., the growth of the human population and the resulting increase of demand for food including fish, especially as income increases in parts of the world. Here, I abstain from presenting a graph: the depressing trends are well known, as are their largely inescapable projections into the future.

Figure 13.2 shows the evolution of global marine fish catches since World War II. Note the rapid increase from the 1960s to 1970s, and the recent flattening of this curve, whose changes are now largely determined by the ups and downs of the population of a few species (e.g., Alaska pollock, *Theragra chalcogramma*; Peruvian anchoveta, *Engraulis ringens*).

Just as some are now trying to anticipate what catches may be in the next decades, attempts were made a few decades ago to predict the world's marine fisheries catches (black dots in Figure 13.2). As might be seen, the fisheries themselves refuted the lowest among these estimates a few years after they were made. The jury is still out on the highest estimates (not shown), which reach into the billions of tonnes per year because they include unconventional species (e.g., large zooplankton such as krill), which humans might still decide to harvest on a large scale. However, one can predict,

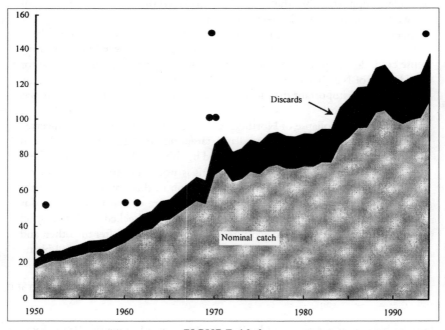

FIGURE 13.2

Marine global fisheries catches in million of tonnes (1950s to 1990s). Based on nominal catch series of the Food and Agriculture Organization of the United Nations. The estimates of discarded by-catch (for the early 1990s) of Alverson et al. (1994) were here assumed proportional to catches for the entire series. The estimates of global potential catch (full dots) plotted against their year of publication are documented in Pauly (1996b).

given the overall shape of the trend in Figure 13.2, and the increasing occurrence of collapses such as in Figure 13.1, that the catch of what is conventionally viewed as "fish" will not keep up with the increasing demand of the next decades. This leads to our second process: given increased demand and a stagnating supply, we can expect price increases on fish products.

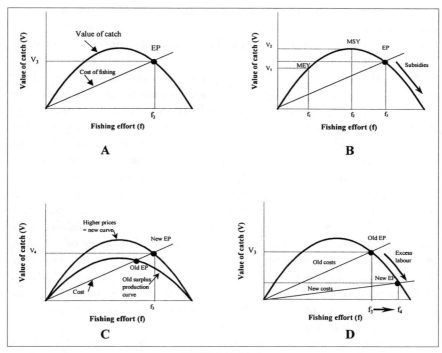

FIGURE 13.3

Schematic representation of the key economic factors affecting open-access fisheries. A: Basic model, in which fishing costs are assumed proportional to fishing effort (f), and gross returns proportional to catches (parabola). B: Under open access, f will increase past Maximum Economic Yield (MEY) at f_1 (where the economic rent, i.e., the difference between total costs and gross returns, is highest), and past Maximum Sustainable Yield (MSY) at f_2, until the equilibrium point (EP) at f_3, where costs and returns are equal, i.e., where the economic rent is completely dissipated. In this situation, subsidies, by reducing costs, increase the level of effort at which EP occurs, and thus decrease catches. C: Price increases, by increasing gross returns, increase the level of effort at which the rent will be dissipated (i.e., from f_3 to f_4), and hence foster overfishing, just as subsidies do. D: In small-scale fisheries, labor is a major cost factor; when its value tends toward zero (as occurs when there is a large excess of rural labor), resources may become severely depleted, leading to Malthusian overfishing (Pauly 1994, 1997).

These, however, have the same effect on fisheries as subsidies, i.e., other things being equal, they tend to foster overfishing (Figure 13.3).

Similarly, a reduction in the value of rural labor (which can be expected for many developing countries, whether or not the dire predictions concerning the future of their agricultural systems come to pass) will have the effect of increasing fishing effort in small-scale fisheries, and thus of fostering overfishing of coastal stocks (Pauly 1997). Indeed, when the price of labor drops to extremely low values, to the extent that mobility *out* of coastal fisheries does not occur, the syndrome I have called Malthusian overfishing (Pauly 1994, 1997) can set in, further depleting coastal resources (Figure 13.3D).

As our third process, we consider an important biological feature of fish stocks that is also likely to shape future fisheries and to strongly impact the integrity of marine ecosystems. Generally, the species that are the first to decline under exploitation are top predators, usually large fish with a low reproductive and/or population growth rate. Thus, in multispecies fisheries (i.e., virtually all bottom-trawl fisheries, especially those targeting shrimps), fishing itself induces replacements, with small, fast-growing species from the lower parts of food webs (i.e., with low trophic levels) gradually replacing (in the landings, and/or in the discarded by-catch) the fish with high trophic levels (Pauly et al. 1998; Figure 13.4). This process of "fishing down marine food webs" sometimes induces a reduction of the value of the catch, given that larger fish are usually more valuable than smaller ones. However, this effect can also be masked by changes in relative market valuations, leading over time toward higher prices for smaller fish (Sumaila 1999), and thus go on until the integrity of the supporting ecosystems is compromised and species are lost (Parrish 1995, 1998).

The fourth process considered here is also a masking effect: the cultural pattern in which successive generations of resource users (and scientists!) tend to forget the ecosystem features and fisheries resources that the generations preceding them took for granted, while continuing to overexploit what is left. The result is what I have called the shifting baseline syndrome (Pauly 1995). It is illustrated in Figure 13.5, and elaborated upon in Pitcher and Pauly (1998).

I see three possible scenarios within which these four processes may act and interact:

1. *Finis mundi.* The apocalyptic scenario that will result if nothing is done to avert the greenhouse effect, and that would probably lead to various resource wars as the warming enters some runaway stage. This is not an impossible scenario, but one that even science fiction authors cannot adequately cover—though they have tried (see Lem 1980 for a critique of the resulting "catastrophism").

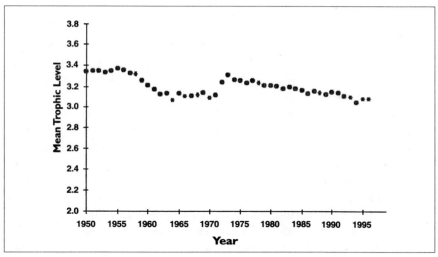

FIGURE 13.4

Mean trophic level of global marine fisheries catches, reflecting increasing targeting of species at the bottom of food webs (i.e., with low trophic levels), and depletion of top predators. Based on nominal catch series of the Food and Agriculture Organization of the United Nations and trophic level estimates in FishBase (see www.fishbase.org; see also Pauly et al. 1998).

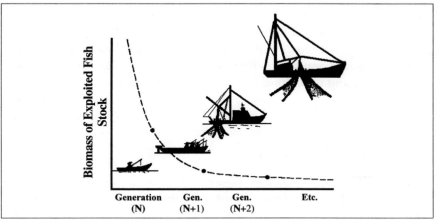

FIGURE 13.5

Schematic representation of the shifting baseline syndrome wherein the rapid decline of sensitive species that occurred in the past, at low levels of fishing effort, is not recalled by the following generations of naturalists or biologists, who tend to use the abundance level prevailing at the start of their careers as the baseline. This leads to a gradual shift of baselines, undermining the very notion of sustainability (Pauly 1995, Pitcher and Pauly 1998).

2. *Benign utopia.* This is the alternative to finis mundi, i.e., a scenario in which all reasonable measures so far proposed to reduce the ecological footprint of humans (Rees, chapter 8, this volume) on the Earth's ecosystems are rapidly implemented. These would include massive investment to foster "decarbonized" and/or otherwise "dematerialized" industrial processes, massive reforestation, and sustainable small-scale farming. For fisheries, this would include the rapid abolition of subsidies for distant and other industrial fleets (Bonfil et al. 1998), the transition to small-scale fisheries wherever possible (see Thomson and FAO 1988, and contributions in Pitcher et al. 1998), the strict enforcement of regulations that limit fishing, and the establishment of large marine protected areas to maintain patches of ecosystem integrity, but also to act as sources of recruitment to the surrounding areas (Bohnsack 1994) and to serve as insurance against recruitment failure (Sumaila 1998a, 1998b). Overall, this would imply a commitment to reregulation, very much at odds with the present trend toward deregulation. Indeed, I am well aware that if we had the institutional capacity for benign utopia, our fisheries would not be threatening the integrity of their resource base, as they are now.

3. *Muddling through.* This likely scenario would consist of doing at the last possible moment what is needed to avoid the immediate consequences of a problem, without necessarily resolving the problem itself (see e.g., Ausubel 1991).

Table 13.1 presents some possible effects on global fisheries of the four processes presented above, in the context provided by these three scenarios.

Three types of approaches have been proposed to deal with the global fisheries crisis and its regional and local manifestations:

1. Market-based approaches

2. Community-based approaches

3. Ecology-based approaches

Market-based approaches are meant to provide an alternative to "open access," the still predominant state of most marine fish stocks, and widely seen as the major cause of the global fisheries crisis and the present trends toward fishing down marine food webs.

The most important tool so far proposed to limit open access is Individual Transferable Quotas (ITQs) (see e.g., contributions in Munro and Pitcher 1996).

The applicability of ITQs to the developing-country fisheries, which

TABLE 13.1

Impact of Key Processes on the Future State of Global Fisheries Resources

Processes/Scenarios	Price Increase	Malthusian Overfishing	Species Replacement	Baseline Shift
Finis mundi	Rapid, then none	Rapid increase, then none	Terminal fauna/flora (if any) determined by temperature and water trends	na
Benign utopia	Countered by abundant supply of alternative food	Solved by rural development and reduced populations	Countered by large marine protected areas	Past populations used as reference for resource rehabilitation
Muddling through	Will cause the loss of numerous fisheries and resources systems	Will cause the loss of numerous fisheries and resource systems, e.g., coral reefs	Will soon cause the loss of many sensitive species	Strong effect, possibly all the way to gradual loss of most wild fauna and flora

nowadays contribute over half of the world catches, has been questioned (Pauly 1996a). Indeed, ITQs do not appear useful under the conditions leading to Malthusian overfishing, which is likely to become more wide-spread in the next decades if tropical agricultural systems indeed make large numbers of rural workers redundant (see earlier text).

Community-based approaches are not new. Communities largely regu-lated the sustainable fisheries of past centuries (e.g., the cod fishery in the early part of the period covered by Figure 13.1).

However, the industrialization of global fisheries in the 1950s and 1960s, which led to the increase of catches shown in Figure 13.2, largely margin-alized small-scale fisheries and the local communities that depended on them. These new industrialized fisheries appear for the most part largely unsustainable (see, e.g., Figure 13.1), however, and their low catch/energy consumption ratio will make them untenable when carbon emissions are taxed (Cairncross 1991). This may enable a market-led reallocation of at least inshore resources to small-scale fisheries, which tend to have lower ecological footprints.

Ecology-based approaches are required to mitigate the damage caused by fishing, and are based on an understanding of what enabled preindustrial (and most small-scale) fisheries to operate sustainably: the fact that a part of an exploited stock (often the large spawners) could not be caught, and hence remained to generate the recruits for that same stock (as was the case for the cod in Figure 13.1 and Box 13.1). However, using modern echolo-cation and geopositioning technology, industrial vessels can locate and catch the last spawners of a fish stock, and thus drive it into extinction (Figure 13.1). Hence our list of marine fish that will not "survive" (Table 13.2). Also note that the fish that can be expected to survive are not particularly appetizing (Table 13.3).

A sensible response to the implications of Tables 13.2 and 13.3 is the es-tablishment of no-take marine protected areas (MPAs), which recreate the natural refuges that sustained fisheries (Bohnsack 1994). MPAs have the ad-vantage that they both reduce risk and accommodate imperfect knowledge (Sumaila 1998b), an advantage that is likely to become worse as global cli-mate changes begin to strongly modify the environments of marine fish-eries.

Moreover, MPAs represent our only answer to the creeping losses of bio-diversity that "muddling through" will cause, given the trend of species re-placement in ecosystems whose integrity has been compromised (see Figure 13.4) and our propensity to allow our biodiversity baselines to shift (see Figure 13.5 and Table 13.1).

Rapid implementation in each country of market-based, community-based, and ecology-based mitigating measures might get fisheries out of the crisis they are in. However, this—in my opinion—is unlikely to happen for the same reasons that make benign utopia unlikely. I will not venture any opinion as to which of the remaining scenarios I think is more likely; I can only hope we will muddle through.

TABLE 13.2

Marine Fish That Will Not Survive, Given Continuation of Present Trends

Large- to moderate-sized, predaceous, territorial reef fishes and rockfishes with late age at maturity, very low natural mortality rates, and low recruitment rates vs. adult stock size	Snappers, sea basses, emperors, rockfishes, sea breams
Large- to moderate-sized shelf-dwelling, soft-bottom predators susceptible to bottom trawling	Cods, flounders, soles, rockfishes, croakers, skates
Large- to moderate-sized schooling midwater fishes susceptible to midwater trawling	Hakes, rockfishes, armorheads, rougheyes
Large- to moderate-sized shelf-dwelling, schooling, pelagic fishes	Bonitos, sierras, capelin, eulachon, salmon, sharks
Any species with exceptionally high monetary value	Bluefin tuna, red snappers, halibuts, medicinal fishes, aquarium fishes, groupers, salmon, red mullets, billfishes

Source: Adapted from Parrish 1995, 1998.

TABLE 13.3

Marine Fishes That May Survive, Given Continuation of Present Trends

Small offshore, nonschooling, mesopelagic, or epipelagic fishes	Lanternfishes, bristlemouths, deep-sea smelts, flying fish
Small, solitary, ugly, shore fishes	Blennies, sculpins, poachers, prickbacks, kelpfish
Small unpalatable, reef and slope bottomfishes	Lizardfish, sand lances, gobies, leatherjackets, toadfish
Small, reef- and slope-dwelling generalists	Cardinalfish, damselfish, soldierfish, wrasses, butterflyfish
Small, early-maturing pelagics with indeterminate spawning	Tropical anchovies, tropical herrings, round herrings, scads, jacks, frigate mackerel

Source: Adapted from Parrish 1995, 1998.

ACKNOWLEDGMENTS

I thank the organizers of The Oceanography Society's 1996 Meeting on the Role of the Ocean in Global Change Research: Highlighting Oceanographic Aspects and Importance of the Global Change Research of WCRP, IGBP and HDP, 8–11 July 1996, held in Amsterdam, The Netherlands, for the opportunity to present an early version of this contribution, and U. R. Sumaila for his suggestions for improving the updated version.

REFERENCES

Alverson, D.L., M.H. Freeberg, S.A. Murawski, and J.G. Pope. 1994. *A Global Assessment of Fisheries Bycatch and Discards.* FAO *Fisheries Technical Paper* 339. 233 p.

Ausubel, J. 1991. A second look at the impacts of global change. *American Scientist* 79(3):210–221.

Beddington, J. 1995. The primary requirements. *Nature* 374:213–214.

Bohnsack, J.A. 1994. Marine reserves: They enhance fisheries, reduce conflicts, and protect resources. *Naga, the ICLARM Quarterly* 17(3):4–7.

Bonfil, R., G. Munro, U.R. Sumaila, H. Valtysson, M. Wright, T. Pitcher, D. Preikshot, N. Haggan, and D. Pauly. 1998. Impacts of distant water fleets: An ecological, economic and social assessment. Pp. 11–111 in *The Footprint of Distant Water Fleet on World Fisheries.* Endangered Seas Campaign, WWF International, Godalming, Surrey. 112 p.

Cairncross, F. 1991. *Costing the Earth.* The Economist Books, London. 256 p.

Christy, F.T. 1997. Economic waste in fisheries: Impediments to change and conditions for improvement. Pp. 28–39 in E.K. Pikitch, D.D. Huppert, and M.P. Sissenwine (eds.), *Global Trends: Fisheries Management.* American Fisheries Society Symposium 20, Bethesda, Maryland.

Hutchings, J.A. and R.A. Myers. 1994. What can be learned from the collapse of a renewable resource? Atlantic cod, *Gadus morhua,* for Newfoundland and Labrador. *Canadian Journal of Fisheries and Aquatic Sciences* 51:2126–2146.

Jamieson, D. 1988. Grappling for a glimpse of the future. Pp. 73–93 in M.H. Glantz (ed.), *Societal Response to Regional Climatic Change: Forecasting by Analogy.* Westview Press, Boulder, Colorado. 428 p.

Lem, S. 1980. *Phantastik und Futurologie.* Vol. 2. Insel Verlag, Frankfurt am Main. 357 p.

MacCracken, M., M.I. Budyko, A.D. Hecht, and Y.A. Izrael (eds.). 1990. *Prospect for Future Climate: A Special US/USSR Report on Climate and Climate Change.* Lewis Publishers, Chelsea, Michigan. 270 p.

Munro, G.R. and T.J. Pitcher (eds.). 1996. Special issue on Individual Transferable Quotas. *Review in Fish Biology and Fisheries* 6(1). 116 p.

Myers, R.A., J. Bridson, and N.J. Barrowman. 1995. *Summary of Worldwide Spawner and Recruitment Data.* Can. Tech. Rep. Fish Aquat. Sci. 2924. 244 p. + appendices.

Parrish, R.H. 1995. Lanternfish heaven: The future of world fisheries? *Naga, the ICLARM Quarterly* 18(3):7–9.

Parrish, R.H. 1998. Life history strategies for marine fishes in the late Holocene. Pp. 524–535 in M.H. Durand, P. Cury, R. Mendelssoln, A. Bakun, C. Roy, and D. Pauly (eds.), *Global Versus Global Change in Upwelling Areas.* Séries Colloques et Séminaires. ORSTOM, Paris.

Pauly, D. 1994. *On the Sex of Fish and the Gender of Scientists: A Collection of Essays in Fisheries Science.* Chapman and Hall, London. 250 p.

Pauly, D. 1995. Anecdotes and the shifting baseline syndrome of fisheries. *Trends in Ecology and Evolution* 10(10):430.

Pauly, D. 1996a. ITQs: The assumptions behind the meme. *Review in Fish Biology and Fisheries* 6(1):109–112.

Pauly, D. 1996b. One hundred million tonnes of fish and fisheries research. *Fisheries Research* 25(1):25–38.

Pauly, D. 1997. Small-scale fisheries in the tropics: Marginality, marginalization and some implication for fisheries management. Pp. 40–49 in E.K. Pikitch, D.D. Huppert, and M.P. Sissenwine (eds.), *Global Trends: Fisheries Management.* American Fisheries Society Symposium 20, Bethesda, Maryland.

Pauly, D., V. Christensen, J. Dalsgaard, R. Froese, and F.C. Torres Jr. 1998. Fishing down marine food webs. *Science* 279:860–863.

Pitcher, T. and D. Pauly. 1998. Rebuilding ecosystems, not sustainability, is the proper goal of fishery management. Pp. 311–329 in T.J. Pitcher, P. Hart, and D. Pauly (eds.), *Reinventing Fisheries Management.* Fish and Fisheries Series 23. Kluwer Academic Publishing, Dordrecht, The Netherlands.

Pitcher, T.J., P.J.B. Hart, and D. Pauly (eds.). 1998. *Reinventing Fisheries Management.* Fish and Fisheries Series 23. Kluwer Academic Publishing, Dordrecht, The Netherlands. 435 p.

Sumaila, U.R. 1998a. Protected marine reserves as fisheries management tools: A bioeconomic analysis. *Fisheries Research* 37(1–3):287–296.

Sumaila, U.R. 1998b. Protected marine reserves as hedge against uncertainty: an economist's perspective. Pp. 303–309 in T.J. Pitcher, P. Hart, and D. Pauly, (eds.), *Reinventing Fisheries Management.* Fish and Fisheries Series 23. Kluwer Academic Publishing, Dordrecht, The Netherlands.

Sumaila, U.R. 1999. Pricing down marine food webs. Pp. 13–15 in D. Pauly, V. Christenson, and L. Coelho (eds.), *Proceedings of the Expo '98 Conference on Ocean Food Web and Economic Productivity.* ACP-EU Research Report No. 5.

Thomson, D. and FAO (Food and Agriculture Organization). 1988. The world's two marine fishing industries—how they compare. *Naga, the ICLARM Quarterly* 11(3):17.

PART IV

Human and Societal Health

This part explores the relationship between loss of ecological integrity and human health.

In chapter 14, "Global Environmental Change in the Coming Century: How Sustainable Are Recent Health Gains?," A. J. McMichael begins by reviewing recent trends in human-induced degradation of ecosystems worldwide and concludes that we are now encountering unprecedented human-induced changes in the composition of the lower and middle atmospheres and worldwide depletion of natural systems (e.g., soil fertility, aquifers, ocean fisheries, and biodiversity).

McMichael next looks at the relationship between human health and degradation of the biosphere's natural systems and concludes that ecological trends are threatening human health because human health depends on maintaining a stable and productive natural environment. Moreover, stresses to the biosphere are causing tensions between human communities that can trigger conflict and its attendant damage to public health. Of particular concern are threats caused by growing scarcity of fresh water because almost 40 percent of the human population is facing water scarcity.

Human-induced climate change, according to McMichael, will affect the survival of humans and species within ecosystems. Climate change will affect rates of mortality and morbidity due to heat waves and thermal stresses in general, the respiratory consequences of change in exposure to aeroallergens, and the direct, often physical hazards of any increases in extreme weather events, including storms, floods, and droughts. The indirect health effects of climate change include alteration in the range and activity of vector-borne infectious diseases (such as malaria, leishmaniasis, and dengue); changes in the transmission of person-to-person diseases (including food poisoning and water-borne pathogens); nutritional and health consequences of local and regional changes in agricultural productivity; and the various consequences of rising sea levels. There would also be more diffuse public health consequences due to population displacement, migration (both "economic" and "distress" migration), and enforced loss of employment due to the disruptive effects of climate change on various economic sectors and vulnerable locations. Climate change would also affect agricultural productivity both because plants are sensitive to temperature and rainfall and because climate change can create land degradation.

Next, McMichael reviews evidence that human health may already be affected by climate change. This includes some suggestive evidence of increases in vector-borne diseases, such as malaria, dengue, and meningitis.

McMichael then goes on to describe why some of the poorest countries in the world are likely to suffer the most from climate change. These countries include Bangladesh, Egypt, Pakistan, Indonesia, and Thailand, which are all threatened by rising sea levels and the loss of fishing mangroves.

McMichael notes that the poorest countries are also at risk from tropical cyclones and droughts.

This topic is followed by a review of the health impacts of stratospheric ozone loss, which include increased sunburn, skin cancer, various eye disorders, and immune suppression. McMichael then examines the health problems caused by growing land degradation that stems from erosion, desertification, nutrient exhaustion, water logging, and salinization. He notes that the poorest countries, including sub-Saharan Africa, the foothills of the Himalayas and the Andes, Haiti and Honduras, and Central and South America, are at the highest risk of land degradation. Poor people in the growing cities throughout the world also experience increased obesity, hypertension, cigarette smoking, sedentism, and traffic-related diseases. McMichael goes on to note that most of the cities in the world rely a on much larger geographical area, sometimes as much as two hundred times greater than their own area, to support their consumption of natural resources.

McMichael concludes his chapter by arguing that recent undeniable positive increases in human health statistics may be misleading to the extent that they hide the growing threats to public health caused by the worldwide degradation of ecosystems. He proposes that public health statistics be augmented by indices of sustainable public health so that the potential damage to public health that may be entailed by these trends will be counted to yield a more realistic picture. McMichael ends these concluding remarks with concerns about shrinking governments in a time when government action is needed to reverse ecological trends.

In chapter 15, "Epidemiologic Methods for Assessing the Health Impact of Diminishing Ecological Integrity," Colin L. Soskolne, Lee E. Sieswerda, and H. Morgan Scott describe the strengths and weaknesses of various epidemiological methods for determining causal relationships between ecological degradation and human health. In the first section of this chapter, there is a discussion of why epidemiological tools should be used to understand cause-and-effect relationships between loss of ecological integrity and human health. The authors state that the purpose of their chapter is to give nonepidemiologists concerned with measuring the human health impacts caused by environmental degradation an understanding of the significance of various epidemiological study designs.

The authors review various epidemiological techniques. First, they note that epidemiological studies can be classified into experiential and nonexperiential studies. The randomized control study is discussed as an experiential method that is rarely used because of ethical restraints on testing humans. Next, the authors review nonexperiential methods, which include cohort studies, case-control studies, cross-sectional (or prevalence) studies, and aggregate data studies. The ability of each of these methods to obtain unbiased or unconfounded estimates of disease risk is reviewed.

Finally, the authors discuss in detail the advantages and disadvantages of aggregate data studies, a method that they believe is the most feasible approach to studying the human health effects of environmental degradation, but one that should be used as an hypothesis–generating step in epidemiological methods that would put conclusions on a firmer scientific basis.

In chapter 16, "Institutionalized Environmental Violence and Human Rights," Laura Westra describes how human health is being damaged by a variety of human activities that are now tolerated by governments around the world. This damage to human health is being caused by: (1) increased exposure to ultraviolet radiation due to loss of stratospheric ozone; (2) physical and disease impacts of climate change; (3) exposure to toxic wastes; (4) exposure to the hazardous by–products of industrial pollution; (5) exposure to chemical food additives and chemical residues; (6) long–term exposure to chemicals; (7) the loss of nature's "goods and services" through loss of biodiversity, fragmentation of natural landscapes, and deforestation; (8) increased presence of particulate and other air pollutants; (9) the loss of safe water; (10) direct contact with pathogens through encroachment with the wild; (11) increased hazards from the presence of bioengineered foods and transgenics; (12) exposure to antibiotic–resistant strains of pathogens; and (13) increases in communicable disease risk through increased human migration.

Westra next notes that the human activities that cause these damages to human health have not been treated in the same way as other forms of violence against which we expect laws and regulations to exist. She argues that not until society sees the activities that are damaging human health in and through the environment as "ecoviolence" are we going to change recent adverse environmental trends. Westra therefore supports an extension of human rights and criminal law to cover what is now institutionalized acceptance of activities that damage human health.

Westra also points out that the poorest people in the world, people who have the least medical resources on which to rely in case of sickness, are most likely to have their health harmed by environmental degradation.

Although Westra is an acknowledged biocentrist in terms of her ethical approach to environmental problems, she notes that because environmentally destructive human activities are degrading human health, anthropocentric ethical systems should also support taking a tougher stand on outlawing environmental degradation that is now accepted.

Finally, Westra argues that the reason environmental violence has become institutionalized is because of the power of some large corporations and their ability to manipulate public perceptions, needs, and political power.

Global Environmental Change in the Coming Century: How Sustainable Are Recent Health Gains?

A. J. McMichael

The global environmental changes now emerging in the world pose a new scale of hazard to human population health (McMichael 1993). The hazard arises because of the systemic strain due to the rapidly increasing aggregate impact of humankind on the biosphere. That aggregate impact reflects the combination of human numbers, consumerist economic "growth," and prodigious waste emissions. It has its roots in the prevailing types of human culture, technologies, social values, and economic systems, and the attendant persistent disparities in material wealth, trading balance, and political power.

We have, for the first time, begun to change the composition of the lower and middle atmospheres—the former via the tropospheric accumulation of heat-trapping "greenhouse gases," the latter via the stratospheric accumulation of ozone-destroying gases (especially the chlorofluorocarbons). There are other signs of planetary overload. These include an apparent recent plateauing in the productivity of our main terrestrial and marine food-producing ecosystems (Doos 1994, FAO 1995), a widespread loss of biodiversity (Pimm et al. 1995), and the global dispersion of various persistent nonbiodegradable pollutants. Much of this damage to various global "commons" is due to the impact of high-throughput consumption in industrial and urban populations, especially in rich countries. Global economic activity increased twentyfold during the twentieth century. Meanwhile, in absolute terms, the human population grew faster than ever in the last quarter-century, capping a remarkable nearly fourfold increase from 1.6 billion to 6 billion. While we remain uncertain of Earth's human "carrying capacity" (Daily and Ehrlich 1992, Holling 1994, Cohen 1995), we expect that world population will approach 9 billion by around 2050.

The upshot of these overload processes is that the world's large biophysical systems that underpin human health are being perturbed or depleted. The resultant global change processes that pose risks to human population health are of two broad types, reflecting the nature of the "globality." At one extreme are changes that transcend their points of origin and that entail change in truly global "commons." This category includes "greenhouse"-mediated climate change and stratospheric ozone depletion. A different type of global change comprises the mosaics of multiple local change, which tend in aggregate to span much of the world. This category includes deforestation, land degradation, the spread of irrigation, the depletion of fresh water (especially aquifers), loss of biodiversity, and depletion or displacement of ocean fisheries.

Large-Scale Environmental Change and Human Health

A basic question for public health science is: In what ways do global environmental changes affect the prospects for human health? This question requires us to think, unusually, within an ecological, and longer-term, framework. The essential task is one of scenario-based health risk assessment (McMichael 1997), and not one of empirically based, retroactive, hypothesis-testing research. Nevertheless, there is also a need to improve this health risk assessment by gathering more empirical data about various poorly researched underlying climate–health relationships.

The sustained good health of a population depends on there being a stable and productive natural environment. Such an environment yields assured supplies of food and fresh water, has a constant climate in which climate-sensitive physical and biological systems do not change for the worse, retains its richness of biodiversity (a source of both present and future value), and promotes secure livelihoods in agriculture, pastoralism, and fishing, along with those in urban professions, trades, and crafts. For the human species, the texture and stability of the social environment is also important to population health—but that is another, albeit related, topic.

The stresses accumulating within the biosphere are likely to cause some tensions between human communities, leading to conflict and its attendant damage to public health (Gleick 1993). For example, Ethiopia, upstream of Nile-dependent Egypt, increasingly needs the Nile's water for its own crop irrigation. Around the world, many other river systems are shared uneasily between neighbors in unstable regions. Around 40 percent of the world's population, living in 80 countries, now faces some level of water shortage. The direct health effects of conflict and warfare are well known. As we look back on the most war-scarred and arms-profiteering century on record, conflict continues to cast a long shadow over the prospects for human health because of the tensions caused by environmental decline, dwindling resources, and ecological disruption (Homer-Dixon 1994). There are increasing tensions between Bangladesh and northeast India over Ganges River water and over arable land and, as mentioned below, land-use pressures and mounting hunger may have contributed to the social collapse and fratricidal conflict in Rwanda in the mid-1990s (King and Elliott 1996).

Because these global changes coexist and share overlapping causes, the net impact upon health will reflect the configuration of environmental changes and the synergies between them. However, given our limited experience and insight in relation to these unfamiliar processes, it is necessary to address them separately.

Global Climate Change and Human Health

The Second Assessment Report of the UN's Intergovernmental Panel on Climate Change (Houghton et al. 1996) points out that the anticipated increase in average world temperature of approximately 2–3 degrees C over the coming century would be more rapid than any temperature change experienced by humans since the advent of agriculture around 10,000 years ago. Climatic conditions and climate-sensitive natural processes are an integral part of Earth's life-supporting mechanisms. Biologists would therefore expect such a change in climate to influence the prospects for survival of populations and species in the affected ecosystems (Houghton et al. 1996). Likewise, the health of *Homo sapiens* would be affected by global climate change.

The direct health effects of climate change would include altered rates of mortality and morbidity due to heatwaves and thermal stresses in general, the respiratory consequences of a change in patterns of exposure to aeroallergens (spores, molds, etc.), and the direct, often physical, hazards of any increases in extreme weather events—including storms, floods, and drought.

The indirect health effects of climate change include alterations in the range and activity of vector-borne infectious diseases (such as malaria, leishmaniasis, and dengue); changes in the transmission of person-to-person infections (including food poisoning and waterborne pathogens); the nutritional and health consequences of local and regional changes in agricultural productivity; and the various consequences of rising sea levels. There would also be more diffuse public health consequences due to population displacement, migration (both "economic" and "distress" migration) and the enforced change or loss of employment due to the disruptive effects of climate change upon various economic sectors.

There are many uncertainties associated with these projected changes in world climate and the resultant impact on biophysical systems. However, far-reaching consequences for human health must be considered as likely.

Some scientists assess that there have been recent signals of changes in health risk in relation to an apparent increased instability in world climatic patterns. For example, the recent concurrence of retreating glaciers, upward migration of alpine plant species, and reports of an increased altitudinal range of malaria and dengue in highlands in several continents may be an early signal of the consequences of global warming (Epstein et al. 1998). Altered patterns of vector-borne diseases have accompanied fluctuations in regional climate associated with heightened ENSO (El Niño Southern Oscillation) activity since the 1970s (Bouma and van der Kaay 1996, Patz et al. 1996). (The ENSO phenomenon entails periodic east–west reversals of warm ocean currents, winds, and atmospheric pressure gradients across the Pacific Ocean.) The World Health Organization (WHO) has reported that the epidemic of meningitis in sub-Saharan Africa in the mid-1990s has coincided with the extension of dry zones—an extension that may have resulted from land-use patterns and regional climatic change.

Climate change would also affect agricultural productivity—not just because plants are sensitive to temperature and rainfall but because of climate-related changes in the pattern of land degradation and in the profile of crop pests and diseases. Meanwhile, if seas rise by around half a meter by 2100 (Houghton et al. 1996), much of the world's coastal arable land and fish-nurturing mangroves would be damaged. Rising seas would salinate fresh-water supplies, particularly under small islands, and may cause sanitation problems for coastal populations. The 10 countries most vulnerable to sea-level rise include Bangladesh and Egypt, with huge river delta farming populations, and Pakistan, Indonesia, and Thailand, all of which have large and relatively poor coastal populations. Other adverse health effects of climate change would result from the social and political instability caused by economic dislocation and demographic dislocations.

Stratospheric Ozone Depletion: A Separate but Related Problem

Stratospheric ozone depletion is essentially a separate phenomenon from greenhouse gas accumulation in the troposphere. Ozone depletion is causing an increase in ultraviolet radiation (UVR) at Earth's surface. Recent evidence from European alpine regions, Toronto, and New Zealand has shown an increase in terrestrial UVR accompanying the amplified decline in winter–spring stratospheric ozone levels (Kerr and McElroy 1993, Basher et al. 1994).

This increase in ultraviolet exposure is expected to peak within about a decade and then decline, in response to the apparently successful phasing out of the major ozone-destroying industrial and agricultural chemicals. For much of the coming century, we can expect an increase in the severity of sunburn, the incidence of skin cancers, and the incidence of various disorders of the eye (especially cataracts). It could also cause some suppression of immune functioning, thus increasing susceptibility to infectious diseases and perhaps reducing vaccination efficacy (WHO/UNEP/ICNIRP 1994, McMichael et al. 1996).

Most interest has centered on the anticipated increase in risk of skin cancer, because of the presumed DNA-damaging effect of UVR. It has been estimated that persistence of the ozone losses of the 1979–92 period for several decades would cause the subsequent annual incidence of basal cell carcinoma (the dominant type) to increase by 1–2 percent at low latitude (50), 14 percent at 55–650 in the northern hemisphere (e.g., the United Kingdom), and 25 percent at that latitude in the south (Madronich and de Gruijl 1993). The estimated percentage increases for squamous cell carcinoma would be approximately twice as great. More detailed, dynamic, mathematical modeling indicates that nonmelanoma skin cancer rates would rise in excess of approximately 10 percent in the United States and Europe around the middle of the twenty-first century (Slaper et al. 1996) and that basal cell carcinoma rates would increase by 8–12 percent in Australia by later in the next century, depending on changes in population age structure (Martens 1997).

A potentially more important, although much more indirect, health detriment could arise from ultraviolet-induced impairment of photosynthesis on land (terrestrial plants) and at sea (phytoplankton). Although such an effect could reduce the world's food production, few quantitative data are yet available.

Health Impacts of Other Forms of Environmental Overload

Next, let us consider the impact of land degradation upon food supplies. During the 1980s, the combination of erosion, desiccation, and nutrient exhaustion, plus irrigation-induced water-logging and salination, rendered unproductive one-fifteenth of the world's 1.5 billion hectares of readily arable farmland (World Resources Institute 1996). The world's per-person production of cereals, the main source of dietary energy, seems to have faltered a little since the mid-1980s (Doos 1994, Kendall and Pimentel 1994)—although there have been economic and commercial influences at work, along with land degradation. The green revolution, which fed much of the expanding human population from the 1960s to the 1980s, depended on laboratory-bred, high-yield cereal grains, fertilizers, groundwater, and arable soils. In retrospect, those productivity gains appear to have come substantially from the depletion of exhaustible ecological "capital"—especially topsoil and groundwater. However, there are competing and complex explanations for these trends (Dyson 1996).

Today, as we continue on the treadmill of having to extract greater food yields to feed ever more people, almost one-tenth of the world population is malnourished in ways that impair health. The absolute numbers of malnourished persons, especially children, are still growing. Meanwhile, at sea, many of the world's great fisheries are now on the brink of being overexploited. The UN's Food and Agricultural Organization estimates that we have neared the sustainable fish-catch limit—around 100 million tonnes per year (FAO 1995).

An even more pervasive problem is the worldwide loss of biodiversity (Dobson and Carper 1993, Pimm et al. 1995). Through our own species' spectacular reproductive "success" and our energy-intensive economic activities, we have occupied, damaged, or eliminated the natural habitat of many other species. Biologists estimate that this fastest-ever mass extinction may cause around one-third of all species alive during the 1900s to be gone before the end of the 2100s (Soulé 1991). The loss of various key species would weaken whole ecosystems, with consequences that would often be adverse to human interests. Those consequences would include disturbances of the ecology of vector-borne infections and reduced yield from food-producing systems. We would also lose a rich repertoire of genetic and phenotypic material. In particular, our major cultivated "food" plants are selectively enhanced descendants of wild strains. To maintain their hybrid vigor and environmental resilience, a diversity of wild plants needs to be preserved as a source of genetic additives. Similarly, a high proportion of modern medicinal drugs in Western medicine have natural origins, and many defy synthesis in the laboratory (Soejarto and Farnsworth 1985). Scientists therefore test many thousands of novel chemicals from nature each year, seeking new drugs to treat HIV, malaria, drug-resistant tuberculosis, cancers, and so on.

Because of the combination of poverty, environmental decline, and hunger with population growth, King and colleagues argue that some of the world's poorest populations are becoming "demographically entrapped": that is, the weight of their current or projected numbers exceeds the carrying capacity of their environment, and, lacking trade and migratory safety valves, they face starvation, disease, or fratricide (King et al. 1995, King and Elliott 1996). They have proposed that certain sub-Saharan African countries illustrate the entrapment dilemma. Rwanda, where population size first exceeded the estimated carrying capacity in the 1980s, may be the prototype; Malawi looks similarly precarious. Last (1995), too, refers to demographic entrapment, and describes how the desperate efforts of such populations "to provide themselves with food, water, and fuelwood can degrade an already fragile ecosystem into a desert that may take centuries to recover." This, he says, is happening in parts of sub-Saharan Africa, in alpine foothills in the Himalayas and the Andes, in crowded small nations such as Haiti and Honduras, and elsewhere in Central and South America. However, a steadying counterexample comes from the experience of the

Machakos district in Kenya, where, since the 1930s, a sixfold increase in population has been accompanied by a substantial regeneration of previously seriously depleted local soils and forested areas (Tiffen and Mortimore 1992)—albeit helped by an abundance of local rains in that location.

The notion of demographic entrapment thus remains controversial—and very difficult to study. Debate about the relationship between carrying capacity and demographic entrapment discomforts some demographers. While we cannot actually prove that entrapment was a (the?) major cause of civil war in Rwanda—or even an important contributor—neither can it be formally disproven. These complex, life-sized problems, afflicting whole regions or populations, are not reducible to simplified linear analysis. We will need to develop a more transdisciplinary, holistic type of scientific assessment, able to integrate across disciplines, sectors, and conceptual planes.

Health Impacts: North versus South

The health impacts from global environmental change will vary around the world. Not only will the attendant environmental stresses vary in intensity in different geographic regions, but, in general, poor populations will be the most vulnerable—whether at the regional, national, or subnational levels. With respect to climate change, the impacts of heatwaves, other extreme weather (e.g., tropical cyclones and droughts), and gradual coastal inundation would affect such populations most. Relatedly, as has been recently foreshadowed by El Niño–associated outbreaks of infectious disease in South Asia, Central America, and Eastern Africa (Bouma and van der Kaay 1996 and Patz et al. 1996), much of the increase in contagious and vector-borne infectious disease would occur in developing country regions.

Likewise, the combined impact of climate change, freshwater shortages, and land degradation is likely to impair agricultural productivity most in those same subtropical and semi-arid regions where food insecurity is currently most prevalent. Meanwhile, the depletion of ocean fisheries—if not offset by unforeseen (Folke et al. 1996) rapid advances in aquaculture—would cause fish prices to rise, and thereby jeopardize the role of seafood as the staple animal protein in many poor countries.

In many African, Asian, and Latin American countries, the average life expectancy is 20–30 years less than in rich Western countries (World Bank 1993). Infectious diseases remain the main killer, particularly in children below age five. Much of this health deficit in poor Third World countries reflects the widespread poverty, the adverse social consequences of export-oriented economic development, and the environmental adversity caused by exploitation of natural resources. In today's increasingly globalized economy, which operates to the general disadvantage of poor countries, the exacerbation of land degradation, rural unemployment, food shortages, and urban crowding all contribute to health deficits for the rural dispossessed, the underfed, and the slum dweller.

In most Third World countries, a mixed profile of health and disease is now emerging. The persistence of widespread poverty, lack of safe water and sanitation, and urban crowding ensure the continuation of infectious diseases, especially as a source of childhood mortality. The recent spread of HIV and other sexually transmitted diseases has added a new and tragic dimension of poor health to many of these poor populations. Rapid increases in extractive and manufacturing industries—often reflecting the largely unregulated spread of transnational companies—cause occupational injuries and diseases (McMichael et al. 1994, Pearce 1996). Meanwhile, the gains in life expectancy and the increase in urbanization are transforming the economy and ecology of Third World populations in ways that are substantially increasing the prevalence of obesity, hypertension, cigarette smoking, sedentism, and urban traffic. All these are contributing to a rise in chronic noninfectious diseases alongside the persistence of infectious diseases.

The "Ecological Footprints" of Urban Populations

Urban living can affect human health directly, via the characteristics of the urban physical and social environment. However, this urbanism also has influence on a much larger spatial-temporal scale, via the wider impact on the productivity and functioning of the huge environmental "hinterland" that is the source of materials and services for an urban population. That wider, total impact is the "ecological footprint" of that city's population.

There are manifest ecological benefits of city living. Cities confer economies of scale, of proximity, and of shared use of resources. Further, there are great but largely unrealized possibilities for reuse and recycling. Equally, though, there are great "externalities." Urban populations do not subsist on their own urban land; they depend on food grown elsewhere, on raw materials (timber, metals, fossil fuels, etc.) extracted from elsewhere, and on having their wastes disposed of elsewhere. Thus, an urban population imports raw materials (thereby causing environmental damage at the source and in transit); makes demands on ecological systems on land and sea to produce food; dumps wastes into rivers, lakes, and oceans; buries wastes on land; and emits wastes as gases and particulates into the atmosphere.

Cities are thus sustained by economic infrastructures and resource supply lines that span vast areas of the world and its ecosystems. Resources are extracted from natural and managed ecosystems often at great distances from the cities. Europeans even celebrate the maximization of "food-miles" as an index of trade liberalization (Lang 1997). Londoners drink wine from southern Australia, South Africa, and Latin America. Our oil supplies come from distant sources. So, too, do the year-round fresh fruits and vegetables that modern affluent Western consumers now take for granted.

Urban populations thus depend on the natural resources of ecosystems that, in aggregate, are vastly larger in area than the city itself. The highly urbanized Netherlands draws in resources from a total surface area 15 times larger than itself. Folke and colleagues (1996) have studied the renewable resource appropriations by the cities of the Baltic Sea region. They estimate that the amounts of resources consumed by 29 cities—wood, paper, fibers, and food (including seafood)—depend upon a total area 200 times greater than the combined area of those cities. That figure of 200 comprises 17 units of forest, 50 units of arable land, and 133 units of marine ecosystems. The sustainability of urban populations and their health thus depends on the continued productivity of those remote ecosystems.

The scale of impact of urban populations is growing, and now includes massive urban contributions to the world's problems of greenhouse gas accumulation, stratospheric ozone depletion, land degradation, coastal zone destruction, and aquifer emptying. Via this scaled-up externalized impact, urbanism is thus jeopardizing the health of current and future generations.

Health as a "Sustainable State"

The fundamental importance of the prospect of global environmental change affecting health is that it bears on the *sustainability* of population health. This requires us to extend our analytic framework—to think prospectively about health. We conventionally measure population health cross-sectionally, in scorecard fashion, as an achieved entity. Yet we are well aware that any such measure reflects recent past activity and experience, including society's recent consumption of natural "capital." It does not measure health as a sustainable property of the population. Rather, this approach resembles how we conventionally assess society's economic performance: we measure accrued wealth and achieved output, rather than ecologically sustainable productivity.

To argue, as some do, that things must actually be getting better since life expectancies are increasing is to misunderstand the nature of the hazard posed by global environmental change. Gains in life expectancy, in nature, tend to happen in circumstances conducive to rapid population growth— that is, when the immediate carrying capacity (supply) of the environment exceeds the number of dependent individuals (demand). These generalized gains in human life expectancy indicate that, currently and recently, the life-supporting capacity of the human-modulated environment has been increasing. But we must ask: At what cost—or at what future risk?

The considerable and widespread gains in health and longevity over the past century have depended primarily on reductions in early-life infectious disease mortality. Basic gains in food security and in sanitation, supplemented by advances in vaccination, antibiotic treatment, and oral rehydration therapy, have changed the profile of infectious disease mortality. These technical and social improvements have been closely allied with the processes of urbanization, industrialization, and increasing material wealth. They and the resultant gains in life expectancy have therefore been positively correlated with increasing levels of physical disruption and of chemical contamination of our ambient environment.

For how long can we expect to maintain these parallel increasing trends in consumption, life expectancy, and environmental impact? At what stage might depletion of the world's ecological and biophysical capital rebound against the health of human populations? As discussed above, many of Earth's vital life-supporting systems are today showing signs of unprecedented systemic stress as, for the first time, the aggregate impact of human numbers and economic activity is overloading the capacity of natural systems to absorb, repair, and provide (McMichael 1993).

In recent history, it is only when the limits of local environmental carrying capacity are reached that the question of sustainable health is seriously addressed (King 1990). Such limits will tend to be reached first in poor, overcrowded populations where environmental infrastructure is consumed or degraded, external sources (accessible via trade or barter) are absent, and food supplies become inadequate. However, it is a more general issue. How can we assess the long-term sustainability of good health in human populations, living in circumstances that have increasingly pervasive and damaging impacts upon local, regional, and global environmental systems (Guidotti 1995)?

Indicators of the Sustainability of Good Health in Populations
In general, indices of the sustainability of population health would need to focus on the integrity and productivity of the biosphere's life-supporting systems. The indices would not directly measure changes in human biology or frank health status, but would assess the extent to which human biological needs are being met by the sustainable consumption of natural resources. Such indices would address dynamic processes, not static conditions. They would measure the balance between population size and available resources, between the production of emissions and wastes and the capacity of environmental sinks. They would monitor selected bioindica-

tors known to be predictive of human disease risk—such as indices of vegetation and groundwater in relation to infectious disease vectors (mosqui-
toes, tsetse flies, etc.), and indices of soil fertility and crop growth. They
would assess the stocks of social capital and patterns of human relations and
community well-being.

We have hardly begun to address this issue yet. There are two main ob-
stacles. First, we are beset with a range of serious and intransigent existing
public health problems. Second, we are bemused about how to reconcep-
tualize our measures of public health within a finite biosphere that, for the
first time, is coming under widespread systemic pressure. We have long in-
dulged the assumption that "progress" is linear and continuing—and that
regularly updated population health scorecards are sufficient. As it becomes
clear that limits are being reached, and that important natural-system components may fail, then we need the ecological equivalent of the clinician's
prognostic indicators.

The Importance of the Long View

The pursuit of good population health makes little sense unless it is sustainable over future generations. Just as short-term economic growth can be attained by imprudent depletion of resources and ecosystems, jeopardizing
future economic welfare, so improvements in population health today may
be gained in ways that jeopardize the continued good health of future generations. This century's gains in life expectancy have derived partly from increasingly intensive, ecologically damaging modes of food production, from
reliance on energy-intensive urban infrastructure and medical technology,
and from overuse of antibiotics and chemical pesticides (causing damage to
the natural pest control services of ecosystems and inducing genetically resistant strains of organisms). Manifestations of this erosion of natural capital
include the increasingly large proportion of the world's net primary (photosynthetic) product being coopted by humans, the loss of productive land,
and reduced biodiversity.

In the past, local human populations could rise and fall without affecting
either distant populations or the sustainability of Earth's large-scale life-support systems. Now, global interconnectedness and the sheer size of the
human population make such segregation of health risk impossible. For example, this interconnectedness has resulted in the introduction to the
United States of a viral-transmitting mosquito, *Aedes albopictus,* from East
Asia in shipments of used car tires. Likewise, in 1991 the seventh pandemic
of cholera reached Latin America in contaminated ship's ballast water—
where dissemination of the bacterium may have been amplified by coastal
blooms of algae, and of the zooplankton that feed on them, nurtured by nu-
trient-rich wastewater runoff and warmer waters (Colwell 1996). That am-

plification theory, entailing a link between planktonic blooms and human cholera, if confirmed, would provide critical new insight into how large epidemics of cholera are initiated.

Risks to health will tend to increase so long as human societies depend upon a linear, waste-generating metabolism that is at odds with the circular metabolism of the rest of nature—wherein every output becomes an input. The high-consumption lifestyle of Western nations depends greatly on continued access to inexpensive inputs from non-Western nations, resulting in depletion of natural resources or the cooption of traditional agriculture into export crop production.

Meanwhile, as developing countries pursue their own economic aspirations, there will be additional strains upon our shared biosphere—and, therefore, increasing risks to population health in countries everywhere. After two centuries of hugely increasing fossil fuel combustion by today's rich countries, further rapid increases in East and Southeast Asia will contribute greatly to the accumulation of greenhouse gases and, hence, to the diverse risks to health. Continual forest clearance brings exposure to new and potentially mobile infective organisms such as hemorrhagic fever viruses (e.g., various arenaviruses in Latin America, Ebola virus in Africa). The overfishing of the oceans is reducing per capita supplies of seafood. Continued pressure on agroecosystems in vulnerable regions, coupled with land degradation and population growth, will increase migratory pressures and their attendant public health risks.

Conclusion

The profile and scale of environmental health hazards is changing. We have previously supplemented our long-standing emphasis upon the effects of local environmental pollution with the recognition that regional phenomena such as acid rain and pesticide bioaccumulation through the food chain can, via various indirect pathways, affect human population health. Today we perceive, within a much greater span of space and time, that large-scale damage to global and regional natural systems may endanger the long-term sustainability of population health (notwithstanding the health gains that have already accrued from our consumption of nonrenewable natural resources). This new perception carries an increased awareness of the ecological dimensions of population health.

The prevailing economic ethos today is shaped by rapid technological change, acquisitive consumerism, a discounting (or ignorance) of distant and deferred environmental impacts, and a pervasive free-market philosophy. Currently, the policy-setting role of national governments is contracting, as trade and financial transactions become globalized and deregulated, as the balance of power between private and public sectors shifts, and as the resultant cost-cutting competitiveness between nations puts a squeeze on social expenditures. Hence, just when coordinated, strong, and far-sighted government is needed to constrain damage to the world's ecological infrastructure and thus to the sustainability of human health, we are instead entrusting ourselves to the limited-vision rationality of the marketplace.

We need, soon, an effective way of collective global decisionmaking. As we acquire a more integrated insight into the world's environment, its ecosystems, and their fundamental role in sustaining population health, so we must think more radically about how best to manage these life-support systems. The public health research agenda is thus broadening, becoming more complex, and extending further into the future. It directs our attention to the notion of the sustainability of population health as a central element in the Sustainability Transition, and hence to recognizing that the implications for social policy are far-reaching. We are entering one of history's great transitional eras (Caldwell 1990)—one that will be played out on a global scale.

REFERENCES

Basher, R.E., Zheng, X., Nichol, S. 1994. Ozone-related trends in solar UV-B series. *Geophysical Research Letters* 21: 2713–2716.

Bouma, M.J. and van der Kaay, H.J. 1996. The El Niño Southern Oscillation and the historic malaria epidemics on the Indian subcontinent and Sri Lanka: An early warning system for future epidemics? *Tropical Medicine and International Health* 1: 86–96.

Caldwell, L.K. 1990. *Between Two Worlds: Science, the Environmental Movement and Policy Choice.* Cambridge: Cambridge University Press.

Cohen, J.E. 1995. *How Many People Can the Earth Support?* New York: Norton.

Colwell, R. 1996. Global climate and infectious disease: The cholera paradigm. *Science* 274: 2025–2031.

Daily, G.C. and Ehrlich, P.R. 1992. Population, sustainability, and Earth's carrying capacity. *Bioscience* 42: 761–771.

Dobson, A., and Carper, R. 1993. Health and climate change: Biodiversity. *Lancet* 342: 1096–1099.

Doos, B.R. 1994. Environmental degradation, global food production and risk of large-scale migrations. *Ambio* 23: 124–130.

Dyson, T. 1996. *Population and Food, Global Trends and Future Prospects.* London: Routledge.

Epstein, P.R., et al. 1998. Biological and physical signs of climate change: Focus on mosquito-borne diseases. *Bulletin of the American Meteorology Society* 78: 409–417.

Folke, C., Larsson, J., Sweitzer J. 1996. Renewable resource appropriation. In: Costanza, R., and Segura, O. (eds.). *Getting Down to Earth*. Washington, DC: Island Press.

FAO. 1995. *State of the World's Fisheries, 1995*. Rome: Food and Agriculture Organization.

Gleick, P. 1993. *Water and Crisis: A Guide to the World's Fresh Water Resources*. Oxford: Oxford University Press.

Guidotti, T. 1995. Perspective on the health of urban ecosystems. *Ecosystem Health* 1: 141–149.

Holling, C.S. 1994. *An Ecologist View of the Malthusian Conflict*. Beijer Reprint Series No. 36. Stockholm: Beijer International Institute of Ecological Economics.

Homer-Dixon, T.F. 1994. Environmental scarcities and violent conflict: Evidence from cases. *International Security* 19: 5–40.

Houghton, J.T., Meira Filho, L.G., Callander, B.A., et al. (eds.). 1996. *Climate Change, 1995—the Science of Climate Change: Contribution of Working Group I to the Second Assessment Report of the Intergovernmental Panel on Climate Change*. Cambridge: Cambridge University Press.

Kendall, H.W. and Pimentel, D. 1994. Constraints on the expansion of the global food supply. *Ambio* 23: 198–205.

Kerr, J.B. and McElroy, C.T. 1993. Evidence for large upward trends of ultraviolet-B radiation linked to ozone depletion. *Science* 262: 1032–1034.

King, M. 1990. Health is a sustainable state. *Lancet* 336: 664–667.

King, M. and Elliott, C. 1996. Averting a world food shortage: Tighten your belts for CAIRO II. *British Medical Journal* 313: 995–997.

King, M., Elliott, C., Hellberg, H., et al. 1995. Does demographic entrapment challenge the two-child paradigm? *Health Policy and Planning* 10: 376–383.

Lang, T. 1997. The public health impact of globalisation of world food trade. In: Shetty, P. and McPherson, K. (eds.), *Diet, Nutrition and Chronic Disease: Lessons from Contrasting Worlds*. Chichester: Wiley, 1997, pp. 173–187.

Last, J.M. 1995. Redefining the unacceptable. *Lancet* 346: 1642–1643.

Madronich, S. and de Gruijl, F.R. 1993. Skin cancer and UV radiation. *Nature* 366: 23.

Martens, W.J.M. 1997. *Health Impacts of Climate Change and Ozone Depletion: An Eco-Epidemiological Modelling Approach*. Maastricht: University of Maastricht.

McMichael, A.J. 1993. *Planetary Overload: Global Environmental Change and the Health of the Human Species*. Cambridge: Cambridge University Press.

McMichael, A.J. 1997. Integrated assessment of potential health impact of global environmental change: Prospects and limitations. *Environmental Modelling and Assessment* 2: 129–137.

McMichael, A.J., Woodward, A.J., van Leeuwen, R.E. 1994. The impact of energy use in industrialised countries upon global population health. *Medicine and Global Survival* 1: 23–32.

McMichael, A.J., Haines, A., Slooff, R., Kovats, S. (eds.). 1996. *Climate Change and Human Health: An Assessment Prepared by a Task Group on Behalf of the World*

Health Organization, the World Meteorological Organization and the United Nations Environment Programme. Geneva: World Health Organization.

Patz, J.A., Epstein, P.R., Burke, T.A., Balbus, J.M. 1996. Global climate change and emerging infectious diseases. *Journal of the American Medical Association* 275: 217–223.

Pearce, N. 1996. Traditional epidemiology, modern epidemiology, and public health. *American Journal of Public Health* 86: 678–683.

Pimm, S.L., Russell, G.J., Gittleman, J.L., Brooks, T.M. 1995. The future of bio-diversity. *Science* 269: 347–354.

Slaper, H., Velders, G.J.M., Daniel, J.S., de Gruijl, F.R., van der Leun, J.C. 1996. Estimates of ozone depletion and skin cancer incidence to examine the Vienna Convention achievements. *Nature* 384: 256–258.

Soejarto, D.D. and Farnsworth, N.R. 1989. Tropical rainforests: Potential source of new drugs. *Perspective in Biology and Medicine* 32: 244–256.

Soulé, M.E. 1991. Conservation: Tactics for a constant crisis. *Science* 253: 744–750.

Tiffen, M. and Mortimore, M. 1992. Environment, population growth and pro-ductivity in Kenya. *Development Policy Review* 10: 359–387.

WHO/UNEP/ICNIRP. 1994. *Ultraviolet Radiation: An Authoritative Scientific Review of Environmental and Health Effects of UV with Reference of Global Ozone Layer Depletion. Environmental Health Criteria No. 160.* Geneva: World Health Organization.

World Bank. 1993. *World Development Report: Investing in Health.* Oxford: Oxford University Press.

World Resources Institute. 1996. *World Resources 1996–97: A Guide to the Global Environment.* Oxford: Oxford University Press.

Epidemiologic Methods for Assessing the Health Impact of Diminishing Ecological Integrity

Colin L. Soskolne, Lee E. Sieswerda, and H. Morgan Scott

In general, life expectancy has been increasing for as long as it has been systematically measured. Especially in rich countries, people are living longer than ever because of increased and more reliable food production, public health and sanitation measures, effective drug therapies, improved standards of living, and better control over their immediate environments (WHO 1995). However, these gains in life expectancy have been achieved at the expense of disrupted, damaged, and sometimes destroyed ecosystems. How one might measure the potential consequences of environmental degradation—past, present, and future—on life expectancy, and human health in general, is the topic of this chapter.

Increasingly, the arguments for preserving ecological integrity (EI) are couched in terms of threats to human health. Ozone layer depletion with consequent increases in ultraviolet (UV) radiation, global warming, predicted food shortages, and biodiversity in its various incarnations have splashed the headlines of newspapers. Alarms about associated dire health consequences have been sounded. Volumes have already been devoted to predicting devastating consequences for human society related to global warming alone.

While these dramatic predictions are at first compelling, scientists, and also the lay public, realize that they are based on models of future events. No shortage of experts exists to argue that the predictions of future health impacts may be erroneous. In a recent article in *Science* (Taubes 1997) that was reported in the lay media, science journalist Gary Taubes challenges the claim that climate change will necessarily lead to adverse human health consequences. In his article, Taubes quotes D. A. Henderson, former leader of the World Health Organization's Smallpox Eradication Program, as saying that the predicted adverse human health impacts of global climate change are based on "a lot of simplistic thinking, which seems to ignore the fact that as climate changes, man changes as well." Many scientists disagree with Taubes and Henderson, and believe that the data do support negative impacts on human health from climate change (McMichael 1995). A role for epidemiology in this controversy would be to develop and apply methods for assessing possible relationships between environmental change and human health.

Causation in general, and particularly in epidemiology, is a complex topic rooted in the philosophy of science. Despite disparate views on the levels and kinds of contributions that epidemiology can make toward an understanding of causation, most scientists would agree that there exists a hierarchy of increasing certainty from various study designs in relating risk factor "exposures" to disease or health outcomes. The hierarchy of evidence generated through different levels of epidemiologic inquiry has a direct bearing on conclusions about causation. Much of the confusion among nonepidemiologists about whether an exposure (i.e., risk factor) will result in a serious health impact arises from a lack of understanding of the epidemiologic process. Understanding each epidemiologic study's attributes, including study design, level of precision, and validity, thus impacts directly on the conclusions that are drawn.

Epidemiology offers an arsenal of techniques for assessing the impact of diminishing EI on human health. Taken literally from its Greek roots, epidemiology means "studies upon the populace." More precisely, it is the study of the distribution and determinants of disease in human populations, with the ultimate aim of controlling those diseases (Last 1995).

The objectives of this chapter are threefold. First, we will outline the multilevel nature of epidemiologic investigation. Second, we will describe the contribution that epidemiology can make, in the near and the long term, to understanding the health consequences of declining EI. In so doing, we will point out that establishing the nature of any relationship between an exposure and a disease is a multiphased process. In particular, we will explore the depths of the cross-sectional aggregate data study design, which, at this stage in the study of EI, is the most feasible. Third, we will provide an overview of the results of our initial attempt to study the relationship between the global loss of EI and selected health outcomes at the aggregated level of countries.

The Epidemiologic Method

We provide the reader concerned with measuring the health impacts of diminishing EI with an overview of epidemiologic study designs. Causal inference from epidemiologic investigations often can be reflected in the hierarchy of study designs at the disposal of the epidemiologist. Thus a basis is provided for understanding when an apparent human health impact is truly an effect, and when we are only pointing toward future testable hypotheses.

The epidemiologic process presented here represents, in simplified form, that which is a complex field. Those wishing to expand their knowledge of epidemiology are advised to consult some of the basic texts on the subject (e.g., Hennekens and Buring 1987).

Epidemiologic studies can be divided into experimental and nonexperimental subtypes. The experimental study called a randomized controlled trial, or RCT, is not generally used in environmental epidemiology, but is worth mentioning here because it provides a benchmark against which to compare the nonexperimental study designs. It is often used as the so-called gold-standard design in epidemiology. It is the analog of the laboratory experiment in other fields, where important aspects of the experiment are under the control of the investigator. Here, randomization is one of the best choices to distribute unknown potential confounders evenly among the study groups. Randomization should result in nearly identical experimental groups where the only factor that should differ among the groups is whether they received the treatment (i.e., a specific level and kind of exposure) or not. Indeed, the degree to which the groups are identical can be verified by comparing them on known attributes. It is important to note that RCTs can be conducted at both the individual and the group level of data aggregation. That is, individuals can be randomly assigned to receive treatments, as can groupings of individuals (e.g., whole communities, families, and schools).

The RCT is, in many ways, the study design of choice because it best provides assurances that any effect seen, positive or negative, is attributable to the treatment and not to some extraneous factor. However, because a research participant should never be exposed to a known or suspected harmful experimental agent, the uses of the RCT are limited, and very strict rules exist to monitor their conduct. The skeptic should note that almost never is a hypothesis in environmental epidemiology tested using this gold-standard approach. Thus the best evidence that epidemiology can produce is not available when testing environmental hypotheses, and other study designs must be employed.

Nonexperimental (or observational) study designs are much more diverse and not only are ethically appropriate, but also are of great utility in environmental epidemiology. Figure 15.1 ranks the various epidemiologic study designs according to their general ability to suggest whether exposure and outcome are linked in a causal relationship. The best nonexperimental study design to help determine cause and effect is the cohort study. In this design, at an individual level of data aggregation, a sample of people (co-

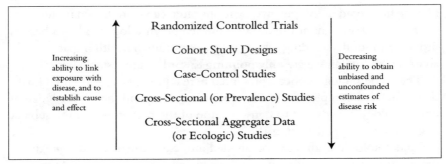

FIGURE 15.1

The hierarchical nature of epidemiologic studies ranked by ability to establish cause and effect.

hort) is drawn from the population of interest and divided into groups based on their exposure status. The groups then are followed up over time to see what disease outcomes manifest. By comparing outcomes for those classified as "exposed" and "unexposed," epidemiologists can obtain estimates about the relative risk of acquiring a disease as a function of whether or not exposure had occurred. Similarly, at a group level of data aggregation, different families or communities can be randomly selected from the population of communities available, their "group-exposure" level determined, and follow-up initiated to determine the subsequent levels of community or family health. An environmental situation that lends itself to the group-level cohort design is that where several geographical units with differing levels of disintegrity are followed up for health effects. Another is where health effect patterns for a single region are known prior to some notable decline in EI; the "notable decline" would be associated or directly attributed to some "intervention." Post-intervention health effects and disease patterns could then be compared with patterns that prevailed prior to the intervention. New advances in biostatistics and epidemiology should permit the modeling of both individual- and group-level environmental risk factors (i.e., multilevel modeling), confounders, and health outcomes in the future (Schall 1991, Kadohira et al. 1997, McDermott et al. 1997).

Unfortunately, prospective cohort studies are generally expensive, time-consuming, and dependent on the continuing involvement of the research participants (or communities). This presents a limitation of this design because those who drop out of the cohort may differ from those remaining, thus injecting a form of bias into the study. In addition, these designs are often not feasible because of the large sample size needed to detect meaningful differences between the cohorts being compared, owing to relatively low levels of exposure. Further, when considering EI, the exposures may be intergenerational, requiring extensive follow-up. Advances in biomarker technology may make this type of study more feasible in the future (Le et al. 1998). More importantly, advances in biostatistics and epidemiologic methods will be necessary to address these multilevel, intergenerational-type research questions.

The next best alternative to help establish cause and effect is the case-control study. In this design, participants (or communities) are chosen based on their health outcome status, and then their exposure status is determined retrospectively. From this, we can determine the relative odds of contracting the disease (outbreak event), having been exposed or not. This is an efficient study design for rare diseases and for diseases with long latency periods because the outcome in question has already occurred. Case-control studies are also relatively quicker and less expensive than cohort studies because there is no long-term follow-up, and fewer people need to be studied. The greatest problem with case-control designs is that accurate exposure measurement is dependent upon the ability of the researcher to determine exposures that may have occurred decades earlier. This is especially tenuous when the exposure assessment is based on a study participant's memory of events that occurred several decades prior. This problem can sometimes be mitigated if there are extant records of individuals' past exposures.

An aggregate data approach to case-control studies is one where two comparable regions are available that have different disease/death patterns; the two regions are then compared to see if they differ on indicators (or actual measurements) of disintegrity. The case-control study thus lends itself nicely to studies of EI, except from the perspective that exposures of current concern may not have occurred sufficiently long ago. As with cohort study designs, the availability of appropriate biomarkers of both exposure and outcome could be helpful. Case-control studies can be conducted "nested" within cohorts. These designs are highly cost-efficient because extensive exposure assessments need be determined for only a subgroup of the cohort.

The third category of nonexperimental study design is the cross-sectional study. In this design, all individuals (or groups) sampled from a defined population (of individuals or groups) are included regardless of whether or not they have the disease (event) in question, and their disease and exposure status are recorded at a single point in time. Consequently, these designs are limited by their inability to establish a temporal sequence between exposure and outcome.

The most readily accomplished nonexperimental design is the cross-sectional aggregate data study (the grouped-data version of the cross-sectional study). This is currently the most important approach for studying EI because the precise "exposure"–disease relationships are, as yet, largely unknown.

The design upon which we focus here is variously called the correlational study, the "cross-sectional aggregate data study," and the ecologic study. All three of these names refer, in epidemiology circles, to the same type of study design. We prefer the term cross-sectional aggregate data study because it correctly alludes to the most salient feature of the type of data to be used, namely that the data are available only for populations and *not* for individuals, and that the analysis is cross-sectional in nature. In addition, it avoids confusion with the discipline of ecology.

In cross-sectional aggregate data studies, we determine the relationship between population characteristics, attributes, or exposures and aggregate outcome statistics at a single point in time. Sometimes these studies can uncover exposure–disease patterns that provide investigators with the justification to move up in the hierarchy of designs and conduct studies more likely to provide information about causality. A well-known example of this approach was toward establishing the relationship between fatal coronary heart disease (CHD) and cigarette smoking. In that study, the investigators found a strong, statistically significant relationship between state-level fatal CHD rates and cigarette sales (Friedman 1967). This finding led researchers to conduct more analytic epidemiologic studies, as well as physiologic studies, which confirmed that smoking indeed is a cause of fatal CHD (Hennekens and Buring 1987).

An example of a cross-sectional aggregate data study in environmental epidemiology is one addressing the relationship between melanoma mortality and latitude. Elwood et al. (1974) studied age-standardized melanoma mortality rates in the United States and Canada and found that mortality from melanoma decreased with increasing latitude. This study supported the hypothesis that exposure to ultraviolet radiation causes malignant melanoma. Noteworthy is that neither of the above two examples of cross-sectional aggregate data studies, by themselves, *proved* that the exposure caused the disease in individuals. The reason for this is that exposure and disease could not have been linked in individuals owing to the absence of individual-level data. Hence, one could not be certain that in these populations, respectively, it indeed was the smoker who was dying of CHD, or that it was the UV-exposed person who was dying of melanoma. Rather, these studies point to where more analytic, individual-level studies should be directed.

Cross-sectional aggregate data studies are generally done because, in using routinely collected or previously collected data, they are relatively quick and inexpensive. Generally speaking, they do not prove exposure–disease relationships; instead, they suggest hypotheses to be explored in more sophisticated study designs. Because diminishing EI, as defined in this book, is a relatively new "exposure" to be subjected to the epidemiologic method, science is still in the hypothesis–generating stage with regard to its potential impacts on human health. Thus the most appropriate study design, given limited knowledge and resources at this time, is the cross–sectional aggregate data study.

All sciences, including epidemiology, have their strengths and limitations. Indeed, despite all of the strengths noted above, it may not be possible by the methods available to epidemiologists to discern the health impacts of disintegrity, especially if they are quite small or sudden.

The Cross–Sectional Aggregate Data Study

The ecologic fallacy, a fundamental problem related to causal inference at the individual level from any type of cross–sectional aggregate data study, was first demonstrated by Robinson (1950). But, while technical literature has existed for some time regarding the special methodological problems of cross–sectional aggregate data studies, it is only recently that guidelines have become widespread in epidemiology. The World Health Organization (WHO) has taken a particular interest in linking aggregate health and environment data, and has published two sets of guidelines intended to disseminate and encourage appropriate methods (Nurminen and Briggs 1996, WHO 1997).

As mentioned above, the cross–sectional aggregate data study uses the group, not the individual, as the basic unit of analysis. The group is most commonly defined by geography, but it may be defined by familial traits, ethnicity, age, sex, time, or any other variable used to categorize groups of people.

Because cross–sectional aggregate data studies are relatively quick to conduct, most often making use of existing data, and are less "analytic" than case–control and cohort designs, some might tend to believe that they are easy. This is not true. In fact, they may be among the most difficult study designs from which to obtain valid results pertaining to individual-level risks for disease. Mainly this is because we cannot be sure that the individuals who are exposed are the same ones who contract the disease. The cross–sectional aggregate data reflect only an aggregated level of exposure and disease for the *group* (e.g., averages), whereas a very different relationship may exist between *individual* exposure and disease. For this reason, we cannot necessarily extrapolate results of cross–sectional aggregate data studies directly to individual risks (i.e., the ecologic fallacy).

Morgenstern (1982) describes four types of cross–sectional aggregate data (ecologic) studies: the exploratory, the multiple-group comparison, the time trend, and the mixed. Each of these designs is of use for studying the relationship between EI and human health.

In exploratory studies, we observe geographic differences in the disease rate among several regions to search for spatial patterns that might suggest an environmental etiology. Essentially, this amounts to descriptive mapping of disease data and is the first type of cross-sectional aggregate data study design. Of course, this mapping could just as well apply to exposure data. Ecologists are familiar with this study design. Recent advances in geographic information system (GIS) technology have made this type of study very useful for setting priorities. For example, Kiester et al. (1996) used GIS data to set priorities for conservation action and research across the state of Idaho. Similar maps have been created for visualizing the distribution of many diseases. Despite the fact that mapping does not, in general, prove cause-and-effect relationships, compelling hypotheses can be generated for subsequent testing.

The second type of cross-sectional aggregate data study is the multiple-group comparison, wherein we observe the relationship between the average exposure levels and the disease or death rates among several groups. In this study design, we quantify our observations and fit the data to a mathematical model. Once we have found areas of heterogeneous EI, we then compare populations living in areas of relatively high integrity to those living in areas of relatively low integrity. Of course, adjustment for confounding (see below) is critically important here to ensure that it is EI that we are comparing and not some other incidental corollary.

In the time trend study, instead of grouping by geographic region, we group by time period. We follow up a single population and observe the relationship between the change in the average exposure levels and the respective changes in the disease or death rates over time. We test for a relationship between the exposure and disease trends, taking into account a possible lag period between a change in the exposure and the subsequent disease or death rate. Figure 15.2 diagrams this method. This is a useful design for studying EI because many of the diseases that we would expect to find associated with disintegrity would be chronic, long-latency diseases like cancer, chronic obstructive pulmonary disease, or diseases associated with ecological changes over time like heat stroke, infectious diseases, or malnutrition. It is also useful because it ensures that we know the temporal sequence of exposure followed by disease. However, this method relies on having data collected over a long time period and is subject to bias owing to migration of individuals into and out of the study area.

A mixed study combines the multiple-group comparison and the time trend study designs. In this design, we follow the relationship between the average exposure levels and the disease or death rates among several groups over time.

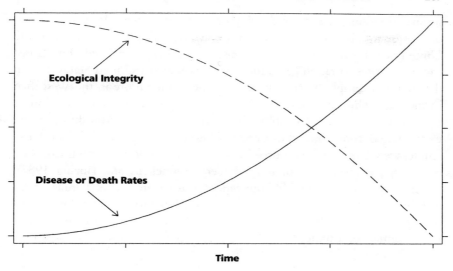

Time

FIGURE 15.2

A hypothetical time trend study. The objective is to test for correlation between integrity or disintegrity and disease or death rates in a single geographical region.

Bias and Confounding

Before we proceed to describe in more detail the unique problems of cross-sectional aggregate data studies, we need to define two terms that appear frequently in that discussion. Those terms are "bias" and "confounding."

Bias

Bias is systematic error introduced into the collection, analysis, interpretation, publication, or review of data by selecting or encouraging one outcome over others (Hennekens and Buring 1987). This is problematic because any observed association between the groups may be not from the covariation between the dependent and independent variables, but instead a result of unseen bias. Results from a biased study lack validity. Once bias has been introduced into the study, there are limited statistical techniques for correcting it. Therefore, the best place to control bias is at any study's design phase.

Confounding

A confounder is a variable that is correlated with the exposure of interest and also contributes to the development of a disease. It cannot be caused by the exposure; however, it can be a common cause of the exposure and the disease. An interesting example of confounding is the relationship between exposure to radon gas and the development of lung cancer. It is well known that smoking also causes cancer, and it is interesting to note that, in the United States, smoking and radon gas exposure are correlated. This is because exposure to radon gas is higher in the western United States than in the East and, simply by coincidence, people smoke more in the West than in the East. Thus, although smoking does not cause exposure to radon or vice versa, they are geographically correlated. The relationships among exposure, confounder, and disease are illustrated in Figure 15.3. In the example, we see that the exposure–disease relationship in question is exposure to radon gas as a cause of lung cancer (Hennekens and Buring 1987). Looking only at tobacco and lung cancer, it is apparent that there is a relationship between the two. However, smoking is a correlate of radon gas exposure and, quite independently of radon, is a cause of lung cancer. Thus it is a potential confounder.

Unique Problems of Cross-sectional Aggregate Data Studies

When cross-sectional aggregate data studies are used to make statements about the potential impacts of declining EI on human health, they should be considered in light of the limitations of such designs. It has been noted earlier that cross-sectional aggregate data study findings, when applied at the individual level of interest, have unique biases not present in individual-level studies. These are called ecologic biases, and are related to the ecologic fallacy.

Ecologic bias arising from data aggregation (also known as aggregation bias or cross-level bias) refers to the failure of relationships at one level of aggregation to reflect either relationships at other levels of aggregation or at the individual level (Greenland and Morgenstern 1989). This means that effects detected using aggregate-level data cannot be directly translated into risks to individuals. Sometimes the effect seen at the aggregate level is, in fact, the reverse of that seen when further individual–level studies are conducted. Essentially, the aggregate-level variable is measuring a different underlying construct than the corresponding individual-level variable.

Choosing the level of aggregation to study requires judgment in balancing between too large and too small a unit of aggregation. First and foremost, the research question being addressed (i.e., the targeted risk assessment or intervention being sought) should determine the level of aggregation being utilized. However, often there is no way of knowing what group size will yield the most informative results. If the group size is too small, we will find too few cases and unstable disease rates, and the esti-

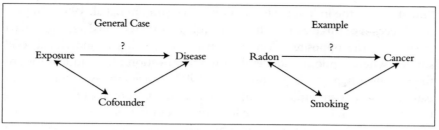

FIGURE 15.3

The general case of confounding and an example. (Adapted from Hayduk 1987.)

mates will be overly affected by migration. If the group size is too large, a small proportion of the population may have a particular exposure such that the effect of the exposure on the disease rates for the group is diluted. Similarly, small increases in disease rates for a community may be the result of a substantially increased relative risk for a small segment of the population of that community.

Ecologic bias arising from model misspecification refers to confounding, or to effect modification by group. Effect modification (or interaction) arises when, across different levels of one factor, estimates of the main effect vary. Confounders or effect modifiers that may not even be present at the individual level can bias estimates of the main effect being studied. More distressing is that individual-level confounders generally cannot be adequately controlled even if they have the same distribution across the groups (Greenland and Morgenstern 1989). The reverse is also true. For example, from individual-level studies, men are at greater risk of bladder cancer than women. However, from the results of cross-sectional aggregate data studies, sex is not very predictive of bladder cancer. Why? This occurs because there are about the same proportion of males and females across all groups (Morgenstern 1982). That is, there is little variability in the sex ratio from region to region. From this, we can see that we could not know from cross-sectional aggregate data studies that sex is predictive of bladder cancer.

Notice, therefore, that we should not attempt to study such individual-level risk factors (where distribution of the variable among groups is uniform) using ecologic-type studies. On the other hand, it is important to acknowledge that a variable such as ecological disintegrity should never be studied other than at the group level of aggregation. The only important issue that remains relates to the level of aggregation (e.g., bioregion, watershed, ecoregion) at which the disintegrity variables should be analyzed.

Cross-sectional aggregate data studies tend to be more sensitive to model misspecification than individual-level studies, and this can lead to nondifferential misclassification, biasing results away from the null hypothesis of "no effect" at the individual level of reference (Brenner et al. 1992). In fact, the direction of this bias away from the null in cross-sectional aggregate data studies has the opposite effect than that which it has in individual-level studies, where random, independent misclassification results in bias toward the no-effect hypothesis (Brenner et al. 1992). Since cross-sectional aggregate data studies are often conducted when little is known of the exact exposure–disease relationship at the level of the individual, model misspecification is probably quite common. This means that many of the results from studies of EI based on cross-sectional aggregate data may be exaggerated when individual effects are the targeted outcome.

Another problem with cross-sectional aggregate data studies is that the investigator generally, by necessity, obtains his or her data from several different sources. Obtaining data from multiple sources can result in an unknown error from multiplying biases owing to the incomparability of covariates from different data sources. In some cases, the data obtained from developing countries, or from countries with political motivations for falsifying their data, may be so poor that United Nations organizations may fail to acknowledge them as "official" data.

In contrast to this seemingly despondent view of the place of aggregate-type studies in a world currently driven by individual risk factor epidemiology, others have begun to call for a more holistic role for epidemiology to truly address public health concerns. Recently Susser published an article decrying the overemphasis on individual risk factor epidemiology that exists in Western science today (Susser 1998). Susser offers, and others concur, that a new paradigm that incorporates the full range of epidemiology, from micro- through to individual—and on to population—(or eco- or socio-) epidemiology, is needed to save epidemiology from imploding. Susser observes: "It is no caricature to say that risk factor epidemiology, while properly described as a population science, nonetheless tends to see its objective as related to a single level of analysis and a congeries of disconnected individuals" (p. 609). Instead, Susser offers hope wherein "the epidemiologist's need [for] hypothesis, design, and analysis would always keep in focus the object of viewing all the relevant levels as a whole. Each level is seen as a system in itself that interacts with those above and below it" (pp. 610–611).

Catastrophic versus Gradual Effects

We have described how epidemiologic methods have been sharpened to deal with large-scale phenomena, but nevertheless remain inadequate for detecting small effects when data are available for only a relatively short time interval. The question of how to relate EI to human health, however, remains. Before we can address this problem, we must distinguish between two distinct phenomena: a catastrophic, high-inertia environmental collapse versus a gradual decline in EI resulting in more subtle health effects.

The health impact of a catastrophic environmental collapse would be enormous, inherently unstable, and impossible to model because there is no prior experience upon which to base such models. Indeed, epidemiologic models are not needed to show that the loss of nature's life-support services, and the consequent period of chaos, would kill millions, if not billions, of people.

On the other hand, if ecospheric declines can be assumed to be a gradual extension of current trends without any sudden collapse, then epidemiology is well equipped to discern which environmental factors currently are most closely associated with human health. The definition of health, in this case, could be as broad or as narrow as the investigator wishes. It could include the biological, emotional, and/or social dimensions of health. The question of how to measure the relationship between EI and human health thus can be answered only if the consequences of a decline in EI would occur in a predictable manner or over a protracted period of time.

Lack of an Integrated Ecological Model

Consider some of the pillars of EI described in the first chapter of this volume: "wildness," autopoiesis, biodiversity, and land protection. Currently, epidemiologists can take these ideas (where data are available) and relate them to general health outcomes. However, a fundamental link in the chain of evidence is missing. A detailed model that integrates humans into Earth's ecological systems is needed which can link elements of EI to human health. With such an integrated model, epidemiologists would have a biological basis that could be used to link specific measures of EI with specific disease outcomes. Fortunately, the Agroecosystem Health Project has attempted to define, describe, and evaluate the health of agroecosystems, including these systems' human components (Smit et al. 1998). This has provided a road map that ecologists, coupled with sociologists and epidemiologists, could use to create an integrated model for much larger natural ecosystems. The role of public health, and its various agencies, then could be reexamined within such an integrated model.

Although research that transcends disciplinary boundaries is rare (Norgaard 1992), it is necessary if an integrated model is to be developed. Disciplines must not simply sit next to one another. Instead, they must go further and generate novel concepts by synthesizing the various disciplinary knowledge bases. More and more in epidemiology, for example, links are made with the social sciences to facilitate research into the social determinants of health (Rosenfield 1992). The synthesis of sociology and epidemiology and the success of this research have greatly advanced the social determinants of health agenda.

Before the relationship between EI and human health could ever be established, the place of humankind within ecosystems and the ecosphere will need to be recognized. In particular, the sustainability of the traditional "goals" of public health, within that framework, will need to be established. Indeed, the continued public health "aspirations" of zero infant mortality and an infinite life span will need to be reconciled with a more ecological viewpoint of humankind's existence on this planet.

Overview of Study Findings

Fortunately, the lack of an integrated ecological model does not paralyze the epidemiologist. Epidemiology is as much an exploratory, descriptive science as one that establishes causality. In fact, we (Sieswerda and Soskolne) have conducted an exploratory, cross-sectional aggregate data study at the international level examining the relationship between some available measures of EI and selected general health indicators (Sieswerda 1999). Measures of ecological disintegrity served as "exposure" in the epidemiologic sense; our variables were chosen according to their plausibility as measures of "intactness" or "wildness" of ecosystems. The lack of an integrated ecological model means that we had no objective criteria for assessing the validity of these choices.

Drawing on our experience with the definition of EI from the Global Integrity Project, we selected the following variables as indicators of EI: percentage of land highly disturbed by human activity; threatened species (%) (total for mammals, birds, higher plants, reptiles, and amphibians); partially protected areas (International Union for the Conservation of Nature [IUCN] categories IV–V) as a percentage of total area; totally protected areas (IUCN categories I–III) as a percentage of total area; forest remaining since preagricultural times (%); and average annual deforestation (%). We modeled these indicators of EI against three health outcomes: life expectancy at birth, infant mortality rate, and percent of low-birth-weight babies. In addition, to ensure that any potential relationships among the EI variables and the health outcomes were not attributable to socioeconomic factors, our analyses controlled for several socioeconomic variables: carbon dioxide emissions per capita (a surrogate for industrial activity), percentage of urbanization, population density, gross domestic product (GDP) per capita (adjusted for cost of living), Gini Index (a measure of income distribution), and adult male literacy.

Despite the shortcomings of having to deal with population-based averages, variable data quality, uncertain causal mechanisms, and the necessity of using surrogates of EI instead of direct measurements, we found a few associations between some of our EI variables and the three human health outcomes that we considered. In the extremely narrow time frame of this cross-sectional study, the conversion of land to permanent human use had a small but stable association with improving health outcomes. Deforestation appeared to have an unstable association with improving health. Neither biodiversity nor land protection had any association with our health indicators. Industrialization was important, but its association varied depending on whether countries were low, middle, or high income. In low- and middle-income countries, industrialization was associated with improvements in the health indicators examined. In high-income countries, further industrialization was associated with negative health impacts.

The results of this study may provide some answers as to why the environment is often a secondary consideration for policymakers. This study shows that ecological disintegrity appears to be "disconnected" from human health. There may exist a trade-off between improving conditions for human life and depleting/destroying the environment. So far, that trade-off has favored continued development at the expense of the environment. In many ways, these findings should not come as a surprise. This interpretation has arisen based on evidence of our species' ability to survive, and even thrive, in "islands" of ecological disintegrity, such as major cities (Rees 1998). This perpetuates the view that humans can survive and achieve high levels of public health independently of nature. In reality, this level of health is maintained by drawing on healthy or productive ecosystems elsewhere. In other words, trade and technology serve to distance human life from its very life source (Rees 1998). An informative way to capture this phenomenon is to utilize ecological footprint analysis (Wackernagel and Rees 1996). Indeed, future epidemiologic studies of this issue will necessarily not only incorporate improvements in methodology, data, and an integrated ecological model for human and public health, but also recognize the realities of global technology and trade in masking the true "connectedness" of human health and EI.

How much integrity is necessary for human health? The ultimate answer must come from ecology because it is the same as whatever amount will forestall the collapse of the biosphere. The models developed for this study are based on past events and are inadequate for predicting catastrophic events. In terms of the less apocalyptic effects on human health, it seems that the current articulation of EI has little relation to human health as studied here. With the help of an integrated ecological model, our model could perhaps be refined with additional variables. Results from this study should therefore be interpreted with great caution.

Conclusion

Solid epidemiologic science is prerequisite to gaining the public trust. If convincing relationships between human health and ecological disintegrity are found, we believe that the potential of epidemiology to impact public policy would be substantial. Most notably, a great leap forward in epidemiologic studies related to EI would require an ecological model integrating natural and human systems. Until then, only weak models will be derivable in the absence of a dramatic shift (i.e., worsening) in any of the relevant health outcomes.

REFERENCES

Brenner H, Savitz DA, Jockel K-H, and Greenland S. 1992. Effects of non-differential exposure misclassification in ecologic studies. *American Journal of Epidemiology,* 135(1):85–95.

Elwood JM, Lee JAH, Walter SD, Mo T, and Green AES. 1974. Relationship of melanoma and other skin cancer mortality to latitude and ultraviolet radiation in the United States and Canada. *International Journal of Epidemiology,* 3:325–332.

Friedman GD. 1967. Cigarette smoking and geographic variation in coronary heart disease mortality in the United States. *Journal of Chronic Diseases,* 20:769.

Greenland S and Morgenstern H. 1989. Ecological bias, confounding, and effect modification. *International Journal of Epidemiology,* 18:269–274.

Hayduk L. 1987. *Structural Equation Modeling with LISREL: Essentials and Advances.* Baltimore: Johns Hopkins University Press.

Hennekens CH and Buring JE. 1987. *Epidemiology in Medicine.* Boston: Little, Brown.

Kadohira M, McDermott JJ, Shoukri MM, and Thorburn MA. 1997. Assessing infections at multiple levels of aggregation. *Preventive Veterinary Medicine,* 29:161–177.

Kiester AR, Scott JM, Csuti B, Noss RF, Butterfield B, Sahr K, and White D. 1996. Conservation prioritization using GAP data. *Conservation Biology,* 10(5):1332–1342.

Last JM. 1995. *A Dictionary of Epidemiology,* 3rd ed. New York: Oxford University Press.

Le XC, Xing JZ, Lee J, Leadon SA, and Weinfeld M. 1998. Inducible repair of thymine glycol detected by an ultrasensitive assay for DNA damage. *Science*, 280:1066–1069.

McDermott JJ, Kadohira M, O'Callaghan CJ, and Shoukri MM. 1997. A comparison of different models for assessing variations in the sero-prevalence of infectious bovine rhinotracheitis by farm, area and district in Kenya. *Preventive Veterinary Medicine*, 32:219–234.

McMichael AJ. 1993 (Canto Edition 1995). *Planetary Overload: Global Environmental Change and the Health of the Human Species*. Cambridge: Cambridge University Press, pp. 143–167.

Morgenstern H. 1982. Uses of ecologic analysis in epidemiologic research. *American Journal of Public Health*, 72(12):1336–1344.

Norgaard RB. 1992. Coordinating disciplinary and organizational ways of knowing. *Agriculture, Ecosystems, and Environment*, 42:205–216.

Nurminen M and Briggs D. 1996. Approaches to linkage analysis: Overview. In: *Linkage Methods for Environment and Health Analysis: General Guidelines*. Briggs D, Corvalan C, and Nurminen M, eds. Geneva: World Health Organization.

Rees W. 1998. Personal communication.

Robinson WS. 1950. Ecological correlations and the behavior of individuals. *American Sociological Review*, 15:351–357.

Rosenfield PL. 1992. The potential of transdisciplinary research for sustaining and extending linkages between the health and social sciences. *Social Science and Medicine*, 35(11):1343–1356.

Schall R. 1991. Estimation in generalized linear models with random effects. *Biometrika*, 78:719–727.

Sieswerda, LE. 1999. Towards measuring the impact of ecological disintegrity on human health. Master's thesis, University of Alberta.

Smit B, Watner-Toews D, Rapport D, Wall E, Wichert G, Gwyn E, and Wandel J. 1998. *Agroecosystem Health: Analysis and Assessment*. Guelph, Ontario: University of Guelph.

Susser M. 1998. Does risk factor epidemiology put epidemiology at risk? Peering into the future. *Journal of Epidemiology and Community Health*, 52:608–611.

Taubes G. 1997. Apocalypse not. *Science*, 278(5340):1004–1006.

Wackernagel M and Rees W. 1996. *Our Ecological Footprint: Reducing Human Impact on the Earth*. Gabriola Island, BC: New Society Publishers.

WHO. 1995. *The World Health Report 1995: Bridging the Gaps*. Geneva: World Health Organization.

WHO. 1997. *Linkage Methods for Environment and Health Analysis: Technical Guidelines*. Corvalan C, Nurminen M, and Pastides H, eds. Geneva: World Health Organization.

Institutionalized Environmental Violence and Human Rights

Laura Westra

We are all familiar with violence and most of us deplore it; many also fight to enact laws and regulations to protect the citizens of all countries from it. We decry it in all its forms: family violence, violence against women, crime in the streets, and all kinds of terrorism. But there are certain other forms of violence that are all-pervasive and as prevalent in Western democracies as they are in the nondemocratic regimes of the developing world. They are *environmental* forms of violence, because they are perpetrated in and through the environment: they represent direct and indirect attacks on our health, our lives, and even on our species and what we are.

Sadly, these forms of violence are hard to proscribe, regulate, and control, for many reasons. Their perpetrators are powerful, their influence is global, but their activities may be said to lack malicious intent, and to be instead deeply entrenched in the very fabric of modern life. As scientific evidence mounts about specific attacks on human health in various parts of the globe, through various means, responsible parties, be they corporate, governmental or other, attempt stalling techniques and use their considerable resources to mount an impressive self-defense. In general, they claim that the *means* of their attacks, either products, processes, or other activities, are "innocent until proven guilty," and that precise proof, in the legal sense, is not available. We saw recently a detailed unfolding of that kind of strategy, as the tobacco industry defended its "innocence" (Cohen 1996).

The difficulties of demonstrating responsibility are compounded, because there are also cumulative effects of toxic substances, where each substance may be at the legal "safe" level, but the result of many such chemicals may be very harmful or even lethal. Then there are the health and other reproductive effects due to low-dose exposure to products and materials that are an accepted part of life in North America. In addition, there are the aggravating effects of global climate change, as well as the effects of environmental racism because too many are disproportionately affected by, and bear burdens far in excess of possible benefits from, practices resulting in environmental pollution.

Institutionalized Environmental Violence

We will examine some of the many forms taken by ecoviolence, starting with the effects of global climate change. The problems we will discuss are interconnected and interrelated, so that most of them are aggravated by the presence of another. Still, it will be helpful to treat them separately, even if they are not really separate, simply to appreciate the magnitude of the problems that we face. We are familiar now with the effects of "holes" in the ozone layer and the corresponding hazards of ultraviolet radiation. These consequences represent an institutionalized attack on our immune system and on our health, and the effects are equally present on all exposed animals, and on crops and vegetation. The attack is "institutionalized," like all other hazards discussed in this chapter, because the activities that produced it were not illegal or proscribed, but were part of a technologically "enhanced" lifestyle that has been supported and even encouraged by corporations and by political institutions intent on pleasing voters. Indeed, the public supports these activities indirectly by their support of these products and the corporations that manufacture them.

Despite the presence of protocols for the mitigation of the present conditions (such as the Montreal Protocol), not only is the time frame more favorable to business than to health protection, but also the efforts aimed at moving forward are hampered precisely by institutionalized democratic practices. The pattern is a familiar one: for instance, multinational automotive corporations threaten job losses with severe impacts on the economy. In December 1997, diplomats from all over the world met in Kyoto, Japan, to hammer out the details of a treaty to show the effects of global warming. This treaty, if enacted, would increase gasoline prices, and the prices of both electricity and automobiles.

I have argued that the corresponding reduction in sales is a necessary part of a first "step-back" to encourage reduced consumption. But corporate interests have been allowed to bring us to this point, where we are all at severe risk from various exposures, including exposure to something that is so much a part of "natural" life—the sun's rays. It is even more disturbing that these corporate giants intend to pursue growth and to discourage additional regulations, rather than prepare themselves to acknowledge their guilt and attempt to make amends.

Scientific evidence mounts about the details of the hazards to which we are exposed, in various measures, according to our geographical location. For instance, not only is short-wavelength UV radiation (UVB) carcinogenic, but new data indicate a carcinogenic role for long-wavelength ultraviolet light (UVA) also. Squamous cell carcinomas and melanomas can be induced in tests by UVA alone or in combination with UVB. In addition, studies on the effects of UV radiation have shown that UVB alters significantly the immunological processes of human and nonhuman animals.

Climate change will have other significant health effects globally, with low-elevation, deltaic, and, in general, less developed countries bearing the heaviest burden of harm. The effects, both present now and envisioned through integrated models, consider both direct and indirect individual biophysical impacts, so that the *indirect* harm caused by changes in horticultural and arable crops, and the *direct* harm caused through the increasing incidence of cyclones, floods, and droughts, particularly for those who are not buffered by the social infrastructures present in affluent countries, become evident (Murray and Lopez 1997). The close relation between the preservation of the environment and the ecological "services" it provides to all life is more visible and better understood in less developed countries, where people live their lives in a state of pervasive poverty and are struggling to survive. The depletion of forests, the loss of medicinal herbs, and other results of climate change, such as flash floods, landslides, soil erosion, and the resulting degradation of agricultural lands, mean that the health of inhabitants is at grave risk.

It is important to keep in mind that the majority of less developed countries have not contributed significantly to the causes of global climate change, and that therefore their greater burden is even more unfair than it would be were it the lot of affluent nations instead. In Africa, environmental disasters escalate and multiply the impact of "Africa's natural hazards," such as epidemics and endemic diseases. Other humanmade disasters—armed conflicts, industrial hazards, the forced movement of populations, food insecurities, and "cultural and political instability"—also interact with climate changes and environmental degradation to make disease and other health emergencies a constant threat (Loretti and Tegegn 1996).

Examples could be multiplied, but the authors of the *World Health Statistics Quarterly* express best the full impact of this deadly interface:

> Disasters occur when hazards and vulnerability meet. Out of 100 disasters reported worldwide, only 20 occur in Africa, but Africa suffers 60 percent of all disaster-related deaths. (Loretti and Tegegn 1996)

In fact, "accident and disaster epidemiology" has become an essential tool to study the health effects of disasters and to emphasize the need for prevention and mitigation of human health effects. Health care preparedness should be made a priority in disaster relief and not brought in only to aid after the fact.

Another familiar area of health hazards is that of toxic waste exposure. A great deal has been done to analyze the impacts on human health of radioactive waste (Shrader-Fréchette 1982).The sheer persistence of radwaste, as well as its toxicity, has shown the wastes of the nuclear industry to be one of the worst threats to humankind today. They represent a clear example of institutionalized ecoviolence: even such democratic countries as Canada or the United States do not offer voters a nonnuclear option as a source of power. Radwaste as well as other toxic agents must be eliminated from waste dumps.

In addition, novel criteria for testing and monitoring must be introduced. For instance, epidemiological studies disclose that the air around such sites is not classified as representative for the possible health burden of exposed persons. But gases emanate from toxic waste sites, and the air at these sites should be studied and compared to "normal" air to detect possible hazardous variations. In contrast, chemical variations in the air may not be sufficient to make a solid case for the affected populations. Another difficulty that must also be addressed is that populations at risk may show only "nonspecific deterioration of health and well-being," rather than "overt clinical disease" (Von Schirnding and Ehrlich 1992).

Toxic waste is also the locus of environmentally racist practices, as it is most often placed in areas populated by people of color in North America and in less developed countries on the other continents (Bullard 1994). In all these cases, the health problems suffered by minorities are aggravated by the lack of health care availability in the areas where they live, and by the insensitive and inadequate legal and institutional infrastructure that does not offer either protection or redress.

Before ending in waste sites, many of these toxic substances are used routinely in industries, especially in agribusiness. Intensive agricultural practices impose risks well beyond carcinogenicity. A recent agricultural health study based in North Carolina and Iowa lists many additional noncancer risks among all persons who have direct contact with pesticides and other agricultural chemicals (e.g., agricultural workers, registered pesticide applicators, and their spouses). Some of the additional risks beyond cancer are neurotoxicity, reproductive effects, immunological defects, nonmalignant respiratory disease, and kidney disease as well as abnormal growth and development in children.

The products that have been shown to cause these health effects are also used in homes, lawns, and gardens and thus provide direct exposure. Indirect exposure may arise from inhaling spray drift, laundering workclothes, or ingesting contaminated food and water. The effects of agricultural business practices and other external uses of these chemicals parallel the internal exposure through ingested foods containing traces and even small quantities of these hazardous products. The general population is exposed to these hazards through accepted legal and regulated practices fully supported by present institutions. But when pesticide residues are ingested, they may be quickly metabolized and eliminated, or may show a strong tendency to accumulate in the body, in which case the worst hazards may be a result of long-term, low-dose exposure. The institutional infrastructure may not recognize the health problems that arise months or even years from the time of exposure. This means that not only are the institutions that support and permit these corporate practices and products morally wrong, but the legal infrastructure of these institutions is equally at fault for requiring victims to carry the burden of proof (Brown 1995).

In another recent study, ambient air was monitored in an Australian town surrounded by banana plantations. Organochlorines and organophosphates were detected, but these were used mostly for nonagricultural purposes. Although the level of the agricultural pesticides used at the plantations did not appear to pose significant health risks (Beard et al. 1995), the synergistic effects of agricultural and nonagricultural chemicals have not been well researched.

Once again, as for toxic wastes, environmental racism also runs rampant in developing countries in the use of pesticides. Pesticides that are banned or restricted in developed countries are routinely used by large groups of agricultural workers in developing countries, and the full range of the health hazards generated by their exposure has not been fully monitored, although fatalities have been recorded. A recent article in the *Journal of Health Services* notes that the unsafe use of increasing amounts of these pesticides has resulted in both acute poisonings and chronic health effects (e.g., neurotoxic and dermatological disorders) in workers (Wesseling et al. 1997). The problem is further aggravated by the fact that malnourished populations are much more vulnerable to the toxicity of pesticide residues. Together with the problem of product misuse, often originating from the lack of instructions in the language of the users, and the presence of restricted or banned pesticides, this should force global institutions and policymakers to rethink all strategies for pest control in the developing world (Dillon 1995). Research indicates that radical rethinking should take place in regard to all agricultural practices and policies that involve chemicals, and there is no need at this time to review the abundant literature available on the topic (Pimentel et al. 1991).

For the purposes of this work, all the evidence shows that the hazardous products and practices are, for the most part, legal, unrestricted, and part of an institutionalized and accepted lifestyle that is never brought into question *as a whole*. At best, studies that identify a specific problem may spur piece-meal legislation, enacted to respond to specific problems. But these sudden grave problems should be viewed as red flags, alerting us to the presence of an unsustainable and violent whole, a society that condones and encourages activities that constitute grave attacks on the physical integrity of individuals and their habitats. When air, water, sun, earth, and food are all contaminated and basically hazardous, then ecoviolence is being perpetrated on a regular basis, and the right to self-defense ought to be invoked to attack the legality of present institutions and eliminate these persistent attacks.

A study published by the *Japanese Journal of Hygiene* proposed using a method similar to the Codex Alimentalius of the WHO/FAO Joint Committee, which established the Recommended Daily Allowances (RDAs) for nutrient intake. The proposed method could be called "Estimated Ecological Daily Intake" (EEDI), and it would calculate the daily intake of food additives and contaminants, based on volunteers' food consumption (Toyokawa and Nishikawa 1994). This sort of research could be repeated at various locations, and it might form the basis for an eventual series of class action suits by groups or even by government institutions on behalf of these groups, similar to the ones brought against the tobacco companies in 1997. If states in the United States can sue tobacco companies to recover the damages arising from health costs incurred because of these companies' practices, then legal actions against other hazardous industries might make a serious impact on the way these corporations conduct their respective businesses, and also on the general uncritical acceptance of those states' institutions.

A similar method might be designed to study the amount of exposure to low-level chemicals and toxics, such as hormone mimics and other endocrine disruptors that are not ingested (Colborn et al. 1996, Westra 1998). These substances and their effects will be discussed in the next section in some detail.

Even more than the specific exposures of agricultural workers or others involved in the manufacture or use of chemical products, low-level exposure is a threat to many in Northwest affluent countries, where the lifestyle is based on the uncritical acceptance of myriad products and processes, all of which may affect us through low-dose exposures. Anyone who uses soft plastics and lives in an area where chemical endocrine disruptors exist (and that is pretty much everywhere) is at risk. As Theo Colborn has it, "Living in a man-made landscape, we easily forget that our well-being is rooted in natural systems. Yet all human enterprise rests on the foundation of natural systems that provide a myriad of invisible life-support services" (Colborn et al. 1996). As seen in animals, endocrine disruptors attack all of us and our future through "widespread disruption in human embryonic development," producing frequent genital abnormalities in infants as well as reduced sperm counts in males and infertility and reproductive difficulties in females (Colborn et al. 1996). Many of these harms are transgenerational, and all are largely invisible and do not produce the clear, "smoking-gun" relations between causes and effects that may move present institutions to curtail or eliminate them (Westra 1998).

We noted earlier some of the effects of global climate change. These changes are already having a significant impact on the spread of vector-borne infectious diseases, and on viral and parasitic infections. All changes in the ecology of a region entail changes in the vector populations. Large-scale movement of human populations contributes to this severe threat as well. The loss of tropical forests, global warming of air and oceans, and all other anthropogenic disturbances all contribute to health threats.

Many believed that infectious diseases had been eliminated through the use of antibiotics; smallpox, whooping cough, diphtheria, paralyzing poliomyelitis, tetanus, and many other diseases are largely extinct. But the majority of "vector-transmitted diseases," such as cholera and several forms of severe respiratory tract infections, will continue to be an important health problem for the twenty-first century. Some of the causes include "lifestyles prone to infectious pathology, such as megacity urbanization," "industrialized foods . . . global commerce and tourism, . . . antibiotic-multiresistant microbial flora; environmental disturbances as a result of global warming, deforestation, the settling of virgin areas, dams, the large-scale use of pesticides, fertilizers and antimicrobials" (Kumate 1997).

Some of the contributing causes cited by Kumate include drug addiction, "sexual liberation," and other nonenvironmental factors. But for the most part, the causes of the emergence and reemergence of life-threatening diseases are environmentally imposed and not subject to individual consent (like sexual orientation). Yet we might want to question this assumption as well. Although no research is available to my knowledge on this aspect of the problem, we might connect the sexual changes imposed by endocrine disruptors to the sexual "choices" that are thought to be freely intended, and cited as contributing factors to the presence of these diseases. If this connection is at least possible, then even sexually transmitted diseases arising from certain choices may not be "chosen," and may thus be listed under environmentally induced threats as well. There has been a general move to grant rights to those with sexual orientations beyond heterosexuality in most Western democracies. Amended laws and regulations are based, for the most part, on the value of individual freedom and on egalitarian considerations. Yet, if the effect of these chemicals is to alter sexual orientation in humans as it often does in birds and marine mammals (Colborn et al. 1996), then granting rights after the fact does not change the impact of the violence that might have been done to these individuals and to their natural functions and sexuality.

The introduction of toxic materials and chemicals not only is a direct form of violence, but also contributes indirectly to the loss of "nature's services" (Daily 1997). When systems are no longer capable of continuing their evolutionary paths, as they are not left unmanipulated or wild, the "services" they provide may be proportionately decreased as our interference with their structure and function eventually eliminates their ability to provide support for all life (Westra 1998). A recent study, for instance, addresses our need for plant life:

> Only green plants can convert the single carbon units of atmospheric carbon dioxide into the multicarbon organic molecules on which all forms of life depend. Only green plants can provide the oxygen required by man and other aerobic organisms (Bell 1993).

Further, the medicinal and nutritive services provided by a vast array of plants are eliminated when these are affected, depleted, or rendered extinct, while so little is known about most of the diversity that still exists. Bell adds, "Nothing or virtually nothing is known about the composition of approximately 250,000 wild and little used species" (Wilson 1991, Harte et al. 1992, Bell 1993). The elimination of biodiversity and of systemic function leads to repeated system collapse: this, in itself, is arguably the most severe threat to human health that we encounter (Jutro 1991, McMichael 1995). Additional impacts on human health arise from two other primary losses that face us: the loss of safe air and the loss of safe water.

Air pollution and the presence of particulates in the air lead to children's asthma in unprecedented numbers, and to the increasing presence of obstructive pulmonary disease in much of the Western world from Europe to North America (Guidotti 1996, Lebowitz 1996). Safe water or at least somewhat uncontaminated water is not available to 40 percent of the population of the world. This represents a factor clearly contributing to the reemergence of vector-borne diseases like cholera, as we saw earlier; the role of unsafe water was evident in the cholera pandemic of January 1991 (Colwell 1996). The cost of providing safe water worldwide, however, would be prohibitive; for instance, a public intervention to supply families with safe water in Latin America would cost between U.S.$1.50 and $4 per family. Globally, although safe water has been taken for granted as an essential public health need, it appears that the time when everyone will have to pay dearly for safe water is almost upon us.

These facts provide ammunition for the thesis of this chapter, and they offer an additional example of the injustice perpetrated by our "ecological footprint" (Rees and Wackernagel 1996), as certain groups are dispropor-tionately affected. For instance, most of the citizens in less developed coun-tries cannot pay the required price for safe water, and infants have special needs in comparison with the rest of the population: they need three times more water than adults if the requirements are calculated according to body weight.

We are also totally vulnerable to pathogens to which animals (such as apes) are routinely exposed, as we encroach on their wild habitats with our expanding populations. The sudden spread of the Ebola virus is a case in point: a disease that might be commonplace for one species may be lethal for another. We are more familiar with another aspect of this phenom-enon—the encroachment on the habitat of one human group by another—as when the first North American colonists arrived in areas previously oc-cupied by peoples native to those regions. In that case, the aboriginal people were the ones affected because they were exposed to pathogens to which they had not developed an immunity. Yet it does not seem as though we have truly understood that lesson, clear as it was. Like that colonizing ex-pansion, our encroachment into habitats of which we are not a part is un-critically accepted and part of "normal" modern life: it has become institu-tionalized.

The newest aliens within ecosystems and habitats, that is, bioengineered and transgenic organisms (both plants and animals), are also a regularly ac-cepted and institutionalized form of ecoviolence perpetrated in various ways against human and nonhuman life (Westra 1998). Altered animals are forced to live in altered conditions, thus requiring food additives including antibiotics in order to survive. This practice in turn gives rise to our own exposure to antibiotic-resistant strains of pathogens (Rissler and Mellon 1993, Westra 1998). Altered foods are also hazardous to the natural systems where they are introduced. Further, they are normally unlabeled, so that another threat to health arises from possible allergic reactions to the hidden components within previously acceptable and safe foods.

Finally, social conditions aggravated by conflicts (Homer-Dixon 1991), as well as the environmental degradation we have briefly detailed here, en-gender the migration of entire groups and populations. Refugees, displaced persons, and legal and illegal immigration all contribute to the spread of health threats to all areas of the globe. We may sum up some of these forms of ecoviolence as follows, although these headings are by no means a com-plete list of all possible harms of this kind:

1. Increased exposure to UVA/UVB because of ozone layer thinning

2. Exposure to direct impacts of global climate change, such as floods, ex-treme temperatures, and other weather changes

3. Exposure to toxic wastes

4. Exposure to toxic/hazardous by-products of industrial production, ranging from nuclear power to high-input agriculture

5. Exposure to food additives and chemical residues in food production

6. Long-term, low-level exposures to various chemicals and processes

7. Exposure to climate-induced health threats from new or renewed infectious diseases

8. The loss of "nature's services" through loss of biodiversity, fragmentation of natural landscapes, and deforestation

9. Increased presence of particulates and other pollutants in the air

10. The diminishing supply of safe water

11. Direct contact with pathogens through encroachment on the wild (Soskolne 1997, personal communication)

12. Increased hazards from the presence of bioengineered foods and transgenics, which may range from unexpected allergic reactions to unlabeled bioengineered food, to exposure to food with unpredictable side effects (as in BSE), to the hidden antibiotics in transgenic fish

13. Exposure to antibiotic-resistant strains of pathogens

14. Increase in communicable-disease risks through migration of persons based on immigration policies of governments and to accommodate refugees, to seek out qualified labor, and to travel

Institutionalized Ecoviolence and Its Ethical Dimensions

Certain common features allow the grouping of all these disparate attacks on our existence. Most of these attacks are viewed as arising out of the "normal" functioning of Western industrialized societies. Another common feature is that, in all cases, there is no candid information available to the public about the "double effects" of products and activities we tend to take for granted. The media (Korten 1995) and certain business practices, such as trade secrets regulations, conspire to keep us in the dark. Many of these products have become "highly desirable," or even "necessities" through clever marketing; in some cases, even planned addiction has been part of the marketing process. Often immense corporate resources promote a product well beyond its intrinsic value, until it becomes a "must-have" icon globally (think of Coca-Cola or McDonald's in this respect).

In contrast, some other features of our list affect Northwest affluent populations in a way that is different from the effects on impoverished minorities in Southeast countries. For instance, low-dosage exposures arise directly from the industrial lifestyle of the Northwest. As Theo Colborn explains, it is the soft plastics, the petrochemical agricultural aids, and other "taken-for-granted" parts of our daily life that cause much of our hazardous exposure: in this regard alone, we are worse off than those who live at or below the poverty level in the developing world (Colborn et al. 1996). But Northwesterners are advantaged in some other ways: our affluence protects us from some of the effects of global climate change, including the resurgence of previous infectious diseases and the emergence of new ones. The siting of hazardous waste facilities, on the other hand, is far more likely to put minority populations at risk, here or in the Southeast.

Although we are assured of protection by our government institutions, such as "security of persons" (Canadian Charter of Rights) or "equal protection" (U.S. constitutional amendments 4 and 15), somehow the harms listed are viewed in a different light. They are not taken to be forms of assaults. They are viewed either as "normal" aspects of modern life or as "acts of God," accidental events beyond our control. What is lacking is the acknowledgment of collective responsibility on the part of the risk imposers themselves, as well as on the part of whole institutions, including the governing bodies that aid and abet these activities. Our politicians accept unrealistic burden-of-proof expectations, as they neglect to factor into their decisions the limits of scientific predictive capabilities, the impact of uncertainty, and the importance of the precautionary principle, particularly in regard to environmental matters.

Aggressions and attacks are still thought of in the narrow sense of direct physical attacks on persons by other persons. I believe that a new approach is necessary, because these "invisible harms" are not acknowledged now: instead, they have become accepted, taken for granted, that is, institutionalized. They are not viewed as unacceptable and abnormal, the way criminal acts are viewed. It is a crime even to carry knives, firearms, or bombs; it is not legal to have them, stockpile them, or use them.

But toxic substances, hazardous chemicals, and even the practices that eliminate biodiversity, reduce and pollute wild habitats, and render clean water a rare resource, are *also* harmful to human life and health. They are even worse than guns, in some sense, as they require neither malice nor intent to be harmful; simple carelessness, negligence, or lack of concern for "nature's services" is sufficient to result in disasters, some of which are irreversible (such as the effects of nuclear waste). Of course, none of the effects I have mentioned are immediate, evident, or even directly causative of the harms they eventually produce. Like the small, cumulative doses of obscure poisons found in the urbane and elegant murder mysteries written by British authors, they do kill, slowly and inexorably. When they do not, they impose disease or they wreak havoc in various ways on the natural functioning of human beings (Longstretch and de Gruijl 1995, McMichael 1995, Colborn et al. 1996, Forbes and Calow 1996).

My approach to environmental ethics is and has been biocentric and holistic: I have defended the intrinsic value of the integrity of systemic wholes (Westra 1998). In my latest work I have also defended the rights of individual organisms (such as human beings) to retain their own microintegrity, as well as the integrity of their habitats. For now, leaving aside the needs of nonhuman animals and the protection of systems *for themselves*, I want to argue that my approach is necessary even if we limit ourselves purely to a consideration of human health, surely an easy goal to defend. What is the relation between ecological integrity and human health? Literature exists about the necessity to establish, respect, or restore wild areas (core areas) in order to reestablish within them the large fauna originally native to each habitat (to the best of our knowledge), and, at the same time, ensure that all the biota necessary to the functioning of each ecosystem are present on each site (Noss 1992, Pimentel et al. 1992). In essence then, our first concern based on respect for others, ourselves, and all life should be the conservation of the resilience of the ecosystems on which human activity depends, and the ability of these systems to continue to provide valued ecological services to *all* biota. To achieve this, not only does the *quality* of ecosystems in the wild need protection, but also their *quantity* (in the sense of the size of the core areas required). A holistic approach is needed so that legislation affecting pollution, agricultural practices, fisheries, or forestry can all be viewed through a perspective that starts from the necessary centrality of integrity, and only then moves on to particularities. Just as it is not possible to save animal species and communities without a primary concern for their habitat, so too, concern for individuals and communities of humans should start with respect for the habitat we share with the rest of the biota.

The difficulty is that disrupting natural processes in large areas not only disrupts the life and health of *their* biota, but also affects *ours:* cutting down forests, for instance, reduces the "services" the trees perform for all air, hence for all forms of life that need to breathe. Introducing toxic and hazardous substances into waterways and oceans not only affects all the wildlife that depends on clean water for its life, but also affects all humans in various ways, as our own food supplies are affected, not only in the water but also through evaporation that distributes the toxins on whatever is grown for food.

We are familiar by now with the almost automatic association between chemicals and their carcinogenic and mutagenic properties. Additional recent research shows no less ominous but different effects of herbicides, fungicides, insecticides, nematocides, and most other "industrial chemicals." Theo Colborn recently sketched a "Toxic Chemical Profile" of these substances and their effects; she shows that they

- Mimic natural hormones
- Antagonize hormone effects by blocking binding sites
- React directly or indirectly with natural hormones
- Alter natural patterns of hormone synthesis, metabolism, and excretion
- Alter hormone receptors' level (Colborn et al. 1996)

These effects are supported by basic research involving wildlife, controlled laboratory toxicology tests, and tests on human epidemiological exposure. Although these substances affect gene expression, however, they are "organizational, activational, not mutational, as they do not affect the integrity of the DNA" (Colborn et al. 1996). What we do see is an almost endless series of sexual and reproductive effects, engendered by very low doses of most of these substances; the loss of structural integrity of male and female reproductive apparatus is followed by the loss of functional (reproductive) capacity, and often by the loss of natural gender orientation and parenting abilities (Colborn et al. 1996).

Many of these effects of low-dose exposure may be found in birds, fish, and mammals, including humans. The increasing frequency of these abnormalities is due to the worldwide exposure to chemicals we are experiencing. Colborn traces the first "wide-scale exposure to manmade chemicals" to the 1940s (after World War II), so that in the 1940s and 1950s a first generation was exposed. In the next 20 years (1950s to 1970s), for the first time, worldwide exposure in the womb occurred, and by the 1990s this generation itself reached reproductive age, thus continuing the pattern of exposure.

But not all the results of these low-dose exposures are clear, observable, sexually related, or representative examples of recognizable diseases. Some are far more subtle and *are not* visible—for example, hyperactivity, reduced head circumference, auditory/verbal deficits, poorer reflex functions, stress intolerance, and reduced average intelligence are just some of the problems increasingly found in populations in the Great Lakes area. Colborn points out that even some economists are beginning to be concerned about the possibility of whole populations "whose intelligence, capacities and reactions are abnormal" (Colborn et al. 1996).

Conclusion

It is clear that we need to find some remedy for these and other such hazardous situations globally, because the list of environmental assaults on the physical integrity of ecosystems and, through them, on our own physical integrity and capacities occurs equally in Northwest affluent and in Southeast developing countries. The global distribution of the threats, from remote islands in the Pacific Ocean to "pristine" areas in the Arctic (Colborn et al. 1996), demonstrates that geographical and political boundaries are not capable of containing and limiting environmental degradation and disintegrity. A careful study of the "hotspots" and locations where the worst hazards persist shows that they are equally global in distribution. We cannot separate democracies from, say, military regimes and other nondemocratic states on the basis of the spread and severity of the environmental threats to which their citizens are exposed (Westra and Wenz 1995).

I have elsewhere proposed arguments for and against criminalizations of these harms (Westra 1998), and space will not permit repeating those arguments now. I will simply conclude that the first step is to become aware of the present institutionalization of ecoviolence—before appropriate measures may be taken to eliminate its impact and to protect human rights.

REFERENCES

Beard, Westley-Wise, V., and Sullivan, G. 1995. "Exposure to Pesticides in Ambient Air," *Australian Journal of Public Health*, 19 (4): 357–362, NSW Health Department, Lismore.

Bell, E.A. 1993. "Mankind and Plants: The Need to Conserve Biodiversity," *Parasitology*, 106: S47–S53.

Brown, D.A. 1995. "The Role of Law in Sustainable Development and Environmental Protection Decisionmaking," in *Sustainable Development: Science, Ethics and Public Policy*, J. Lemons and D.A. Brown, eds., Kluwer Academic, Dordrecht, The Netherlands, 64–76.

Bullard, R. 1994. *Dumping in Dixie (Race, Class, and Environmental Quality)*, Westview Press, Boulder, CO.

Cohen, J. 1996. "Tobacco Money Lights Up a Debate," *Science*, 272 (5261): 488–494.

Colborn, T., Dumanoski, D., and Myers, J.P. 1996. *Our Stolen Future*, Dutton, Penguin, New York.

Colwell, R. 1996. "Global Climate and Infectious Disease: The Cholera Paradigm," *Science*, 274: 2025–2031.

Daily, G., ed. 1997. "Introduction," in *Nature's Services*, Island Press, Washington, DC, 3–4.

Dillon, J.C. 1995. "Risks Associated with Pesticide Residue Contamination of Foods in Developing Countries," *Cahiers de Nutrition et de Dietetique*, 30 (5): 294–299.

Forbes, V. and Calow, P. 1996. "Costs of Living with Contaminants: Implications for Assessing Low-Level Exposures," *Belle Newsletter*, 4 (3): 1–8.

Grantstein, R.D. 1990. "Photoimmunology," *Seminars in Dermatology*, 9 (1): 16–24.

Guidotti, T.L. 1996. "Ambient Air Quality and Human Health: Current Concepts," part 2, in *Canadian Respiratory Journal*, 3 (1): 29–39.

Harte, J., Torn, M., and Jensen, D. 1992. "The Nature and Consequences of Indirect Linkages between Climate Change and Biological Diversity," *Global Warming and Biological Diversity*, R.L. Peters and T. Lovejoy, eds., Yale University Press, New Haven, CT.

Homer-Dixon, T. 1991. "On the Threshold: Environmental Changes as Causes of Acute Conflict," *International Security*, 16, (2): 76–116.

Jutro, P.R. 1991. "Biological Diversity, Ecology, and Global Climate Change," *Environmental Health Perspective*, 96: 167–170.

Korten, D. 1995. *When Corporations Rule the World*, Kumarian Press, Berret Koehler, West Hartford, CT.

Kumate, J. 1997. "Infectious Diseases of the 21st Century," *Archives of Medical Research*, 28 (2): 155–161.

Lebowitz, M.D. 1996. "Epidemiological Studies of the Respiratory Effects of Air Pollution," *European Respiratory Journal*, 9 (5): 1029–1054.

Longstretch, J.D., de Gruijl, F.R., et al. 1995. "Effects of Increased Solar Ultraviolet Radiation on Human Health," *Ambio*, 24 (3): 153–165.

Loretti, A. and Tegegn, Y. 1996. "Disasters in Africa: Old and New Hazards and Growing Vulnerability," *World Health Statistics Quarterly*, 49 (3–4): 179–184.

McMichael, A.J. 1995. *Planetary Overload*, Cambridge University Press, Cambridge.

Murray, C.J.L. and Lopez, A.D. 1997. "Global Mortality, Disability, and the Contribution of Risk Factors: Global Burden of Disease Study," *Lancet*, 349 (9063): 1436–1442.

Noss, R.F. 1992. "The Wildlands Project: Land Conservation Strategy," *Wild Earth*, Special Issue: 10–25.

Pimentel, D. et al. 1991. "Environmental and Economic Effects of Reducing Pesticide Use," *BioScience* 41 (6): 402–409.

Pimentel, D. et al. 1992. "Conserving Biological Diversity in Agricultural/Forestry Systems," *BioScience*, 42 (5): 747–757.

Rees, W.E. and Wackernagel, M. 1996. "Urban Ecological Footprints: Why Cities Cannot Be Sustainable and Why They Are a Key to Sustainability," *Environmental Impact Assessment Review*, 16: 223–248.

Rissler, J. and Mellon, M. 1993. *"Perils Amidst the Promise": Ecological Risks of Transgenic Crops in a Global Market*, Union of Concerned Scientists, Cambridge, MA.

Shrader-Fréchette, K. 1982. *Nuclear Power and Public Policy*, Kluwer Academic, Dordrecht, The Netherlands.

Toyokawa, H. and Nishikawa, H. 1994. "A New Estimation of the Intake of Contaminants, Based on Daily Consumption Data," *Japanese Journal of Hygiene,* 49 (2): 606–615.

Von Schirnding, Y.E.R. and Ehrlich, R.I. 1992. "Environmental Health Risks of Toxic Waste Site Exposure—an Epidemiological Perspective," *South African Medical Journal,* 81 (11): 546–549.

Wesseling, C., McConnell, R., Powtanen, T., and Hogstedt, C. 1997. "Agricultural Pesticides Use in Developing Countries: Health Effects and Research Needs," *International Journal of Health Services,* 27 (2): 273–308.

Westra, L. 1998. *Living in Integrity: A Global Ethic to Restore a Fragmented Earth.* Rowman and Littlefield, Lanham, MD.

Westra, L. and Wenz, P. 1995. *Faces of Environmental Racism: The Global Equity Issues,* Rowman & Littlefield, Lanham, MD.

Wilson, E.O. 1991. "Biodiversity, Prosperity and Value," in *Ecology, Economics and Ethics,* Yale University Press, New Haven, CT.

PART V

The Economics and Ethics of Achieving Global Ecological Integrity

B elieving that values and ethical assumptions of society are important considerations for determining whether a concept is implementable, the Global Integrity Project examined the ethical basis for protecting ecological integrity. This part explores some of the economic and ethical issues that need to be considered to protect global ecological integrity. It also examines the prospects for greater protection of ecological integrity in light of the way our economic institutions work and how governments have responded to international agreements.

In chapter 17, "The Cost of the Wild: International Equity and the Losses from Environmental Conservation," Ted Schrecker examines tensions between environmental protection and equitable economic development goals. This analysis is made to question the claim that environmental conservation always deserves ethical priority when conflicts arise with economic development.

Among other observations, Schrecker shows that those who advocate that environmental goals should always trump economic development interests wind up supporting programs that ensure the largest burdens will be paid by the poorest people. Through a thought experiment, Schrecker demonstrates how programs that pursue protection of biodiversity without considering questions of distributive justice are likely to make things worse for the poor or most vulnerable. In making this demonstration, Schrecker examines three commonly heard justifications for the priority of environmental over economic policy. These include positions that justify giving priority to environmental policy on the basis that: (1) all human activity depends on the life support provided by the biosphere; (2) there are no ultimate conflicts between environmental and economic objectives; and (3) environmental objectives are entitled to higher ethical standing than economic goals.

Schrecker goes on to review several decision rules that have been proposed for resolving conflicts between human and environmental needs. These rules include those that make distinctions between basic human needs and nonbasic needs, subsistence emissions versus luxury emissions, and levels of per capita income. Schrecker notes that given the wide disparities between the richest and poorest nations, strict application of these rules might lead to kicking the development ladder out from under those poor nations trying to catch up to richer nations.

Schrecker next argues that the best strategy for resolving the dilemma of conflicting economic and environmental goals is to recognize the obligations of the international community and, in particular, the richer nations to compensate those that are generating the environmental benefits. Schrecker acknowledges that such a strategy means accepting that some economic aspirations and claims of distributive justice may compete with environmental protection. Schrecker offers and answers some objections to establishing a compensation regime.

This discussion is concluded by a recognition of the current political improbability of the compensation regime being accepted by the national governments, multinational institutions, and the private investors and investment managers who dominate the emerging global economy. Schrecker foresees a future in which there is further strengthening of environmentally and socially destructive policies worldwide. In the meantime, he argues that further research on economic development policy options and their environmental and distributive consequences on scales ranging from local to transnational is needed. It is Schrecker's belief that such research will generate support for a global regulatory framework "that is people-centered rather than capital-driven," in Richard Falk's words, and that such a framework is a necessary condition for any convincing and ethically defensible vision of environmentally sustainable development.

In chapter 18, "A Complex Systems Approach to Urban Ecosystem Integrity: The Benefit Side," Philippe Crabbé provides an analysis of the human welfare benefits of cities. He claims that increasing urbanization cannot and should not be stopped because human culture has greatly benefited from cities, and cities develop in accordance with rules contained in systems theories.

According to Crabbé, cities are healthy when they are able to learn from their history and create a better quality of life for their inhabitants, for the ecosystems they are located in, and for the people and ecosystems they affect. Principles that follow an ecosystem approach to the city require that cities must be clean (i.e., not impair the uses of ecosystems), green (i.e., protect natural ecosystem functions), usable by people according to diversified tastes, open (i.e., physically accessible and aesthetically inviting), accessible to all, continuous so as not to break the ecosystem artificially, affordable, and attractive, while at the same time valorizing, nature.

Next, Crabbé analyzes the city through the theoretical lens of complex systems theory and then from an urban economics perspective. He believes that both disciplines have important insights on how and why cities prosper and produce benefits.

Against those who argue for limiting the growth of cities, Crabbé argues that as long as private benefits in cities exceed private costs, large migrations to cities will continue. By the year 2000, some 45 percent of the developing world and 75 percent of the developed world were living in cities; reversing this trend is both unfeasible and undesirable, according to Crabbé.

Crabbé notes that economists believe that urban sprawl is the result of hidden subsidies and the consequence of the automobile. The way to control sprawl, according to Crabbé, is road pricing and investments in alternative modes of transportation, such as trains and buses.

Crabbé asserts that people live in cities because of the benefits of living there, which can be great but are not necessarily so. An ecosystem approach to city government requires quite a bit of government intervention through official plans, zoning, protection of essential functions of ecosystems, building codes, investment in transit systems and pollution prevention, taxes and subsidies, education, and so on. Protecting urban ecosystem structure is what can contribute to urban ecosystem integrity.

Finally, Crabbé reacts to those who implicitly criticize cities through a discussion of their ecological footprint. He argues that to the extent that a city's footprint describes an area of a city much larger than the city needs to meets its consumption needs, such description does not, by itself, carry normative consequences given the benefits that are accruing to humans from the existence of cities. Crabbé believes that the footprint, if it is to have normative significance beyond efficiency, must have ethical dimensions of dominance and inequity, whether intergenerational, intragenerational, or spatial.

In chapter 19, "A Biocentric Defense of Environmental Integrity," James P. Sterba develops a biocentric ethical justification of protecting ecosystem integrity. He argues that both humans and nonhuman species and their members count morally. To count morally, Sterba argues, entails that the good of the thing that has moral significance should at least in some circumstances restrain the pursuit of an individual's interest.

Because humans and nonhumans count morally, Sterba argues that protecting ecosystem integrity is instrumentally good for humans because it promotes the good of human and nonhuman species.

As far as moral duties directly to ecosystems, Sterba believes that the moral significance of ecosystems as ecosystems depends on whether one follows the beliefs of those who see ecosystems as: (1) integrated stable wholes that are at or moving toward mature equilibrium states, or (2) subject to constant change and disturbance as the norm. If this latter ecology of disequilibrium is true, Sterba argues that ecosystems do not meet conditions of being morally considerable in themselves even though their protection is justified on moral grounds because of their benefits to humans and nonhuman species.

Sterba therefore agrees that ecosystem integrity should be protected from the perspective of biocentric ethics because ecosystems promote the good of humans, plants, and animals.

In chapter 20, "Commodity Potential: An Approach to Understanding the Ecological Consequences of Markets," Jack P. Manno examines the processes that work to assure that individual and social welfare have been tied increasingly to high levels of material and energy consumption and its accompanying waste products. He goes on to describe the process, termed "commoditization," through which commodities, or commercial goods and services, are systematically privileged over noncommodity, noncommercial means of satisfying human needs and aspirations. This systematic preference amounts to a selection process following Darwinian principles. The process rewards innovations that promote commoditization with investments and research and development funds, and does not reward those innovations that are less commoditized. It drives the evolution of the human economy toward increasing commoditization and a corresponding increase in the mobilization of the Earth's material and energy resources, a trend in the exact opposite direction from what is typically recommended as the path toward sustainable development. Manno's chapter describes the social and political implications of commoditization and offers a definition of oppression as the systematic denial of attention and resources to noncommodity, noncommercial goods and the people who provide them as well as those that depend on them. Manno suggests that by better understanding these dynamics, political theorists and activists can adopt practical strategies and policy tools to move societies toward sustainable development.

Manno stresses that governments must intervene in markets to effectively counterbalance commoditization pressures, and he recommends that policy instruments be designed in the following categories: (1) increased public investment in research and development for noncommodity products; (2) taxes and fees for energy and materials that internalize environmental and social costs; (3) laws that protect ecological integrity; (4) more investment in social and natural capital; (5) tax reforms on labor; (6) abolishing harmful subsidies; (7) protecting workers' rights; and (8) empowering local and indigenous communities.

In chapter 21, "The State of the Planet at the Five-Year Review of Rio and the Prospects for Protecting Worldwide Ecological Integrity," Donald A. Brown reviews the prospects for protecting global ecological integrity in light of recent environmental trends and international cooperation. This chapter first describes the deal struck between the rich and poor countries at the 1992 Earth Summit in Rio de Janeiro. The heart of the deal was the promise on the part of the rich countries to contribute 0.7 percent of gross domestic product to assist the poor countries in complying with the environmental and development provisions in Agenda 21. Other important elements of the North's commitments to the South were provisions that deal with poverty alleviation, reduction of unsustainable consumption patterns, and technology transfer.

Next, Brown discusses positive and negative environmental, economic, and social trends at the five-year review of the Rio summit. This discussion concludes that despite some positive economic and social trends, increasing globalization of the economy was speeding up global deterioration of water resources; land degradation; food production; deterioration of forests, coastal ecosystems (including wetlands, tidal flats, saltwater marshes, mangrove swamps, and coastal nursery areas), fisheries, and biodiversity; waste production; chemical contamination; greenhouse gas buildup; and stratospheric ozone. In summary, increased global economic activity is degrading local, regional, and global ecosystems worldwide.

Brown goes on to assert that a bitter North–South fight over who will pay for sustainable development has been responsible for not only lack of progress since the Rio summit but increasing global ecological degradation. Moreover, the rich countries continue to contribute larger shares of pollution loading at a time when differences in income between rich and poor countries are getting worse.

Brown concludes that unless the North assumes greater responsibility for its unsustainable consumption and production patterns and agrees to help the South financially and technically, degradation of global ecosystems is likely to continue and get worse. Brown states that an honest analysis of worldwide progress made since the Rio summit leads to pessimistic conclusions about the prospects for protecting global ecological integrity.

The Cost of the Wild: International Equity and the Losses from Environmental Conservation

Ted Schrecker

> I am not an exporter. I am a cultivator. I farm rice. These days,
> I don't make enough money from that. . . . So, to me, I can do
> one of three things with these boas. I can leave them alone, and
> not have enough to eat. I can eat them. Or I can sell them to
> people. I make enough from selling one snake to eat for a
> month—or more. What would you choose?
>
> —*Julien, a young Madagascan farmer and collector of endangered*
> *ground boas, quoted by Webster 1997, p. 32*

Julien's situation illustrates tensions between environmental sustainability[1] and the economic aspirations of large numbers of people around the world. Most often, those economic aspirations involve nothing more than the desire either for an adequate money income or for another, comparable source of livelihood. In this chapter I focus on these tensions as they affect the conservation of biological diversity in situ, for several reasons.

Biological diversity is both a crucial component and an indicator of environmental sustainability (see e.g., Holdgate 1996, Smith 1996). Strategies for conserving biological diversity, like those for slowing the pace of global climate change, are likely to entail substantial economic losses to certain groups and regional economies. Concern is in order about justice in the distribution of those losses.

> In general, while there is growing recognition that many of the
> benefits from conserving biodiversity go to the world as a whole,
> in many cases the costs are borne at national and local levels. The
> heaviest burden tends to be borne by poorer countries, and especially by impoverished people living in remote rural areas of these
> poor countries in the proximity of protected areas. (Wells 1992, p.
> 237)

Finally, protection of biological diversity in situ, as distinct from protection in zoos, experimental farms, or gene banks, is a necessary, although not a sufficient, condition for the maintenance of ecological integrity (see e.g., Norton and Ulanowicz 1992, pp. 246–47). Ecological integrity is a considerably more demanding concept than the preservation of biological diversity, because of its "foundational role" (Westra 1995, p. 16) and the restrictions it implies on land use. Thus observations about the tension between economic aspirations and the protection of biological diversity apply with even greater force if ecological integrity is the environmental desideratum of concern. I have used the generic phrase "environmental conservation" to describe efforts to achieve either objective.

In this chapter, I first explore possible tensions between economic aspirations and environmental conservation by way of a hypothetical example, representing a provocative composite of the environmental and economic situations of a number of real countries outside the industrialized world. I then suggest that global economic winners may have an obligation to compensate the losers from environmental conservation, and explore a few objections to this position. I conclude with a rather pessimistic view of the prospects for equitable environmental conservation policies in the current international economy. Although some of my argument is presented in oversimplified form, my objective is not to defend specific answers, but rather to suggest that tensions between economic development and environmental conservation are real, and would present difficult questions of distributive justice even in a world considerably less flawed than the one we live in.

Although I am primarily concerned with economic inequalities between nations, many of the same considerations apply to the distributional implications of environmental conservation measures within nations. Exploring ethical tensions between the two levels of analysis—for example, when environmental protection measures also protect the earnings of workers in the United States against competition from their Mexican counterparts, who can never realistically expect to enjoy either comparable incomes or comparable levels of environmental quality—would unfortunately require a separate paper.

A Revealing Thought Experiment

Consider a hypothetical low-income country, or a region within such a country, which has recently emerged from a period of corrupt and autocratic rule. It is impoverished, lacks hard currency reserves, and has little to offer the international economy apart from (a) cheap labor and (b) rich deposits of copper, substantial tropical forest reserves, or some other resource whose commercialization involves substantial land use and land cover change. The new government is committed both to rapid, broadly shared improvements in human welfare and to being environmentally conscientious. It must therefore simultaneously develop and implement strategies for economic growth, which is urgently needed in order to raise the nutritional, health, and educational status of its population, and for environmental conservation. Cities are growing rapidly, as a result of overall population growth and rural–urban migration. Urbanization goes along with an increased demand for employment and also exacerbates environmental problems that would be considered health emergencies if they occurred in the cities of the industrialized world, as indeed they once did. The money to reduce the severity of these problems, or just to keep them from getting worse, must come from somewhere. In the countryside, deteriorating agricultural productivity as the result of soil degradation has combined with the uncertain state of crop and commodity markets to generate vulnerabilities like the one described in the epigraph to this chapter.

Our hypothetical government is quite correctly committed to the idea that it owes Julien's counterparts answers, and opportunities. How should it reconcile this commitment with conserving biological diversity?

First, it might simply invoke the ultimate dependence of all human activity on the resources and life-support systems provided by the biosphere. Although popularized by the Brundtland Commission (World Commission on Environment and Development 1987), this level of abstraction will be singularly unhelpful, and fails to consider important distributional issues. The poor and otherwise vulnerable are often hurt first, and worst, by environmental damage. However, they may well be hurt even more seriously by policies aimed at preventing it. Thus the mistake made by environmentalists resembles one often made by proponents of cost-benefit analysis of environmental policies. Potential Pareto improvement, defined as the ability of winners to compensate losers while still leaving themselves better off, provides the basic philosophical underpinning for the criterion of economic efficiency (Rescher 1980, Schrecker 1987). Just as demonstrating that a given policy will generate potential welfare gains provides no assurance that the transfers needed to prevent any net loss from the policy will ever actually take place, so presuming that in an ideal world environmental conservation would be compatible with social and economic policies that improve the lot of the poor and vulnerable provides no reason to think that such a happy convergence will actually happen.

Second, our hypothetical government might generalize about the absence of conflicts between environment and development based on numerous individual cases of exhausted fisheries, soils ruined as a result of ill-advised irrigation schemes, and so on. Unfortunately, it would quickly realize that it is an error of logic to infer the absence of such conflicts from any number of specific cases; each case must be considered on its own. Neither can such cases illuminate two critical questions: (a) whether the revenues available from nondestructive land uses such as ecotourism, biodiversity prospecting, or complete preservation could ever compare with those from mining copper or harvesting timber, and (b) how to make such environmentally sensitive management actually happen. Our hypothetical government would need to ask such questions with some urgency while simultaneously learning from past environmental management disasters.

A third approach, environmental absolutism (Schrecker 1998), simply rejects a priori the proposition that the economic aspirations of low-income people might be more pressing than the environmental imperative. Robert Goodland and Herman Daly (1996), for example, proclaim environmental sustainability "universal and nonnegotiable" as a constraint on public policy, although their other work suggests that they might not apply the principle as inflexibly as this formulation would imply. Eric Katz and Lauren Oechsli (1993) concede the importance of distributional considerations, as between the industrialized and developing worlds, but only within the constraints that follow from an "obligation of preservation to nature and its ecosystems," which in turn "makes many of the issues about trade-offs of human goods irrelevant" (Katz and Oechsli 1993, pp. 57–58). In asserting the foundational nature of ecological integrity as an ethical principle, Laura Westra argues that "*all* competing economic, social, and developmental claims should be understood in the context of the primary necessity of large wilderness preservation" (Westra 1995, p. 16, emphasis added) and that "[i]ntegrity must be viewed as the core measure. *Nothing* can be either moral or appropriate to public policy that contravenes the requirements of noninterference and the protection of wild areas and appropriately sized buffers" (Westra 1995, p. 20, emphasis added).

Can one argue that no exceptions exist to the rule that the copper reserves should be simply left in the ground, or the forests left undisturbed, if commercialization would compromise the ecological integrity of the region or imply some reductions in biological diversity? I think not, and if proponents of ecological integrity as an ultimate binding ethical principle do not mean to preclude such developments under all circumstances, some clarification of their position is in order. Indeed, the need for clarification is suggested by Westra's own comment that the principle of integrity "makes the ecosystem both morally considerable and primary, at least in respect to other human preferences and rights, beyond the right to life" (Westra 1993, p. 125). If it is to be ethically meaningful, the right to life means more than the right to be born, move around for a while, and then starve. This means that livelihood and quality of human life have some kind of ethical claim, at least some of the time, against the absolute primacy of ecological integrity.

Perhaps a defensible approach to ethics and public policy should incorporate environmental sustainability as paramount, but only on a prima facie basis. If so, then some criterion is needed for identifying circumstances under which economic aspirations, and the activities that satisfy them, may take precedence over environmental sustainability. Such an approach is embodied in Richard Bishop's proposal for safe minimum standards (SMSs) for conservation of biological diversity. He argues for "avoiding extinction in day-to-day resource management decisions. Exceptions would occur only when it is explicitly decided that costs of avoiding extinction are intolerably large or that other social objectives must take precedence." Biodiversity protection is placed "beyond the reach of routine tradeoffs, but not beyond the reach of all tradeoffs" (Bishop 1993, p. 72).

Many proponents of a biocentric approach to environmental ethics would abhor Bishop's approach, but there is substantial support for it in the philosophical literature. Kristin Shrader-Fréchette (1994, p. 67; see also Donner 1996, p. 65) has noted that "it is impossible to maximize two variables and hence impossible to give priority position both to the biotic community and to human rights." To resolve this problem, she suggests "giving priority to strong human rights over environmental welfare, and to environmental welfare over weak human rights" (Shrader-Fréchette 1994, p. 69). The phrase "human rights" is here used in a broader sense than is customary, to refer to any elements of human welfare that are ethically significant. Shrader-Fréchette's argument becomes more compelling if we define a certain minimum material standard of living, perhaps including environmental quality and adequate income, as a human right in the narrower, more familiar sense. Within a decisionmaking framework of the kind I am suggesting, it is also necessary to distinguish the gravity of various kinds of environmental harms, based in part on their distribution. Avoiding some such harms should command a higher priority than avoiding others. However, my principal concern here is with the question of what might distinguish strong and weak human rights (in Shrader-Fréchette's terminology) or intolerably large costs from tolerable ones (in Bishop's) in the context of environmental policy.

Priority for Basic Needs . . . and More?

The distinction between basic and nonbasic needs occurs frequently within the environmental ethics literature. James Sterba distinguishes between actions necessary for self-defense or for the meeting of basic (human) needs, which he considers justifiable on grounds of preservation "even when they require aggressing against the basic needs of animals and plants," and actions "that meet nonbasic or luxury needs," which are impermissible "when they aggress against the basic needs of animals and plants" (Sterba 1994, pp. 231–32). Henry Shue invokes a distinction between "subsistence emissions and luxury emissions" for purposes of determining how fairly to allocate the costs of slowing global warming and mitigating its consequences, and argues "that it is not equitable to ask some people to surrender necessities so that other people can retain luxuries" (Shue 1993, p. 56). "One person's desire for an additional jar of caviar is not equal in urgency to another person's need for an additional bowl of black beans" (Shue 1996, p. 10). Although skeptics might wonder what should be taken to constitute a basic need, there is more than a hint of sophistry in such queries. Surely we can clearly identify those hundreds of millions of people worldwide whose basic needs, including not only adequate income but also an environment that is not actively destructive of human health, are *not* being met (see e.g., UNDP 1996, pp. 38–42).

Goodland and Daly have quantified the economic dimension of any concept of basic needs, arguing that the aim of development policy should be to provide per capita annual income levels in the lowest-income countries of U.S.$1,500–$2,000, which "may provide 80 percent of the basic welfare provided by a $20,000 income—as measured by life expectancy, nutrition, education and other measures of social welfare" (Goodland and Daly 1996, p. 1004).[2] Their observations might provide the foundation for a basic needs exception to the principle of ecological integrity. That exception would demand a lower standard of environmental care in situations where economic activities that are not environmentally sustainable are essential to raising per capita income to the levels specified by Goodland and Daly, provided (a) that the activities in question do not directly threaten to undermine provision for those needs in the future *and* (b) that there is no other feasible and environmentally preferable way of doing so *within a comparable time frame.*

The first proviso is the conventional definition of sustainable development à la Brundtland, and has been the focus of considerable debate about the extent to which humanmade capital should be taken to substitute for natural capital.[3] The italicized component of the second proviso guards against the rhetoric of short-term pain for long-term gain, recalling Keynes to the effect that in the long run we are all dead, and against the prospect that the interests of today's most vulnerable populations will be sacrificed in order to provide for their counterparts tomorrow.

Critics of such a basic needs exception might reply that averages are misleading, and a per capita annual income of $1,500–$2,000 does not necessarily ensure that basic needs will be met in situations where the distribution of income and wealth is highly unequal. I will return to this point later. First, however, it is worth asking whether basic needs constitute the only economic aspirations that can claim an ethical status in conflicts with desiderata such as environmental sustainability or the protection of ecological integrity. If basic needs of the kind familiar to users of the United Nations Development Program's Human Development Index are being met, then can no further case be made on grounds of economic inequality against keeping the copper reserves or the tropical forest off-limits on environmental grounds? More polemically: having been lifted a bit, should the environmental conservation lid slam shut on economic aspirations once a national income level of $2,000 per capita has been reached, or in countries that are already above that level?

Despite Mark Sagoff's (1996, pp. 6–7) claim that surveys show little connection between income and happiness once basic needs are met, abundant *behavioral* evidence suggests that money matters. People would not be indifferent as between the levels of per capita income in the United States and, say, Mexico (which is a relatively high-income country in the global context) even if the educational status, longevity, and nutrition of the countries' populations were magically to be equalized (Schrecker 1997). The transition to environmental sustainability will, in any economy and society, probably imply some eventual limit on economic output and therefore on income: in other words, some notion of economic sufficiency. It is less clear whether, in the interests of environmental care, Mexicans (or Jamaicans, or Algerians, or Indians) may justifiably be asked to content themselves with incomes a fraction of those in the industrialized world.

We in the industrialized countries can legitimately be accused of wanting to kick the economic ladder down behind us if we demand of others a standard of environmental care that was seldom, if ever, met as the industrialized countries attained their present level of affluence. In the case of global climate change, such questions of fairness arise as they relate not only to the present environmental situation and global distribution of income, but also to the relative contribution of rich and poor countries to the global warming that has already occurred. "The most important contributors to global warming are gases produced by the industrial activities that have made the rich rich. How much should the poor contribute to the solution of a problem caused by activities from which they have not benefitted nearly as much?" (Shue 1996, pp. 13–14).

The argument about kicking the ladder down is extremely difficult to counter, at least until and unless judgments about patterns of consumption and sources of growth in countries outside the industrialized world are "guided by a decreased lifestyle goal that we ourselves are willing to adopt" (Westra 1995, p. 20) and until "we" have shown that willingness in behavior as well as rhetoric. This is not an easy test to meet. The alternative is either (a) to return to the absolutist position that environmental sustainability, ecological integrity, or the conservation of biological diversity is so important that it trumps all concerns about income and wealth distribution, or (b) to presume that existing global inequalities of income and wealth are justified. The policy consequences of the former presumption are unpalatable; the latter presumption converts accidents of birth into the basis for economic entitlements, or exclusion from access to economic entitlements. Such presumptions should always be viewed as suspect, whether they are invoked intra- or internationally (Westra 1993, p. 127; Shue 1996, pp. 11–12).

The Obligations of the International Community

Perhaps the most constructive strategy for responding to the problems raised in my hypothetical case changes the level of analysis, and asks whether the imperative of global environmental conservation may create obligations on the part of the rich countries, individually and as key players in multilateral economic and political institutions. For example, if the benefits from conserving biological diversity are to be pursued as a matter of policy, then "the international community must develop institutions that will channel compensation to those generating these benefits" (Swanson 1992, p. 250), on grounds both of fairness and of political feasibility. The amount of compensation required to make those strategies attractive will vary directly with the stringency of the conservation measures that are contemplated—a point of particular significance in the context of ecological integrity because of the critical role of land-use restrictions (Westra 1995).

The imaginary government in my example is not justified in tolerating gratuitous destruction of the natural environment. It is, however, entitled, perhaps even obligated, to articulate the goals of its environmental conservation policy primarily in economic terms. In other words, although every effort would be made to reconcile conservation priorities with economic development, environmental conservation would need to generate economic returns roughly comparable to those available from other competing land uses, such as mining, over a time frame short enough to be meaningful in terms of improving the lives and life chances of people now alive.

The ethical case for compensating countries outside the industrialized world for economic losses associated with environmental conservation is distinct from the argument that calculations of the total economic value of biological diversity or ecosystem services in a particular region should be incorporated into conservation policy. If they are sufficiently comprehensive, such calculations are both intellectually and strategically valuable because they direct attention to the fact that protecting natural systems and the services they provide, such as watershed protection and carbon sequestra-tion, benefits "the entire global community" (Swanson 1992, p. 250; see also Ehrlich and Ehrlich 1992, Costanza et al. 1997). At the same time, the results are highly indeterminate and probably subject to manipulation. From another perspective, we are intuitively uncomfortable with exercises that attempt such calculations as the "viewing value of elephants" (Brown and Henry 1993, pp. 146–55), and may view these as a cognitively irre-sponsible compression of the priceless, or at least the incompensable, into a framework of monetary values. Such criticisms have considerable ethical force. At the same time, the hard choices that arise when environmental conservation policies may deny substantial numbers of people access to ad-equate livelihood, or may slow their progress out of impoverishment, cannot be wished away.

On this point, "valuation by itself is of little interest to a country owning environmental assets unless they can be turned into revenue flows" (Adger et al. 1995, p. 286; see also Pearce 1991, pp. 48–49). Resistance to intro-ducing any element of economic valuation into environmental policy, based on the claim that elephants (or Siberian tigers, or the remaining forests of Amazonia or British Columbia) are priceless, may just mean that advocates of environmental conservation want to shift its costs to other people rather than sharing in them. Defining the rich countries' obligations to share those costs with reference to *forgone income or revenues* (the opportunity cost of conservation) when the poor or otherwise vulnerable are the economic losers, rather than to the outcomes of academic calculations of total eco-nomic value, brings this issue into focus. The opportunity cost approach does not imply intellectual acceptance of total economic value as a criterion of the worth of protected environments. It does mean accepting that some economic aspirations, and some instances of distributive injustice, generate ethical claims that compete with those of environmental conservation and that include claims on the resources of the rich countries.

What amounts might actually be involved in a policy of compensating the losers from environmental conservation? One recent study on a local scale estimated the annual economic losses to the local subsistence economy following the establishment of a protected area in eastern Madagascar at an average of $49 per household, "which amounts to 18 percent of their total gross income in 1991," or $305,590 in total (Shyamsundar and Kramer 1997). This may be an overestimate of net losses, in that it did not consider the value to local residents of the environmental services provided by the park's forests, but this omission is arguably in keeping with the present chapter's emphasis on equity. Even if such benefits are substantial, surely some of the poorest households in the world should not bear the cost of pre-serving them.

On a national scale, David Pearce (1991) calculated that stopping all mining, mineral processing, logging, and ranching activity in the Brazilian Amazon would have meant forgoing income of $5.8 billion in 1980. Because much economic activity in the Amazon was heavily, and notoriously, subsidized by the Brazilian government, the actual loss in national income associated with putting the tropical forest off-limits would have been substantially lower. On the other hand, increases in the market value of mineral products and tropical timber would increase the opportunity costs of forest preservation, unless comparable increases occurred in the anticipated revenue flows from alternative uses.

Similar calculations for other kinds of land-use restrictions would be extremely useful, for two reasons. First, they would underscore the point that fair worldwide application of any demanding regime of environmental conservation, in the context of a wildly unequal distribution of income and wealth, requires very substantial economic transfers from rich to poor. Second, they would provide a basis for provocative comparisons between the costs involved and such figures as the amounts that national governments routinely spend on weapons and preparations for war.[4]

Objections to Compensation

The logistical and administrative problems of establishing a compensation regime, and ensuring compliance with the terms of compensation agreements, are formidable. In this section, I make the (perhaps heroic) assumption that they could be dealt with adequately, and instead outline a few conceptual objections and try to respond to them.

First, it could be said that my focus on forgone income simply replicates the environmentally destructive short-termism exemplified by Canada's destruction of the North Atlantic cod fishery; neglects all the lessons learned in the process; and disregards options for environmentally sustainable economic development that would simultaneously improve the lot of the poorest people in a particular economy. For reasons already outlined, development policy cannot assume that such win-win outcomes are achievable. Consequently, the presumption against environmentally damaging activity cannot defensibly be regarded as absolute. Short-termism—including widespread destruction of natural capital during the early stages of industrialization—has paid very well indeed for most people in the industrialized economies. Quite apart from the wealth of individual households, it has financed the creation of a tremendously valuable infrastructure. We in the industrialized world have not so far been noticeably eager either to share the spoils or to participate in the creation of comparable infrastructure elsewhere in the world on anything other than a strictly self-interested basis. Since the global distribution of income and wealth now generates "an extreme inequality in life prospects that cries out for either change or justification" (Shue 1996, p. 12), the reply that lurks as a subtext in a lot of contemporary environmental discourse is: it's not a fair world, but we got there first. This is simply not good enough. Indeed, rejecting this reply is at the heart of the argument for compensation, and is why the primary focus should be on preventing environmental damage *and* compensating for forgone income streams.

Second, the entire theme of compensation might be objected to, on the grounds that no compensation is owed those who engage in environmentally destructive activities in order to earn an income; many people do not do so, and they (we?) are simply better people. This objection is a variant of the "let them work in ecotourism" (at lower wages) position of affluent urban environmentalists, whose commitment to stopping industrial projects that represent a major potential source of employment is unmatched by a commitment to alternative economic development strategies that would generate comparable opportunities. Such claims of moral authority are tenuous even as applied to environmental politics in rich countries, and even more tenuous in the global context. This is not to say that ethical judgments about the ways income is earned are off-limits. We may and must condemn the global weapons trade as a source of livelihood, although this is not the same as condemning all its employees. We may and must distinguish revenues from resource development projects that would flow to residents of nearby communities, or be invested in a universally accessible national health and education infrastructure, from those that would swiftly return to foreign corporate treasuries or be appropriated by local elites. However, just as "we got there first" is an unsatisfactory response to concerns about international economic inequality, so "there are better ways to earn a living" is an unsatisfactory justification for cutting off the livelihoods of people with few real choices.

Third and most compelling is an objection based on intranational inequalities in income and power. Although the well-meaning think about countries outside the industrialized world as relatively homogeneous collections of the poor, with a few desperate exceptions nothing could be further from the truth. Income inequalities are often even more pronounced than in the industrialized world, reflecting and reinforcing concentrations of political and military power. In the world as it now is, compensation paid to national governments for revenues lost through the adoption of conservation strategies might just invite the establishment of a high-stakes protection racket. The money might quickly find its way into the investment portfolios of political elites, as is often the case with transfers of other kinds, while no protection would be provided for the livelihoods of those beneficiaries whose situation gives the argument for compensation its ethical force.

The argument for compensation, as made here, is rooted in an egalitarianism that assigns highest priority to the meeting of basic needs. This objection therefore leads us into a more general discussion of the responsibilities of governments rulers and the context in which they operate. Ideally, all governments would resemble the imaginary one described earlier in this chapter in their commitment to widely shared improvements in living standards. However, my imaginary government was exactly that. Outcomes in real political systems emerge from an ongoing series of exchanges between governments and various actors in the societies they rule, in which the primary (although not the only) motivation is self-interest. The actors' importance depends on the resources they command; the resources that are most important vary, but money is consistently at or near the top of the list. Furthermore, the basic process of exchange is remarkably constant across time, space, and variations in political institutions. Even in formally democratic states, "[p]oliticians generally know whom they must regard as important and whom they can afford to neglect" (Caldwell 1990, p. 88).

Environmentally destructive development need not be countenanced, and offers to compensate for forgone revenues probably should not be made, when most of the revenues from development will be appropriated by gangster rulers, extremely large-scale landowners, or corporate shareholders half a world away. Compensation should be contingent on a credible case that substantial and widely shared improvements in the conditions of life, with special emphasis on the meeting of basic needs, would have been associated with the development that is being restricted in the pursuit of conservation objectives. Tragically, stating the issue in these terms risks setting the standard for compensation so high that few governments could meet it, meaning that they would simply opt for business as usual. This is a particularly serious problem unless some way can be devised of incorporating negative as well as positive reinforcement into an international conservation regime—for example, by combining compensation for income lost as a result of environmental conservation measures with environmental conditions attached to other forms of development assistance, or with trade sanctions against nations whose stance toward conservation is particularly recalcitrant. Even to state these options is to suggest the magnitude of the political task that would be involved. Furthermore, as when trade sanctions are linked to environmental or social performance standards, the risk is that the most vulnerable people in a jurisdiction will be the ultimate losers from the actions of rulers they did not choose and cannot safely resist.

Conclusion: Fragile Prospects
for Environmental Conservation

The basic weakness of the approach I have outlined here is not ethical, but rather political. The recent policies of national governments, multinational institutions, and the private investors and investment managers who dominate the emerging global economy have been generally hostile to concerns for distributive justice. Almost two decades of "structural adjustment" often lowered the incomes of the poor and eroded their already precarious nutritional and health status (Cornia 1987, Stewart 1991), but succeeded in imposing a market discipline consistent with the needs and norms of the global economy. Countries that survived structural adjustment are now open for business; they have few other choices.

As fluid, high-velocity, cross-border networks of trade and capital flows start to create a global labor market (World Bank 1995), analogous competitive pressures are transforming the economies of many industrialized countries. Consequently, economic inequality is increasing both within and among nations (UNDP 1999, pp. 25–76). In the future, distinctions between rich and poor countries may be blurred (Mead 1992; Freeman 1997, p. 142). Relentless downward pressure on wages, working conditions, and social safety nets will be the rule for much of the population. Simultaneously, the rich, regardless of where in the world they live, will become truly cosmopolitan as transnational corporations reorganize production across national borders and high-income households allocate their assets among financial markets with comparable ease.

The probable drift in public policy can be inferred from welfare "reforms" that reduce or eliminate access to income outside the labor market, and that are justified with reference to keeping costs down in a global economy (see e.g., Sachs 1996). Politically significant constituencies for policies of making up the income losses associated with environmental conservation are unlikely to emerge in the industrialized countries. More probable is the further strengthening of quietly self-interested support for environmentally and socially destructive, but profitable, policies elsewhere in the world. The repeated repudiation of efforts to link the industrialized countries' trade and investment policy with human rights concerns, even when the governments in question are singularly brutal, dramatically illustrates the importance of the "what's in it for me?" test in explaining both political allegiances and public policy. We all need to be reminded of this fundamental principle of political economy in all its variants, because at least two prerequisites exist for achieving environmental sustainability on equitable terms.

Ethically, distributions of economic and political power that lead to the

valuation of ground boas in terms of their price on the collector market and
to the valuation of people in terms of their worth in the emerging global
labor market must both be viewed as obscene, and for similar reasons. Politically, effective support needs to be found for "a regulatory framework for
global market forces that is people-centered rather than capital-driven"
(Falk 1996, p. 13). In the foreseeable future, neither set of commitments appears likely to command support among those who must, in Caldwell's formulation, be regarded as important. This category currently leaves out most
of the world's population.

NOTES

1. In this chapter I follow Goodland and Daly (1996) and Westra (1995, p. 15) in
   distinguishing environmental sustainability from social or economic sustainability. I use "environmental conservation" as a general term to describe policy
   measures that are aimed at maintaining, or moving toward, environmental sustainability.
2. By way of providing context, a per capita annual income of $1,500–$2,000
   falls into the lower middle income range in the World Bank's most recent statistical tables; in 1994 Jamaica, Paraguay, Algeria, Ukraine, and Namibia fell
   into this income range. Peru was just above it, but $2,000 is less than half Mex-
   ican per capita annual income in 1994 (World Bank 1996, pp. 188–89, all figures unadjusted for purchasing power).
3. For a succinct review see Pearce and Atkinson (1995).
4. For example, the U.S. stealth bomber program *alone* will cost over $44 billion,
   for 21 warplanes that cannot be left out in the rain (United States General Accounting Office 1997).

ACKNOWLEDGMENTS

Research was partly supported by Social Sciences and Humanities Research
Council of Canada grant 806-93-0002.

REFERENCES

Adger, W.N., K. Brown, R. Cervigni, and D. Moran. 1995. "Total Economic
    Value of Forests in Mexico." *Ambio* 24: 286–296.
Bishop, R. 1993. "Economic Efficiency, Sustainability, and Biodiversity." *Ambio* 22
    (no. 2–3, May): 69–73.
Brown, G. and W. Henry. 1993. "The Viewing Value of Elephants." In *Economics
    and Ecology: New Frontiers for Sustainable Development,* edited by E. Barbier,
    146–155. London: Chapman and Hall.
Caldwell, L. 1990. *Between Two Worlds: Science, the Environmental Movement, and
    Policy Choice.* Cambridge: Cambridge University Press.
Cornia, G. 1987. "Economic Decline and Human Welfare in the First Half of the

1980s." In *Adjustment with a Human Face,* vol. 1, *Protecting the Vulnerable and Promoting Growth,* edited by G. Cornia, R. Jolly, and F. Stewart, 11–47. Oxford: Clarendon Press.

Costanza, R. et al. 1997. "The Value of the World's Ecosystem Services and Natural Capital." *Nature* 387: 253–260.

Donner, W. 1996. "Inherent Value and Moral Standing in Environmental Change." In *Earthly Goods: Environmental Change and Social Justice,* edited by F. Hampson and J. Reppy, 52–74. Ithaca, NY: Cornell University Press.

Ehrlich, P. and A. Ehrlich. 1992. "The Value of Biodiversity." *Ambio* 21: 219–226.

Falk, R. 1996. "An Inquiry into the Political Economy of World Order." *New Political Economy* 1: 13–26.

Freeman, R. 1997. "Does Globalization Threaten Low-Skilled Western Workers?" In *Working for Full Employment,* edited by J. Philpott, 132–150. London: Routledge.

Goodland, R. and H. Daly. 1996. "Environmental Sustainability: Universal and Non-negotiable." *Ecological Applications* 6: 1002–1017.

Holdgate, M. 1996. "The Ecological Significance of Biological Diversity." *Ambio* 25: 409–416.

Katz, E. and L. Oechsli. 1993. "Moving beyond Anthropocentrism: Environmental Ethics, Development, and the Amazon." *Environmental Ethics* 15, Spring: 49–59.

Mead, W.R. 1992. "Bushism, Found: A Second-Term Agenda Hidden in Trade Agreements." *Harper's Magazine,* September: 37–45.

Norton, B. and R. Ulanowicz. 1992. "Scale and Biodiversity Policy: A Hierarchical Approach." *Ambio* 21: 244–249.

Pearce, D. 1991. "Deforesting the Amazon: Toward an Economic Solution." *Ecodecision* 1: 40–49.

Pearce, D. and G. Atkinson. 1995. "Measuring Sustainable Development." In *The Handbook of Environmental Economics,* edited by D. Bromley, 166–181. Cambridge, MA: Blackwell.

Rescher, N. 1980. "Economics versus Moral Philosophy: The Pareto Principle as a Case Study." In *Unpopular Essays on Technological Progress,* 69–78. Pittsburgh: University of Pittsburgh Press.

Sachs, J. 1996. "The Social Welfare State and Competitiveness." In *The Global Competitiveness Report 1996,* 20–26. World Economic Forum, Geneva.

Sagoff, M. 1996. "On the Value of Endangered and Other Species." *Environmental Management* 20 (no. 6): 1–16.

Schrecker, T. 1987. "Risks versus Rights: Economic Power and Economic Analysis in Environmental Politics." In *Business Ethics in Canada,* edited by D. Poff and W. Waluchow, 265–285. Scarborough, ON: Prentice-Hall Canada.

Schrecker, T. 1997. "Money Matters: A Reality Check, with Help from Virginia Woolf." *Social Indicators Research* 40: 99–123.

Schrecker, T. 1998. "Sustainability, Growth and Distributive Justice: Questioning Environmental Absolutism." In *Sustainability and Ecological Integrity: Concepts and Approaches,* edited by J. Lemons, L. Westra, and R. Goodland, 218–234. Dordrecht: Kluwer.

Shrader-Fréchette, K. 1994. "Sustainability and Environmental Ethics." In *The Notion of Sustainability*, edited by G. Skirbakk, 57–78. Oslo: Scandinavian University Press.

Shue, H. 1993. "Subsistence Emissions and Luxury Emissions." *Law and Policy Quarterly* 15: 39–59.

Shue, H. 1996. "Environmental Change and the Varieties of Justice." In *Earthly Goods: Environmental Change and Social Justice*, edited by F. Hampson and J. Reppy, 9–29. Ithaca, NY: Cornell University Press.

Shyamsundar, P. and R. Kramer. 1997. "Biodiversity Conservation—At What Cost? A Study of Households in the Vicinity of Madagascar's Mantadia National Park." *Ambio* 26: 180–184.

Smith, F. 1996. "Biological Diversity, Ecosystem Stability and Economic Development." *Ecological Economics* 16: 191–203.

Sterba, J. 1994. "Reconciling Anthropocentric and Nonanthropocentric Environmental Ethics." *Environmental Values* 3: 229–244.

Stewart, F. 1991. "The Many Faces of Adjustment." *World Development* 19: 1847–1864.

Swanson, T. 1992. "Economics of a Biodiversity Convention." *Ambio* 21: 250–257.

UNDP (United Nations Development Program). 1996. *Human Development Report 1996*. Oxford and New York: Oxford University Press.

UNDP (United Nations Development Program). 1999. *Human Development Report 1999*. Oxford and New York: Oxford University Press.

United States General Accounting Office. 1997. *B-2 Bomber: Cost and Operational Issues*, GAO/NSIAD-97-181. Washington, DC: U.S. GAO.

Webster, D. 1997. "The Looting and Smuggling and Fencing and Hoarding of Impossibly Precious, Feathered and Scaly Wild Things." *New York Times Magazine*, February 16: 26–33, 48–53, 61.

Wells, M. 1992. "Biodiversity Conservation, Affluence and Poverty: Mismatched Costs and Benefits and Efforts to Remedy Them." *Ambio* 21: 237–243.

Westra, L. 1993. "The Ethics of Environmental Holism and the Democratic State: Are They in Conflict?" *Environmental Values* 2: 125–136.

Westra, L. 1995. "Ecosystem Integrity and Sustainability: The Foundational Value of the Wild." In *Perspectives on Ecological Integrity*, edited by L. Westra and J. Lemons, 12–32. Dordrecht: Kluwer.

World Bank. 1995. *World Development Report 1995: Workers in an Integrating World*. New York: Oxford University Press.

World Bank. 1996. *World Development Report 1996: From Plan to Market*. New York: Oxford University Press.

World Commission on Environment and Development (the Brundtland Commission). 1987. *Our Common Future*. New York: Oxford University Press.

A Complex Systems Approach to Urban Ecosystem Integrity: The Benefit Side

Philippe Crabbé

City benefits, the focus of this chapter, are interpreted here in an anthropocentric perspective. Hierarchical holism (Shrader-Fréchette 1997) is difficult to apply to cities because most of the benefits of the city result from weak human rights (unrelated to human survival). Rural migrations to cities, however, are influenced by labor-saving technological progress that forces people out of rural employment into the manufacturing or service sectors, which are located in cities. Other city benefits are diversity (a weak human right) as a manifestation of self–organization, and some spillover effects, i.e., benefits that cannot be appropriated by individuals.

Cities are ecosystems. They exchange energy, matter, and information with their environment. They are high–density human settlements in built environments. They are healthy when they are able to learn from their history and create a better quality of life—as judged by humans—for their inhabitants, for the ecosystems they are located in, and for the people and ecosystems they affect. Ecosystem health is what connects cities to nature. They grow, decay, and become extinct out of competition for survival with the qualitative properties of predator–prey ecological models and exhibit dampened oscillatory motion about their carrying capacity, which may change abruptly for cities endowed with relatively old infrastructures. Their survival depends upon their endowed resources and the population (labor) they are able to attract through the incomes they are able to provide. Incomes grow through innovations, and otherwise decline (Jacobs 1969, Dendrinos 1983). The degree of connectedness of urban ecosystems is relatively independent of the size of their population (Lees and Hohenberg 1988). The reasons for their location are sometimes obvious, by necessity—a natural harbor, for example—and sometimes fortuitous, by chance. Urban economics tends to focus on the first—necessity—at least since von Thünen (1826), while complex systems thinking tends to focus on the latter—

chance—at least since A. Weber (1909) (Arthur 1995). The systems concepts of central place (Christaller 1933) or gateway city (Burghardt 1971), which originated in the geography literature, belong to the urban economics paradigm, while the network concept (Braudel 1966) overlaps with both systems thinking and urban economics (Lees and Hohenberg 1988).

The prejudice that cities develop at the expense of the countryside finds its origin in the physiocrats. It was carried to North America by the agrarian movements, which wanted farmers to cooperate, thereby avoiding supporting "unproductive" urban classes, "monopolies," and "middlemen." The agrarian movements failed to some extent because of lack of understanding of the concepts of "central place" or "network" (Cronon 1991, pp. 360–64).[1]

Cities are part of nature. "A city's history must also be the history of its human countryside, and of the natural world within which city and country are both located"(Cronon 1991, p. 19). In the United States, the "Boosters" tradition emphasized the "symbiotic relationship" between cities and their environment (Cronon 1991, p. 34). The location of cities depends upon the availability of natural capital: natural resources, transportation routes, and favorable climatic conditions, factors to which one might add demographic trends and some gravitational interpretation (Cronon 1991, pp. 36–41).

We have in Canada a splendid illustration of the ecosystem approach as applied to cities in the report *Regeneration* (Royal Commission 1992). A city is located in an ecosystem and interacts with air (pollution, noise), land (alternative agricultural uses and landfills) and water (drinking, wastewater), and the local flora and fauna. Urban and nearby parks, forests, greenbelts, rivers, and lakes are what connects the city to the wild. *Regeneration* refers to integrity both in the definition of the ecosystem approach and in its definition of the endpoints for rehabilitation. The principles for an ecosystem approach to the city are that cities must not impair ecosystem functions and must be usable by people according to diversified tastes, physically accessible, affordable, and attractive while valorizing natural beauty (Royal Commission 1992). Ecological integrity, besides ecosystem health, also means the ability for the ecosystem to withstand stress and to continue to self–organize (Kay and Schneider 1994).

This chapter will focus on the benefit side of cities viewed from two complementary perspectives. The first one is the complex systems perspective, which emphasizes the roles of both chance and necessity in urban systems: processes, creative random factors, path-dependence (history matters), hierarchical structures, positive feedbacks, adaptation, learning, and innovation; the second one is the urban economics perspective, which emphasizes the deterministic aspects of city formation and growth while focusing on equilibrating mechanisms (negative feedbacks), optimization, economies of scale, and spillover effects.

Attempts at stopping the growth of large cities go back at least to Plutarch and failed without exception. Schemes to make agriculture more attractive through subsidies led to more migration to the cities because they led to more labor-saving agricultural improvements (Montroll and Badger 1974). Moreover, rural people tend to migrate "for the reason that all the opportunities for rising in the world are in the cities" (Weber 1899).

As projected, in the year 2000, 45 percent of the population of the less developed world and 75 percent of the developed one live in cities (Alberti and Susskind 1996). Reversing this trend is both unfeasible and undesirable.

As long as benefits of city living exceed its costs, whether actual or perceived, migration to cities will continue. Both benefits—in terms of consumption of private goods and services and in terms of income—and costs—in terms of search for jobs and commodities—may be private. Benefits and costs may no longer be privately borne by individuals but may also become social benefits and costs when other individuals may not be prevented from sharing in these benefits and are able to shirk the costs. Thus, even though private benefits may not exceed costs, net benefits of city living might still be positive if social benefits or amenities exceed these costs. This may explain why cities, through their social amenities, attract a marginal population that is not earning income but that reaps higher net benefits than it would if it were living elsewhere.

Higher incomes earned by firms in large cities are indications that firms obtain some cost advantage in an urban environment. Since incomes seem to be correlated with the size of the city, there appear to be competitive advantages for firms based on city size (Bradfield 1988).

Complex and Mechanical Approaches to the City as a Human System

Human systems are neither mechanical nor statistical systems. They are middle number systems, the domain of organized complexity (Weaver 1948, Weinberg 1975), purposeful systems (Ackhoff 1972), soft systems (Checkland 1981). Urban systems are therefore complex systems in which one emphasizes processes (urbanization), behavior (change), and positive feedbacks (growth). Complex systems thinking acknowledges that the world, the city, is too rich to be understood by one approach only, say, urban economics. Complex systems thinking emphasizes hierarchical systems, i.e., systems composed of stable (observable) subsystems unified by some ordering relationships through echelons. Upper echelons control or offer the context for lower echelons; the former coordinate the goals of the latter. Context or structure remains relatively constant while the system exhibits behavior. Context is the main source of the system's integrity. Hierarchical systems require communication or information transfers among echelons. Complex systems thinking requires fine details at the low-level echelons because small details end up being amplified to have large outcomes (chaotic behavior and positive feedbacks); in other words, low-level detail can exert an influence on high echelons, thereby affecting the behavior of the whole system. Details do not disappear through averaging. Complexity involves relating structure and processes that are observed at different scales. The scale of observation depends upon the spatial and temporal measurement protocols (Ahl and Allen 1996).

One way to handle the difficulty of human systems is to deny the reality of choices and use the mechanistic analogy of classical physics. This is what neoclassical economics does with *Homo oeconomicus*. If one knows an individual's utility function, one can predict that person's behavior; behavior is deterministic. Since we cannot observe utility functions, one must infer the latter from observed behavior, and "circularity" creeps into the reasoning: individuals behave in a certain way because they maximize utility, and utility must be such because a certain behavior has been observed. When human systems are treated as mechanical systems, their components are classified by average types, i.e., within a given type, all individuals are assumed identical. Predictions are made by simply running the model forward in time, and the unique final state of the system is deemed inevitable. It is the point attractor of the system that expresses some optimum (a state of maximum per capita consumption). Economics focuses on equilibrium (a negative feedback) and its stability and optimality properties (Allen 1982).

The German industry location school since von Thünen still provides the standard neoclassical explanation for the formation of cities (the bid rent function). Cities are by necessity the consequence of geography, transportation costs, factor endowment, industry needs, and the induced spatial distribution of prices and rents; they are point attractors. Cities shape their countryside landscape by the values their inhabitants confer to the products of the soil and by the cost of bringing these products to markets (Cronon 1991, p. 50). However, according to neoclassical economics, history is irrelevant to explain their formation.

Ecological and human systems are in constant dialogue with their environment. They maintain their capacity to evolve, even if they are not evolving, drawing on the diversity of their components. The focus for these systems is on change, evolution, and instability rather than on rest, equilibrium, and stability, the central concern of economics. While economics focuses on efficiency (optimization), actual human agents do focus on learning, i.e., on generating new information. Complex systems are unable to be optimal because of random elements that cannot be averaged out. Economics focuses on negative feedbacks (dampening mechanisms), while complex systems thinking concentrates on positive feedbacks (reinforcing mechanisms), which are essential to insure persistence, survival, and growth in an unstable world. While economics pursues the positivistic epistemology of reductionist sciences, the epistemology of complex systems is definitely constructivist; there is no separation between the observer and the observed (recursiveness), and the approach is definitely teleological and process oriented.

Another way to handle the difficulty of human systems is to acknowledge that choices are equivalent to bifurcations in nonlinear dynamic systems, i.e., that identical environments may lead to different possible structures represented by an evolutionary tree. The evolution is neither totally deterministic, as assumed in neoclassical economics and classical physics, nor totally stochastic, but a composite of the two. When the system is near a bifurcation, it may become relatively unstable. Weak perturbations that may be random will bring the system on one branch rather than on another one. While moving along a branch, the system behaves in a deterministic fashion and is predictable, but only for an unpredictable time; when it faces a bifurcation point, it behaves stochastically because of "historical accidents" and is unpredictable (Prigogine et al. 1977). According to Nicolis and Prigogine,

> Starting from a space where variables are initially distributed at random, we observe the gradual emergence of an organized pattern with its own administrative and business centers, its industrial zones, its shopping centers and its residential neighbourhoods of varying qualities. In the absence of massive disturbances, the pattern remains stable indefinitely. The spontaneous symmetry breaking is very similar to the formation of spatial structures in hydrodynamics and chemical kinetics. . . . A very interesting result from the model is the following. If a new activity is launched at a certain time, it will grow and stabilize. If the place is well chosen, it may even prevent the success of similar attempts made nearby at a later time. However, if the same activity is launched at a different time, it need not succeed; it may regress and represent a total loss. (1989, pp. 241–42)

Macrostructures such as cities are no longer explained in a reductionist fashion by the simple aggregation of microstructures such as economic agents. Cities are emergent structures. Moreover, the city performs a function: it is a problem–solver (Tainter 1988).[2] Cities and economic agents are rather mutually consistent entities. Cooperative structures can emerge from competitive behavior among individuals, as in Axelrod's indefinitely repeated prisoner's dilemma (Axelrod 1984). Economic competitive behavior is analogous to political conflict resolution resulting from differential economic success, while cooperative behavior is analogous to political integration, which is concerned with the well-being of the total populace (Tainter 1988). Increasing cooperation and complementarity rather than competition leads to a successful community. Cooperation concentrates people and activities, while competition spreads things out spatially (Arthur 1995).

Branches of an evolutionary tree are qualitatively different from each other in terms of characteristics and dimensionality. Therefore, even if the initial state of organization of the city is quite simple, it may become extremely complicated through several bifurcations generated by successive instabilities. Since branches of an evolutionary tree are qualitatively different, they will be perceived differently by various components of the system. Various parts of the system will evaluate branches differently, and their evaluations cannot be aggregated.

The complex systems approach requires that we plan the city as a generic model since various bifurcations will represent various structures which are part of the possible futures of the city. The actual city is one possible future or structure of the city. These structures might be new centers for the city, new congestion points, or new transportation roads. Instability at the bifurcation points will be of a spatial nature. The model is a nested hierarchy. It has fractal qualities; it will form a hierarchy of spatial scales from the world all the way down to the neighborhood. The hierarchical levels interact according to economic conditions, whether of a competitive or complementary nature. Cities are systems within a hierarchical system of cities (Berry 1964). This does not mean that cities keep occupying the same level in the hierarchy over time, as the central place theory would have it; the hierarchy may change according to circumstances (Cronon 1991). Two important concepts for understanding the city as a problem–solving complex system are unequal access to resources and heterogeneity under the guise of multiple hierarchies, which both tend to increase with information needs and diversification (Tainter 1988).

Therefore, evolution is understood as a dialectical relationship between the deterministic equations of movement that express the average behavior of individual agents and a series of perturbations coming from outside the model. Stochasticity is no longer a minor deviation from the average, from the prediction; it changes the state of organization of a structure. Stochasticity is the "Élan vital" (Bergson 1907) of change. In human systems, stochasticity results from "bounded rationality," irrationality, uncommon local conditions (fire, flood), and simply from the desire to be different. Therefore, the adaptive potential of a system is bound by its heritage of variety. Innovation results from the momentary occurrence of the uncommon leading the system to completely new average behaviors. Unusual, irrational, creative behaviors from individuals may lead to the long-run survival of the system. Without them, the system becomes fossilized and crumbles. Evolution may not necessarily be progress, though (Allen and Sanglier 1979; Allen 1982, 1986, 1990, 1992, 1994; Allen and McGlade 1987). On the other hand, stochasticity can be excessive and exceed the ability of the city to cope with stress. To the extent that a city is hierarchical, it will not collapse completely under excessive stress but will simply regress to a previous stage of organization (Simon 1962, Ahl and Allen 1996).

The city is no longer the outcome of economic necessity—the "Boosters" compared a city to an organism subject to natural laws of origin and growth (Cronon 1991, p. 35)—but the outcome of the more or less random location of early industries to which others are attracted because of complementarities and positive feedbacks. History of random events has become all important. The actual city is a nonunique strange attractor; had history been different, the actual city could have located somewhere else at another strange attractor (Arthur 1995). Both chance and necessity contribute to the city's ability to self-organize even as a subsystem of an ecosystem. Which ecosystem changes due to the presence of the city are acceptable are ultimately a matter of human judgment (Kay and Schneider 1994). The ecosystem itself, in the complex systems approach, reflects the values and mental maps of its modeler.

The Main Economic Characteristics of the City

There are three strands of economic literature dealing with the city. First, there is the competitive market theory of neoclassical economics, which sees the expansion of the city as the result of market forces and looks favorably upon the spread effects of large cities upon their periphery. Second, there is the dominant firm theory, which leads to the growth pole development theory. Finally, there is the core-periphery dependency theory with a Marxian perspective, which rejects the neoclassical analysis (Bradfield 1988).

The first strand of literature explains what is happening on the branches of the urban system evolutionary tree. The second and third may contribute to the explanation of what happens at bifurcation points.

The neoclassical literature considers the city as part of a network system.

The city serves international trade mainly through economic specialization. Specialization occurs because of economies of scale, i.e., decreasing per-unit costs with increased production. Several specialized activities are located in the same city because of agglomeration, urbanization, and localization economies, and because of complementarities among products (see *infra*; Lees and Hohenberg 1988).

The growth pole theory views dominant industries as transforming the cities in which they are located. They become the development poles of their region through positive feedbacks. For Perroux (1955), dominance consists of an irreversible or only partially reversible influence exercised by one economic unit on another because of its dimension, its negotiating strength, the nature of its activity, or because it belongs to a zone of dominant activity. The dominant firm tends to be large and oligopolistic (a few producers only in an industry) and exerts considerable influence on the activities of the suppliers and clients. Dominance is exerted in economic space, i.e., on the set of linked industries rather than on geographical space. In other words, growth centers (geographical space) should not be confused with growth poles (economic space). Growth centers, according to neoclassical theory, result from linked industries (industrial complexes) and because of urban(ization) scale economies generated by unrelated firms (Bradfield 1988).

Finally, there is the third strand of literature, which holds that core regions are able to impose organized dependency on their periphery. The development of core regions leads to the underdevelopment of the periphery (Bradfield 1988).

Therefore, economic specialization, dominance, and dependency effects, with their positive feedbacks in terms of power, all play a role on both the cost and the benefit side of cities. For example, the ability of firms located in big cities to pay higher wages may be due to economies resulting from specialization and to unions that are able to share in the oligopoly profits of dominant firms (Bradfield 1988) as well as in the ability of the core to weaken the periphery.

A city has eight main economic characteristics:

1. A city is located on land at one location only, and land, though it is a commodity, is immobile; therefore, economic agents hold preferences on locations; they select either one or another but cannot select several at the same time. This trivial remark has important consequences for economic analysis. While economic analysis focuses on decreasing returns and negative feedbacks, it must now, when applied to cities, focus on increasing returns and positive feedbacks, as is done in complex systems. In order to handle the mathematical difficulties of the problem,

two assumptions are made. First, each household selects one and only one location. Second, as is typical in mechanical models, there are many households of each type. These two assumptions allow the use of the bid rent function, which transforms the usual commodity space into urban space (with dimensions, location, and land rent). The bid rent function represents the ability to pay per unit of land.

When an economic activity takes place in a city, it generates direct revenues (employment) to those who partake in the activity and indirect ones to those from whom those who partake in activities have purchased. This so-called multiplier effect is subject to leakages according to the proportion of income spent in the city and the balance that is spent elsewhere. The more one spends in the city, the more closed the city economy is. Regional growth is demand determined. Supply, when factors are freely mobile, adjusts to demand (Armstrong and Taylor 1985, p. 65).

2. Economic activities in cities will endure as long as their private benefits exceed their private costs. Regional policies are an amalgam of subsidies to firms and other actors, of controls and investments. Without a full-fledged input–output model, it is difficult to evaluate social benefits and costs of regional policies because of their multiplier effect throughout the economy. Increased output is the main benefit and forgone output the main cost of a regional policy. Another benefit of a regional policy is the decrease in external diseconomies (see *infra*). Reduced migration is yet another benefit.

3. The city is a network of complementary activities that may be described by an input–output table. The structure of the table describes the structure of the economy. An interesting case is one in which the table is nearly a block diagonal. Activities within the block have some relations with activities outside the block, but they are sparse. This could explain the concept of an economic neighborhood within a city. Another case would be one where the input–output table is triangular—one activity interacts with all others in a strictly hierarchical fashion. A one-industry town would be of this type. All activities would ultimately depend on the one industry, but the industry would, for example, export its products outside the city. The city would be highly vulnerable to the vagaries of this industry. A final case is that of a highly connected network (the input–output table has almost no zero element) of activities in which all activities could depend on nearly all others. This is a more realistic description of the large modern city.

Modern technology has made bunched-up complementary activities the basis for the definition of an industry. For example, the information industry, the entertainment industry, the tourism industry, and the finance industry all have in common a shared infrastructure. These industries are like multiproduct firms. Therefore, an industry is now a set of firms that produce complementary products.

4. The city generates positive and negative network effects and externalities (agglomeration, localization, and urbanization) as well as club goods (defined below). Externalities are interactions among economic agents that are not the object of market transactions or for which agents are not fully compensated, such as the availability of a wide choice of goods and services (positive externality) or crowding, noise, and other forms of pollution (negative externality). Externalities often result from economies of scale that are external to firms. For example, a large concentration of computer-literate workers in a city results from the large number of computer firms located in the city.

Public goods are indivisible goods from the consumption of which no agent can be excluded and whose consumption does not decrease their availability to others. Public goods may confer benefits (availability of a wide choice of goods and services) or costs (noise) like externalities. Public goods, however, affect all economic agents, while externalities could be limited to just one. A sonic boom versus a loud apartment sound system could illustrate the difference. Public goods may harm some individuals while providing benefits to others. Billboards advertising smoking may be of this nature.

Club goods have all the characteristics of public goods except that their consumption is purely voluntary; they are unable to harm anybody because one can avoid them by moving out of the location in which the (local) public good is provided. Club theory is concerned with the formation of spatially optimal consumption (sharing) and production groups, their characteristics, and their sustainability under a competitive market regime. A club is defined as a voluntary group deriving mutual and excludable benefit from sharing production costs, members' characteristics, and/or excludable goods. Urban economics nowadays represents urban structures as systems of independent spatial–club agglomerations at specific locations along a strip of land. By doing so, it merges the local public goods tradition with the economic theory of central places (Hekila 1993).

Network externalities (not to be confused with network effects) are externalities that depend upon the number of participants in the network. For example, a large population allows for a good public transportation network and for esoteric activities that appeal to a small number of customers.

Network effects are ordinary externalities that may not depend upon the number of participants but may depend upon the economies of scale resulting from geographical proximity in the network. For example, the concentration of economic activities (shops) in one place (the shopping mall) reduces the transaction costs of searching for a particular item.

Three types of external economies of scale can be distinguished: agglomeration, localization, and urbanization economies. Agglomeration economies are economies of scale in production internal to the firm, which can be achieved as a result of locating in a large urban area. These firms may need large inputs of labor. In turn, they may need a large demand for output if the product is subject to large transportation costs (cement). The city does not generate these economies internal to the firm but allows the firm to reap them.

Localization economies (network effects) result from the spatial concentration of plants in the same industry, plants that have input–output linkages with each other. These economies are external to the firm but internal to the industry. Nodes for transportation networks where distribution and assembly costs can be minimized are examples. Localization externalities allow much greater specialization. Localization concentration facilitates research and development. It also creates a pool of labor and services (banking) with required skills and experience. This pool is not costlessly mobile. This avoids the payment of monopsony (one-purchaser industry) wages (Glaeser et al. 1992). Transportation costs among firms are minimized. Customers save shopping time and comparative shopping is made easier. The shopping activity itself is subject to indivisibilities: indivisibility of the shopper, of the automobile, and of the commodities themselves (Eaton and Lipsey 1982). These indivisibilities explain multipurpose shopping and, therefore, the existence of the shopping mall. Of course, the costs of these infrastructures may be publicly supported while, outside the city, they would have to be privately supported. Energy efficiency can also be greater in cities because of built forms and higher densities (Alexandre and De Michelis 1996).

Urbanization economies (network externalities) result from the association of a large number of unrelated economic activities such as transportation, well-organized labor markets, large pools of skilled workers with differentiated skills, provision of social overheads and government services, legal and commercial (accounting and financial) services, market-oriented activities, and cultural and social facilities. These externalities result from the sheer volume of economic activities. When an industry grows, it raises local payrolls and local demand for unrelated

products. Cities are good breeding grounds for research and development. The latter seems positively related to the size and growth of
cities (Bradfield 1988). The limit to urbanization economies is
crowding, which raises wages and rents and, thereby, slows down the
growth of unrelated industries.

The benefits of cities reside, therefore, mainly in scale economies,
network externalities, and effects. These are club goods benefits since,
if the costs of city living exceed the benefits, citizens will move to other
locations.

In monocentric cities, the cost of transportation increases more than
proportionately to population. Their benefits must, therefore, exceed
the increase in the cost of transportation. Resource endowment of the
city may confer a comparative advantage. Economies of scale frequently
result from infrastructure indivisibility, i.e., from their public good
nature. Economies of scale affect public services (schools, hospitals, etc.)
as well. Household indivisibility creates new job opportunities. The
greater the variety of consumer goods available in a city, the higher the
real income of each customer. The greater the variety of inputs available
in a city, the higher the productivity of a firm. Complementary effects
among output goods may result in economies of joint production. If,
moreover, economies may result from production of these complementary goods at the same location, one speaks of economies of scope.
Joint location will save on transportation costs for intermediate inputs
(Fujita 1989).

5. Population moves among cities according to deterministic factors such
    as employment opportunities, amenities, and net benefits, and ac-
    cording to random factors. Employment opportunities are in turn de-
    termined by local population increases, which increase demand
    through positive feedbacks. With local public goods (club goods), effi-
    ciency can be achieved if individuals are allowed to vote with their feet.
    In other words, they may move from one city to another (Tiebout
    1956). Efficiency requires that the number of household types be small
    with respect to the number of cities and that local governments behave
    as profit maximizers (Fujita 1989).

6. Producers of local goods are in a relatively monopolistic situation. A
    model of monopolistic competition essentially replicates the positive
    results of an external economy model, but with entirely different nor-
    mative implications. Monopolistic competition with increasing returns
    (internal to the firm) in the service industry is not efficient, while it can
    be shown that the externality (internal to an industry) model leads to an
    efficient outcome (Fujita 1989).

7. Urban infrastructures are highly durable club goods. Infrastructures are replaced when they wear out (water pipes), when their operation and maintenance costs are too expensive, and when competing infrastructures become available that are cheaper or less polluting. Some infrastructures exceed their planned life and, generally, the sites on which infrastructures are located are permanent (Maryland and Weinberg 1988).

8. Dynamic externalities generate innovations through cross-sectoral spillovers. Urban sprawl and renewal are dynamic phenomena. The recent theory of economic growth views dynamic externalities (especially the ones associated with knowledge spillovers) as the engine of growth. This theory deals with technological externalities, i.e., innovations and improvements occurring in one firm increase the productivity of other firms without full compensation. The theory of dynamic externalities explains why cities grow. It does not explain why cities form and specialize. This is the domain of static externality theories. Spillovers may happen within one industry: "Through spying, imitation, and rapid interfirm movement of highly skilled labor, ideas are quickly disseminated among neighboring firms" (Glaeser et al. 1992, p. 1127). Local monopoly within this industry is better than local competition, according to some, because it allows externalities to be internalized by the innovator, thereby allowing innovation and growth to speed up. Others, including Porter and Jacobs, argue the reverse because the alternative to innovation is demise in a competitive environment. Competition fosters imitation and innovation. Jacobs maintains that spillovers among varied but geographically proximate industries speed up the adoption of new technologies. Cross-fertilization of ideas across different lines of work, rather than specialization, is key to city growth. Empirical evidence seems to favor the latter hypothesis (Glaeser et al. 1992).

Urban sprawl, or decreasing urban density, is frequently the result of hidden subsidies. It is also the consequence of the automobile. The economist's way of controlling urban sprawl is road pricing; investments in alternative modes of transportation, such as buses and rail (more subject to economies of scale than buses), are another way of braking urban sprawl (Beesley and Kemp 1987).

Conclusion

Generally speaking, human culture has reached its high moments in cities. Human culture, through cross-fertilization of ideas, diversity, and spillover effects, has had a beneficial impact on innovation and, thus, on economic welfare of both cities and their hinterland. The city's relations to nature (natural capital availability and nature's intrinsic value) are an essential feature of its integrity because ecosystem health is a necessary condition for ecological integrity. The benefits of living in cities result from the opportunity cost of living elsewhere. Cities create numerous benefits that result from togetherness and living in human communities, some benefits resulting from the sheer number of people (network externalities). As long as the net private and social benefits of living in cities are positive, and agricultural employment continues to decrease through labor-saving technological progress, possibly magnified by protective agricultural policies, cities will continue to grow.

An ecosystemic approach to city growth requires quite a bit of government intervention through official plans, zoning, protection of essential functions of ecosystems, building codes, investment in transit systems and pollution prevention, taxes and subsidies, education, etc. These tools help the city reach its ecologically desirable endpoints. Protecting urban ecosystem structure contributes to urban system integrity and thus to ecosystem integrity, each in a hologrammatic relationship with the other. Urban system integrity buttresses ecosystem integrity, and the latter is a mainstay for urban system integrity. Wilderness access in the vicinity of the city is also important for nurturing the relationships between nature and culture.

Urban economics and the complex systems methodology are two complementary approaches contributing to city understanding and its ecosystemic relationships. The former emphasizes the deterministic aspects of city formation and growth, including emergent properties such as diversity and spillover effects, while the latter emphasizes the city's hierarchical structure, the nonlinearity and chaotic behavior of its dynamics, and the essential role of random factors that complement deterministic ones.

Cities' system integrity results from the stability or cohesion of their component subsystems and from the ordering principle of their hierarchies (Ahl and Allen 1996). Since both spillover effects and products and factors diversity play a crucial role as ordering principles in an urban system, the cohesion of cities results from the benefits they confer to the people who live in their zone of influence (externalities) and from the values these people confer to the surrounding landscape and its products. Cohesion does not mean absence of change of position within the hierarchy. Cities go up and down the hierarchy according to competition (predator–prey) principles and random events. System integrity results from the stability of context, from the stability of slow-moving upper echelons. If changes in upper echelons result in disintegration of the lower ones, the system lacks integrity. If, on the other hand, changes in the lower echelons result in a new organizing principle for the hierarchy, the system exhibits integrity (Ahl and Allen 1996).

ACKNOWLEDGMENTS

Detailed comments from James Kay have improved this chapter, the remaining shortcomings of which are mine.

NOTES

1. I owe this reference to Mark Sagoff.
2. I owe this reference to James Kay.

REFERENCES

Ackhoff, R.L. 1972. Towards a System of Systems Concepts, in J. Beishon and G. Peters, eds. *Systems Behavior*, London: Harper, 83–90.

Ahl, V. and T. Allen. 1996. *Hierarchy Theory: A Vision, Vocabulary and Epistemology*, New York: Columbia University Press.

Alberti, M. and L. Susskind. 1996. Managing Urban Sustainability: An Introduction to the Special Issue, *Environmental Impact Assessment Review*, 16:4–6.

Alexandre, A. and N. De Michelis. 1996. Environment and Energy: Lessons from the North, in *Managing Urban Sustainability*, 249–57.

Allen, P. 1982. Evolution, Modeling and Design in a Complex World, *Environment and Planning*, 9:95–111.

Allen, P. 1986. Vers une science nouvelle des systèmes complexes, in *Science et pratique de la complexité*, Paris: La Documentation Française, 307–40.

Allen, P. 1990. Why the Future Is Not What It Was, *Futures*, 22:555-70.

Allen, P. 1992. Modeling Evolution and Creativity in Complex Systems, *World Futures*, 34:105–23.

Allen, P. 1994. Coherence, Chaos and Evolution in the Social Sciences, *Futures*, 26:583–97.

Allen, P. and M. Sanglier. 1979. A Dynamic Model of Growth in a Central Place System, *Geographical Analysis*, 11:256–72.

Allen, P. and J. McGlade.1987. Modeling Complex Human Systems: A Fisheries Example, *European Journal of Operations Research*, 30:147–67.

Armstrong, H. and J. Taylor. 1985. *Regional Economics and Policy*, Oxford: Philip Allan.

Arthur, W.B. 1995. Urban Systems and Historical Path Dependence, in W.B.

Arthur, *Increasing Returns to Scale and Path Dependence in the Economy,* Ann Arbor: University of Michigan Press, ch. 6, 99–110.

Axelrod, R. 1984. *The Evolution of Cooperation,* New York: Basic Books.

Beesley, M.E. and M.A. Kemp. 1987. Urban Transportation, in P. Nijkamp, ed., *Handbook of Regional and Urban Economics,* vol. 2, *Urban Economics,* Amsterdam: North-Holland, ch. 26.

Bergson, H. 1907. *L'évolution créatrice,* Paris: Payot.

Berry, B.J.L. 1964. Cities as Systems within Systems of Cities, *Regional Science Association, Papers and Proceedings,* 13:147–63.

Bradfield, M. 1988. *Regional Economics,* New York: McGraw-Hill.

Braudel, F. 1966. *La Méditérranée et le monde méditerranéen à l'époque de Philippe II,* 2nd ed., Paris: Colin.

Burghardt, A.F. 1971. A Hypothesis about Gateway Cities, *Annals of the Association of American Geographers,* 61:269–85.

Checkland, P. 1981. *Systems Thinking, Systems Practice,* New York: Wiley.

Christaller, W. 1966. *Central Places in Southern Germany,* transl. from German 1933, Englewood Cliffs, N.J.: Prentice Hall.

Cronon, W. 1991. *Nature's Metropolis: Chicago and the Great West,* New York: W.W. Norton.

Dendrinos, D.S. 1983. Epistemological Aspects of Metropolitan Evolution, in R.W. Crosby, *Cities and Regions as Nonlinear Decision Systems,* Boulder, Colo.: Westview Press, 143–54.

Eaton, B.C. and R.G. Lipsey. 1982. An Economic Theory of Central Places, *Economic Journal,* 92:56–72.

Fujita, M. 1989. *Urban Economic Theory,* Cambridge: Cambridge University Press.

Glaeser, E.L., E.D. Kallal, J.A. Scheinkman, and A. Shleifer. 1992. Growth in Cities, *Journal of Political Economy,* 100:1122–52.

Hekila, E.J. 1993. *Are Municipalities Non-Tieboutian Clubs?,* draft, University of Southern California, Los Angeles, School of Urban and Regional Planning.

Jacobs, J. 1969. *The Economy of Cities,* New York: Random House.

Kay, J. and E. Schneider. 1994. Embracing Complexity: The Challenge of the Ecosystem Approach, *Alternatives,* 20:32–38.

Lees, L.H. and P.M. Hohenberg. 1988. How Cities Grew in the Western World: A Systems Approach, in J.H. Ausubel and R. Herman, *Cities and Their Vital Systems,* Washington, D.C.: National Academy Press, 71–84.

Maryland, G. and A.M. Weinberg. 1988. Longevity of Infrastructure, in J.H. Ausubel and R. Herman, *Cities and Their Vital Systems,* Washington, D.C.: National Academy Press, 312–32.

Montroll, E. and W. Badger. 1974. *Introduction to Quantitative Aspects of Social Phenomena,* New York: Gordon and Breach.

Nicolis, G. and I. Prigogine. 1989. *Exploring Complexity: An Introduction,* New York: Freeman.

Perroux, F. 1955. Note sur la notion de pôle de croissance, *Économie appliquée,* 7:307–20.

Prigogine, I., P. Allen, and R. Herman. 1977. Long-Term Trends and the Evolution of Complexity, in E. Laszlo and J. Bierman, *Goals in a Global Community,* vol. 1, *Studies on the Conceptual Foundations,* New York: Pergamon, 1–63.

Royal Commission on the Future of the Toronto Waterfront. 1992. *Regeneration,* Minister of Supply and Services Canada.

Shrader-Fréchette, K.S. 1997. Sustainability and Environmental Ethics, in L. Westra and J. Lemons, *Perspectives on Ecological Integrity,* Dordrecht: Kluwer, ch. 4.

Simon, H. 1962. The Architecture of Complexity, *Proceedings of the American Philosophical Society,* 106:467–82.

Tainter, J.A. 1988. *The Collapse of Complex Societies,* Cambridge: Cambridge University Press.

Tiebout, C.M. 1956. A Pure Theory of Local Expenditures, *Journal of Political Economy,* 64:416–24.

von Thünen, J.H. 1966. *Von Thünen Isolated State,* transl. from German 1826, 1842, New York: Pergamon Press.

Weaver, W. 1948. Science and Complexity, *American Scientist,* 36:536–644.

Weber, A. 1929. *Theory of the Location of Industries,* transl. from German 1909, Chicago: University of Chicago Press.

Weber, A.F. 1899. *The Growth of Cities in the 19th Century,* New York: Greenwood Press.

Weinberg, G.M. 1975. *An Introduction to General Systems Thinking,* New York: Wiley.

CHAPTER 19

A Biocentric Defense
of Environmental Integrity

James P. Sterba

In her book *An Environmental Proposal for Ethics: The Principle of Integrity,* Laura Westra defines (ecosystem) integrity in terms of four features:

1. The health and present well-being of an ecosystem

2. The ability of an ecosystem to deal with outside interference and, if necessary, regenerate itself following upon it

3. An ecosystem's undiminished optimal capacity for the greatest possible ongoing developmental options within its time/location

4. The ability of an ecosystem to continue its ongoing changes and development unconstrained by human interruptions past or present[1]

More recently, however, Westra has proposed defining ecosystem integrity simply as the property of being essentially wild, that is, being free as much as possible from human interference.[2] This latter definition, which focuses exclusively on the fourth feature of the earlier definition, is virtually identical with James Karr's definition of (ecological) integrity as the condition at sites with little or no influence from human actions.[3] In this chapter, I propose to defend this latter notion of environmental integrity as captured by the principle of environmental integrity:

> Other things being equal, we ought not to interfere with nonhuman living nature.

★   ★   ★

To defend the principle of environmental integrity, it is necessary to show that the principle is morally required, that is, to show that, other things being equal, we are morally required not to interfere with nonhuman living nature. This requires showing that nonhuman living nature or nonhuman living beings should count morally. Now to say that something should count morally is to say that the good of that thing should constrain the pursuit of our own good in certain ways. Thus, to say that other human beings should count morally is to say that the good of these other human beings should constrain the pursuit of our own good in certain ways, for example, by our not killing them whenever it just happens to serve our interest to do so. Likewise, to say that other living beings should count morally for us is to say that the good of these other living beings should constrain the pursuit of our own good in certain ways, for example, by our not killing them whenever it just happens to serve our interest to do so.

But how do we establish that human beings and/or other living beings should count morally? Clearly, there is only one way we can do so, and that is by means of a good argument. So what we are looking for is a good argument that humans and/or other living beings should count morally. Now a good argument, by definition, must be a non-question-begging argument. So what we are looking for is a non-question-begging argument that humans and/or other living beings should count morally.

Is there such an argument? Let us first consider whether there is such an argument with respect to our fellow humans and then consider whether there is such an argument with respect to other living beings.

An Argument That All Human Beings Should Count Morally

Now with respect to our fellow humans, we have the capacity of entertaining and acting upon both self-interested and moral reasons, and the question we are seeking to answer is what sort of reasons for action it would be rational for us to accept.[4] This question is not about what sort of reasons we should publicly affirm, since people will sometimes publicly affirm reasons that are quite different from those they are prepared to act upon. Rather, it is a question about what reasons it would be rational for us to accept at the deepest level—in our heart of hearts.

Of course, there are people who are incapable of acting upon moral reasons. For such people, there is no question about their being required to act morally or altruistically. Yet the interesting philosophical question is not about such people but about people, like ourselves, who are capable of acting self-interestedly or morally and are seeking a rational justification for following a particular course of action.

In trying to determine how we should act, we would like to construct an argument that does not beg the question against egoism.[5] The question at issue here is what reasons each of us should take as supreme, and this question would be begged against egoism if we propose to answer it simply by assuming from the start that moral reasons are the reasons that each of us should take as supreme. But the question would be begged against morality as well if we proposed to answer the question simply by assuming from the start that self-interested reasons are the reasons that each of us should take as supreme. This means, of course, that we cannot answer the question of what reasons we should take as supreme simply by assuming the general principle of egoism:

> Each person ought to do what best serves his or her overall self-interest.

We can no more argue for egoism simply by denying the relevance of moral reasons to rational choice than we can argue for pure altruism simply by denying the relevance of self-interested reasons to rational choice and assuming the following principle of pure altruism:

> Each person ought to do what best serves the overall interest of others.[6]

Consequently, in order not to beg the question against either egoism or altruism, we have no other alternative but to grant the prima facie relevance of both self-interested and moral reasons to rational choice and then try to determine which reasons we would be rationally required to act upon, all things considered.[7]

In this regard, there are two kinds of cases that must be considered. First, there are cases in which there is a conflict between the relevant self-interested and moral reasons. Second, there are cases in which there is no such conflict.

Now it seems obvious that where there is no conflict and both reasons are conclusive reasons of their kind, both reasons should be acted upon. In such contexts, we should do what is favored both by morality and by self-interest.

Needless to say, defenders of egoism cannot but be disconcerted with this result since it shows that actions that accord with egoism are contrary to reason, at least when there are two equally good ways of pursuing one's self-interest, only one of which does not conflict with the basic requirements of morality. Nevertheless, exposing this defect in egoism for cases where moral reasons and self-interested reasons do not conflict would be but a small victory for defenders of morality if it were not also possible to show that in cases where such reasons do conflict, moral reasons would have priority over self-interested reasons.

Now when we rationally assess the relevant reasons in such conflict cases, it is best to cast the conflict not as a conflict between self-interested reasons and moral reasons but instead as a conflict between self-interested reasons and altruistic reasons.[8] Viewed in this way, three solutions are possible. First, we could say that self-interested reasons always have priority over conflicting altruistic reasons. Second, we could say just the opposite, that altruistic reasons always have priority over conflicting self-interested reasons. Third, we could say that some kind of compromise is rationally required. In this compromise, sometimes self-interested reasons would have priority over altruistic reasons, and sometimes altruistic reasons would have priority over self-interested reasons.

Once the conflict is described in this manner, the third solution can be seen to be the one that is rationally required. This is because the first and second solutions give exclusive priority to one class of relevant reasons over the other, and only a completely question-begging justification can be given for such an exclusive priority. Only by employing the third solution—sometimes giving priority to self-interested reasons, and sometimes giving priority to altruistic reasons—can we avoid a completely question-begging resolution.

Notice also that this standard of rationality will not support just any compromise between the relevant self-interested and altruistic reasons. The compromise must be a nonarbitrary one, for otherwise it would beg the question with respect to the opposing egoistic and altruistic views. Such a compromise would have to respect the rankings of self-interested and altruistic reasons imposed by the egoistic and altruistic views, respectively. Since for each individual there is a separate ranking of that individual's relevant self-interested and altruistic reasons, we can represent these rankings from the most important reasons to the least important reasons as follows:

Individual A		Individual B	
Self-interested reasons	Altruistic reasons	Self-interested reasons	Altruistic reasons
1	1	1	1
2	2	2	2
3	3	3	3
.	.	.	.
.	.	.	.
.	.	.	.
n	n	n	n

Accordingly, any nonarbitrary compromise among such reasons in seeking not to beg the question against egoism or altruism will have to give priority to those reasons that rank highest in each category. Failure to give priority to the highest-ranking altruistic or self-interested reasons would, other things being equal, be contrary to reason.

Of course, there will be cases in which the only way to avoid being required to do what is contrary to one's own highest-ranking reasons is by requiring someone else to do what is contrary to that person's highest-ranking reasons. Some of these cases will be "lifeboat cases." But although such cases are surely difficult to resolve (maybe only a chance mechanism can offer a reasonable resolution), they surely do not reflect the typical conflict between the relevant self-interested and altruistic reasons that we are or were able to acquire. Typically, one or the other of the conflicting reasons will rank significantly higher on its respective scale, thus permitting a clear resolution.[9]

Now it is important to see how morality can be viewed as just such a nonarbitrary compromise between self-interested and altruistic reasons. First, a certain amount of self-regard is morally required or at least morally acceptable. Where this is the case, high-ranking self-interested reasons have priority over low-ranking altruistic reasons. Second, morality obviously places limits on the extent to which people should pursue their own self-interest. Where this is the case, high-ranking altruistic reasons have priority over low-ranking self-interested reasons. In this way, morality can be seen to be a nonarbitrary compromise between self-interested and altruistic reasons, and the "moral reasons" which constitute that compromise can be seen as having priority over the self-interested or altruistic reasons that conflict with them.[10]

It might be objected that this defense of morality as compromise could be undercut if in this debate we simply give up any attempt to show that any one view is rationally preferable to the others. But we cannot rationally do this, for we are engaged in this debate as people who can act self-interestedly and can act altruistically, and we are trying to discover which way of acting is rationally justified. To rationally resolve this question, we must be committed to finding out which view is more rationally defensible than the others. So as far as I can tell, there is no escaping the conclusion that morality as compromise is more rationally defensible than either egoism or altruism, which means that we have a non-question-begging argument that all human beings should count morally.

An Argument That All Living Beings Should Count Morally

But do we also have a non-question-begging argument that all living beings should count morally? Well, just as we allowed that with respect to our fellow human beings, we have the capacity of entertaining and acting on both self-interested and altruistic reasons, so likewise with respect to all living beings, we have the capacity of entertaining and acting on anthropocentric reasons that take only the interests of humans into account as well as entertaining and acting on nonanthropocentric reasons that take into account only the interests of other living beings. And here too we are looking for a non-question-begging argument to determine which way we should act.

Now right off we might think that we have non-question-begging grounds for taking only the interests of humans into account, namely, the possession by human beings of the distinctive traits of rationality and moral agency. But while human beings clearly do have such distinctive traits, the members of nonhuman species also have distinctive traits that humans lack, like the homing ability of pigeons, the speed of the cheetah, and the ruminative ability of sheep and cattle. Nor will it do to claim that the distinctive traits that humans possess are more valuable than the distinctive traits that members of other species possess because there is no non-question-begging standpoint from which to justify that claim. From a human standpoint, rationality and moral agency are more valuable than any of the distinctive traits found in nonhuman species, since, as humans, we would not be better off if we were to trade in those traits for the distinctive traits found in nonhuman species. Yet the same holds true of nonhuman species. Generally, pigeons, cheetahs, sheep, and cattle would not be better off if they were to trade in their distinctive traits for the distinctive traits of other species.[11]

Of course, the members of some species might be better off if they could retain the distinctive traits of their species while acquiring one or another of the distinctive traits possessed by some other species. For example, we humans might be better off if we could retain our distinctive traits while acquiring the ruminative ability of sheep and cattle.[12] But many of the distinctive traits of species cannot be even imaginatively added to the members of other species without substantially altering the original species. For example, in order for the cheetah to acquire the distinctive traits possessed by humans, presumably it would have to be so transformed that its paws became something like hands to accommodate its humanlike mental capabilities, thereby losing its distinctive speed and ceasing to be a cheetah. So possessing distinctively human traits would not be good for the cheetah.[13] And with the possible exception of our nearest evolutionary relatives, the same holds true for the members of other species: they would not be better off having distinctively human traits. Only in fairy tales and in the world of Disney can the members of nonhuman species enjoy a full array of distinctively human traits. So there would appear to be no non-question-begging perspective from which to judge that distinctively human traits are more valuable than the distinctive traits possessed by other species. Judged from a non-question-begging perspective, we would seemingly have to grant the prima facie relevance to rational choice of both anthropocentric and nonanthropocentric reasons and then try to determine which reasons we would be rationally required to act upon, all things considered.[14]

In this regard, there are two kinds of cases that must be considered. First, there are cases in which there is a conflict between the relevant anthropocentric and nonanthropocentric reasons. Second, there are cases in which there is no such conflict.

Now it seems obvious that where there is no conflict and both reasons are conclusive reasons of their kind, both reasons should be acted upon. In such contexts, we should do what is favored both by anthropocentrism and by nonanthropocentrism.

Needless to say, defenders of anthropocentrism cannot but be disconcerted with this result since it shows that actions that accord with anthropocentrism are contrary to reason, at least when there are two equally good ways of pursuing anthropocentrism, only one of which does not conflict with the basic requirements of nonanthropocentrism. Nevertheless, exposing this defect in anthropocentrism for cases where nonanthropocentric reasons and anthropocentric reasons do not conflict would be but a small victory for defenders of nonanthropocentrism if it were not also possible to show that in cases where such reasons do conflict, nonanthropocentric reasons would have priority over anthropocentric reasons.

Now when we rationally assess the relevant reasons in such conflict cases, three solutions are possible. First, we could say that anthropocentric reasons always have priority over conflicting nonanthropocentric reasons. Second, we could say just the opposite, that nonanthropocentric reasons always have priority over conflicting anthropocentric reasons. Third, we could say that some kind of compromise is rationally required. In this compromise, sometimes anthropocentric reasons would have priority over nonanthropocentric reasons, and sometimes nonanthropocentric reasons would have priority over anthropocentric reasons.

Once the conflict is described in this manner, the third solution can be seen to be the one that is rationally required. This is because the first and second solutions give exclusive priority to one class of relevant reasons over the other, and only a completely question-begging justification can be given for such an exclusive priority. Only by employing the third solution—sometimes giving priority to anthropocentric reasons, and sometimes giving priority to nonanthropocentric reasons—can we avoid a completely question-begging resolution.

Notice also that this standard of rationality will not support just any compromise between the relevant anthropocentric and nonanthropocentric reasons. The compromise must be a nonarbitrary one, for otherwise it would beg the question with respect to the opposing anthropocentric and

nonanthropocentric views. Such a compromise would have to respect the
rankings of anthropocentric and nonanthropocentric reasons imposed by
the anthropocentric and nonanthropocentric views, respectively. Since for
each individual there is a separate ranking of that individual's relevant anthropocentric and nonanthropocentric reasons, we can represent these
rankings from the most important reasons to the least important reasons as
follows:

Individual A		Individual B	
Anthropocentric reasons	Nonanthropocentric reasons	Anthropocentric reasons	Nonanthropocentric reasons
1	1	1	1
2	2	2	2
3	3	3	3
.	.	.	.
.	.	.	.
.	.	.	.
n	n	n	n

Accordingly, any nonarbitrary compromise among such reasons in
seeking not to beg the question against anthropocentrism or nonanthropocentrism will have to give priority to those reasons that rank highest in
each category. Failure to give priority to the highest-ranking anthropocentric or nonanthropocentric reasons would, other things being equal, be
contrary to reason.

It might be objected that this defense of morality as compromise could
be undercut if, in this debate, we simply give up any attempt to show that
any one view is rationally preferable to the others. But we cannot rationally
do this, for we are engaged in this debate as people who can act anthropocentrically and can act nonanthropocentrically, and we are trying to discover which way of acting is rationally justified. To rationally resolve this
question, we must be committed to finding out which view is more rationally defensible than the others. So as far as I can tell, there is no escaping
the conclusion that morality as compromise is more rationally defensible
than either anthropocentrism or nonanthropocentrism, which means that
we have a non-question-begging argument that all living beings should
count morally.

★   ★   ★

But how is this compromise to be specified? Put another way, to what degree should nonhuman living nature count morally? In earlier work, I have
defended a set of principles that I think appropriately captures the compromise that is required.[15] The first of these principles is the principle of human
defense:

> Actions that defend oneself and other human beings against harmful aggression are permissible even when they necessitate killing or harming nonhumans.[16]

This principle of human defense allows us to defend ourselves and other human beings from harmful aggression, first against our persons and the persons of other human beings that we are committed to or happen to care about, and second against our justifiably held property and the justifiably held property of other human beings that we are committed to or happen to care about.[17]

This principle is analogous to the principle of self-defense that applies in human ethics[18] and permits actions in defense of oneself or other human beings against harmful human aggression.[19] In the case of human aggression, however, it will sometimes be possible to effectively defend oneself and other human beings by first suffering the aggression and then securing adequate compensation later. Since in the case of nonhuman aggression, this is unlikely to obtain, more harmful preventive actions such as killing a rabid dog or swatting a mosquito will be justified. There are simply more ways to effectively stop aggressive humans than there are to stop aggressive nonhumans.

The second principle is the principle of human preservation:

> Actions that are necessary for meeting one's basic needs or the basic needs of other human beings are permissible even when they require aggressing against the basic needs of nonhumans.[20]

Clearly our survival requires a principle of preservation that permits aggressing against the basic needs of at least some other living things whenever this is necessary to meet our own basic needs or the basic needs of other human beings. Here there are two possibilities. The first is a principle of preservation that allows us to aggress against the basic needs of both humans and nonhumans whenever it would serve our own basic needs or the basic needs of other human beings. The second is the principle, given above, that allows us to aggress against the basic needs of only nonhumans whenever it would serve our own basic needs or the basic needs of other human beings. The first principle does not express any general preference for the members of the human species, and thus it permits even cannibalism provided that it serves to meet our own basic needs or the basic needs of other human beings. In contrast, the second principle does express a degree of preference for the members of the human species in cases where their basic needs are at stake. Happily, this degree of preference for our own species is still compatible with granting moral status to all species because favoring the members of one's own species to this extent is characteristic of the members of nearly all species with which we interact and is thereby legitimated. The reason it is legitimated is that we would be required to sacrifice the basic needs of members of the human species only if the members of other species were making similar sacrifices for the sake of members of the human species.[21] In addition, if we were to prefer consistently the basic needs of the members of other species whenever those needs conflicted with our own (or even if we did so half the time), given the characteristic behavior of the members of other species, we would soon be facing extinction, and, fortunately, we have no reason to think that we are morally required to bring about our own extinction. For these reasons, the degree of preference for our own species found in the above principle of human preservation is justified within morality as compromise.

Nevertheless, preference for humans can go beyond bounds, and the bounds that are required by morality as compromise are expressed by the principle of disproportionality:

> Actions that meet nonbasic or luxury needs of humans are prohibited when they aggress against the basic needs of humans.

This principle is strictly analogous to the principle in human ethics mentioned previously that prohibits meeting some people's nonbasic or luxury needs by aggressing against the basic needs of other people.[22]

Without a doubt, the adoption of such a principle with respect to nonhuman nature would significantly change the way we live our lives. Such a principle is required, however, if there is to be any substance to the claim that the members of all species count morally. We can no more consistently claim that the members of all species count morally and yet aggress against the basic needs of some nonhumans whenever this serves our own nonbasic or luxury needs than we can consistently claim that all humans count morally and aggress against the basic needs of some other human beings whenever this serves our nonbasic or luxury needs.[23] Consequently, if the claim that all species count morally is to mean anything, it must be the case that the basic needs of the members of nonhuman species are protected against aggressive actions that serve only to meet the nonbasic needs of humans, as required by the principle of disproportionality.[24]

★   ★   ★

Now reflecting on the principles of human defense, human preservation, and disproportionality all together, you can see how they are related to the principle of environmental integrity, which, you recall, holds that, other things being equal, we ought not to interfere with nonhuman living nature. The principles of human defense, human preservation, and disproportionality are concerned with the permissibility or impermissibility of interference with nonhuman living nature. The principles of human defense and human preservation tell us when interference *is* permissible, which is when things *are not* equal according to the principle of environmental integrity. The principle of disproportionality tells us when interference *is not* permissible, which is when things *are* equal according to the principle of environmental integrity. Put another way, the principles of human defense, human preservation, and disproportionality, taken together, explain how the principle of environmental integrity is to be understood and applied.

Nevertheless, a considerable debate continues over whether the notion of environmental integrity can be usefully applied in ecology or in environmental ethics leading to the determination of social policy. Philosopher Mark Sagoff, in his most recent contribution to the debate, writes:

> Many of us recognize important moral and aesthetic differences between, say, the wild spontaneity of Nature and the rather gruesome and unattractive goings-on in factory farms. The genius of theoretical ecology today lies in its attempt to provide an objective basis for these moral and aesthetic differences. Theoretical ecologists today argue that Nature in its spontaneous course has an order and entelechy that it loses when subverted by human beings.[25]

But Sagoff argues that these theoretical ecologists have failed to uncover this order, entelechy, or environmental integrity possessed by pristine environments but absent from human-managed environments. Ecologist Robert McIntosh reaches a similar conclusion. Noting that environmental integrity has been variously defined, he writes, "In many ways, integrity seems to turn more on political change or relevance than on [the] scientific understanding of ecology. It is rhetorically powerful but scientifically unclear."[26]

So let us consider again how this defense of the principle of environmental integrity relates to the debate between theoretical ecologists, their philosophical allies, and their critics such as Sagoff and McIntosh. The principle of environmental integrity is supported by a non-question-begging argument as to who should count morally and how much they should count. Of course, this argument presupposes that nonhuman living nature has a good of its own, at least in the sense that individual organisms and maybe species have a good of their own, but all this is presumably common ground between theoretical ecologists, their philosophical allies, and their critics. It should also be common ground that nonhuman living nature can be more or less free of human interference. Maybe nowadays nonhuman living nature can never be completely free of human interference, but clearly some parts of nonhuman living nature are more interfered with than

others, e.g., an area that is turned into a professional golf course is more interfered with than one that is preserved as a national park. If, then, having
environmental integrity means being free of human interference, surely
nonhuman living nature can possess this quality to a greater or lesser degree.
Moreover, the principle of environmental integrity goes further and spec-
ifies when nonhuman living nature should possess this quality, specifically
when the principle of disproportionality prohibits that interference—that
is, when the interference would aggress against the basic needs of animals
and plants in order to meet nonbasic or luxury needs of humans. It is just
this type of human noninterference that should characterize nonhuman
living nature whether or not it happens to do so. But all of this should also
be common ground between theoretical ecologists, their philosophical
allies, and their critics. They all should agree that nonhuman living nature
can be characterized as being more or less free of human interference, and
further, they should agree that it should be free of particular kinds of
human interference.

What they presumably can legitimately disagree about is who or what it
is that is harmed by these particular kinds of human interference. Theoretical ecologists think that it is ecosystems or larger biotic communities as well
as individual organisms and their species that are harmed. By contrast,
critics like Sagoff and McIntosh deny that we can sufficiently identify and
reidentify entities such as ecosystems or larger biotic communities to be able
to legitimately claim that they have a good of their own and, therefore,
should be free of certain types of human interference.[27] But presumably
critics like Sagoff and McIntosh have no difficulty granting that individual
nonhuman organisms or species should be free of certain types of human interference, and since interferences with ecosystems or larger biotic communities would surely translate into interferences with individual nonhuman
organisms or species, there need not be any practical difference between
their views.[28] In fact, as far as I can tell, if they all accept the principle of environmental integrity, supported as it is by a non-question-begging argument, there should not be any practical difference between their views, that
is, they all should support the same practical policies of eliminating certain
kinds of interferences with nonhuman living nature, specifically those that
are prohibited by the principle of disproportionality, that is, those interferences that would aggress against the basic needs of nonhumans in order to
meet nonbasic or luxury needs of humans.

NOTES

1. Laura Westra, *An Environmental Proposal for Ethics: The Principle of Integrity*
   (Lanham: Rowman & Littlefield, 1994), pp. 24–25.

2. Laura Westra, "Ecosystem Integrity and Sustainability: The Foundational Value of the Wild," in *Perspectives on Ecological Integrity,* edited by Laura Westra and John Lemons (Dordrecht: Kluwer, 1995), p. 12.

3. J.R. Karr, "Ecological Integrity and Ecological Health Are Not the Same," in *Engineering within Ecological Constraints,* edited by P. Schultze (Washington, DC: National Academy Press, 1996), pp. 97–109.

4. "Ought" presupposes "can" here. So unless people have the capacity to entertain and follow both self-interested and moral reasons for acting, it does not make any sense asking whether they ought or ought not to do so. Moreover, moral reasons here are understood to necessarily include (some) altruistic reasons but not necessarily to exclude (all) self-interested reasons. So the question of whether it would be rational for us to follow self-interested reasons rather than moral reasons should be understood as the question of whether it would be rational for us to follow self-interested reasons exclusively rather than some appropriate set of self-interested reasons and altruistic reasons, which constitutes the class of moral reasons.

5. Of course, we don't need to seek to construct a good argument in support of all of our views, but our view about whether morality or egoism has priority is an important enough question to call for the support of a good argument.

6. I understand the pure altruist to be the mirror image of the pure egoist. Whereas the pure egoist thinks that the interests of others count for them but not for herself except instrumentally, the pure altruist thinks that her own interests count for others but not for herself except instrumentally.

7. Self-interested reasons favor both relational and nonrelational goods for the self, while altruistic reasons favor both relational and nonrelational goods for others.

8. This is because, as I shall argue, morality itself already represents a compromise between egoism and altruism. So to ask that moral reasons be weighed against self-interested reasons is, in effect, to count self-interested reasons twice — once in the compromise between egoism and altruism and then again when moral reasons are weighed against self-interested reasons. But to count self-interested reasons twice is clearly objectionable.

9. It is important to point out here that this defense of morality presupposes that we can establish a conception of the good, at least to the degree that we can determine high- and low-ranking self-interested and altruistic reasons for each agent.

10. It is worth pointing out here an important difference between these self-interested and altruistic reasons that constitute moral reasons. It is that the self-interested reasons render the pursuit of self-interest permissible, whereas the altruistic reasons require the pursuit of altruism. This is because it is always possible to sacrifice oneself more than morality demands and thus act supererogatory. Yet even here there are limits and one can sacrifice oneself too much, as presumably the pure altruist does, and consequently be morally blameworthy for doing so.

11. See Paul Taylor, *Respect for Nature* (Princeton: Princeton University Press, 1987), pp. 129–135, and R. and V. Routley, "Against the Inevitability of

Human Chauvinism," in *Ethics and Problems of the 21st Century,* edited by K.E. Goodpaster and K.M. Sayre (Notre Dame: University of Notre Dame Press, 1979).

12. Assuming God exists, humans might also be better off if they could retain their distinctive traits while acquiring one or another of God's qualities, but consideration of this possibility would take us too far afield. Nonhuman animals might also be better off if they could retain their distinctive traits and acquire one or another of the distinctive traits possessed by other nonhuman animals.

13. This assumes that there is an environmental niche that cheetahs can fill.

14. Self-interested reasons favor both relational and nonrelational goods for the self, while altruistic reasons favor both relational and nonrelational goods for others.

15. Most recently in *Justice for Here and Now* (New York: Cambridge University Press, 1998), chapter 6.

16. For the purposes of this article, I will follow the convention of excluding humans from the class denoted by "animals."

17. For an account of what constitutes justifiably held property within human ethics, see *Justice for Here and Now,* chapter 3.

18. By human ethics, I simply mean those forms of ethics that assume without argument that only human beings count morally.

19. Of course, one might contend that no principle of human defense applies in human ethics because either "nonviolent pacifism" or "nonlethal pacifism" is the most morally defensible view. However, I have argued in *Justice for Here and Now,* chapter 7, that this is not the case, and that still other forms of pacifism more compatible with just war theory are also more morally defensible than either of these forms of pacifism.

20. The principle of human preservation also imposes a limit on when we can defend nonhuman living beings from human aggression. According to this principle, the preservation of nonhumans is limited by the preservation of humans.

21. Notice that this is not an argument that since the members of other species aren't sacrificing for us, we don't have to sacrifice for them, but rather an argument that since the members of other species are not sacrificing for us, we don't have to sacrifice *our basic needs* for them. (A strictly analogous principle holds in human ethics with regard to when humans should be willing to sacrifice their basic needs for other humans.) Now it may be objected that the members of most other species are incapable of making this kind of sacrifice. This is true for most species, but irrelevant here because to reasonably ask this much altruism from humans just requires comparable altruism from the members of other species benefiting those humans. Actually, this degree of altruism toward humans may be found in some species of domestic animals, e.g., dogs and horses.

22. This principle is clearly acceptable to welfare liberals, socialists, and even libertarians. For arguments to that effect, see my *How To Make People Just* (Totowa: Rowman & Littlefield, 1988), and the special issue of the *Journal of Social Philosophy,* Vol. 22 no. 3, devoted to *How To Make People Just,* including my "Nine Commentators: A Brief Response."

23. Of course, libertarians have claimed that we can recognize that people have equal basic rights while, in fact, failing to meet, but not aggressing against, the basic needs of other human beings. However, I have argued in *Justice for Here and Now* that this claim is mistaken.

24. It should be pointed out that although the principle of disproportionality prohibits aggressing against the basic needs of animals and plants to serve the non-basic needs of humans, the principle of human defense permits defending oneself and other human beings against harmful aggression of animals and plants, even when this serves only the nonbasic needs of humans. The underlying idea is that we can legitimately promote our nonbasic needs *by defending* our persons and our property against the aggression of nonhuman others but *not by aggressing against* them. In the case of human aggression, a slightly weaker principle of defense holds: We can legitimately promote our nonbasic needs by defending our persons and property except when humans are engaged in aggression against our nonbasic needs because it is the only way to meet their basic needs. This weaker principle is grounded in the reciprocal altruism we can reasonably expect of humans.

25. Mark Sagoff, "Concepts of Nature's Integrity in Historical Context," p. 10.

26. Robert McIntosh, "Ecological Science, Philosophy and Ecological Ethics" (forthcoming), pp. 10–11.

27. Thus, when Sagoff claims that there are important moral and aesthetic differences between "the wild spontaneity of Nature and the rather gruesome and unattractive goings-on in factory farms," the claim of moral difference presupposes that the good of nonhuman nature is better served by the wild spontaneity of Nature than it is by typical factory farms. And while the good involved here need not be the good of ecosystems or larger biotic communities, it must at least be the good of individual organisms or species. So when Sagoff contrasts the view he favors with the view of theoretical ecologists who claim to find order and entelechy in nonhuman nature, the contrast cannot be as sharp as he suggests. Anyone who morally values something must find order and entelechy in it at least to some degree. What is at issue between Sagoff and theoretical ecologists, therefore, is whether ecosystems or larger biotic communities have a good of their own, not whether individual organisms or even species have such a good.

28. So instead of talking about what is harmful to ecosystems or larger biotic communities, we can talk about what is harmful to at least some of their members, just as instead of talking about what is good for ecosystems or larger biotic communities, we can talk about what is good for at least some of their members, and possibly bad for others, e.g., the individual deer that are culled from a herd that has become too large for its environmental niche.

Commodity Potential: An Approach to Understanding the Ecological Consequences of Markets

Jack Manno

Much of the prevailing discourse on sustainable development and global ecological integrity includes a critique of the spread of Western patterns of consumption and production and the burden such resource use places on planetary ecological systems. This chapter provides a means for understanding the process by which individual and social welfare has become tied to increasingly high levels of material and energy consumption and accompanying waste products. It explores the process, termed "commoditization," by which commodities or commercial goods and services are systematically selected over noncommodity, noncommercial means of satisfying human needs and aspirations.

Commoditization works against the apparent solutions to global environmental degradation that have most often been proposed: that we need to live more lightly on the Earth (Miller 1996), utilize technology that is optimally appropriate to the task and least productive of waste (Ausubel 1996), drastically reduce our consumption of material inputs per unit of service (Schmidt–Bleek 1993, 1994), reduce the energy embodied in our products (Odum 1996), reduce our ecological footprint (Wackernagel and Rees 1994), and so on.

There are many possible approaches to satisfying human needs and aspirations. Commoditization acts as a selection pressure that disproportionately selects those approaches which can be most readily and effectively packaged into a commodity (see Table 20.1).

The line distinguishing high from low commodity potential is permeable, the differences a matter of degrees. Goods and services more or less have the qualities of a commodity. They are more or less mobile, alienable, marketable, and centralizable. Noncommodities are less alienable (more com-

TABLE 20.1

Commoditization Favors Those Goods That Have the Quality of a Commodity (see Table 20.2).

Sector	High Commodity Potential (Commercial Goods)	Medium Commodity Potential (Artisan Goods)	Low Commodity Potential (Common Goods)
Children's play	Barbie dolls, action figures, packaged entertainment	Handicrafts, child care, live entertainment	Direct child-led interaction with natural surroundings, group play, interpersonal goods
Food production	Commercial fertilizers, pesticides, engineered seeds, mechanization tools, genetic material	Commercial manure, stored seeds, farm animals, tools for small farms, agricultural extension and research services	Knowledge of soil, locally coevolved skills and techniques
Health care	Mass-marketed drugs, diagnostic equipment, hospital supplies, insurance	Doctor-provided services, hands-on therapies and treatments	Knowledge of healing, personal health maintenance and illness prevention, lifestyle adaptations, sense of well-being
Energy	Grid-dispersed electricity, power plant equipment, fossil and nuclear fuels	Renewable energy sources, energy conservation services, wage labor	Personal energy conservation strategies, passive solar design, cooperative sharing activities
Transportation	Personal transport vehicles and the infrastructure of roads, etc., that supports them	Public transportation	Transportation reduction strategies (such as cluster housing near workplaces, etc.), walking
Environmental protection	Pollution control equipment, waste-to-energy incinerators and equipment	Recycling, pollution reduction/prevention services	Pollution prevention redesign, materials and energy use reduction strategies
Mental health	Mind-altering drugs	Therapists, fitness clubs	Peer counseling and mutual help, friendship, exercise
Finance/credit	Options, junk bonds, credit cards	Neighborhood banking, credit unions	Personal loans, gifts

Note: Goods and services with low commodity potential (LCP) involve direct and cooperative relationships between human beings or between humans and the natural world. Goods and services with medium commodity potential (MCP) involve a direct exchange relationship between the purveyor of the goods and the end-user. High commodity potential (HCP) goods and services involve highly abstracted and usually distant relationships between producers and consumers.

munal), less mobile (attached to local ecosystems or local culture), less marketable (being communal and attached), and less centralizable. Most things are some of each. Even noncommodities like "friendship" have their commoditized service version in "psychic friends networks," personal ads, etc. There is no aspect of human life that has not been commoditized to some extent. The selection pressures that favor commodities over noncommodities involve a gradual "survival of the fittest" where what is fit is by definition what is marketable.

Consider, for example, children's need for play. At one end of the scale of commodity potential are such mass-marketed toys as Barbie dolls, superhero action figures, and the packaged entertainment that accompanies them. These products are inexpensive, marketed worldwide, and involve immense sums invested in product research and development, packaging, and marketing. Their production is energy intensive and fossil fuel dependent and involves the highly publicized exploitation of cheap labor and mountains of industrial and postconsumer waste. In the middle of the commodity scale lie locally produced, handcrafted dolls, toys, and games usually made from renewable materials and with local or culturally idiosyncratic designs. These are the goods of the crafts market and bazaar. Also in the mid-scale are all the services for sale: child care, playgroups, clowns for hire, etc. At the far end of the commodity potential range are things that are not for sale such as making angels in the snow, play with found objects, group play, sing-alongs and all the goods of interpersonal contact.

The point here is *not* that less commodity-intensive goods are morally preferable or even always more benign. It is most likely that a sustainable society would have a healthy, balanced development between both commercial and noncommercial goods and services. Given the selection pressures of commoditization, however, unless public policy intervenes, commercial goods inevitably outcompete common and personal goods for social allocations of time, attention, and the means of material survival. Commoditization pressures act over time to gradually and inexorably expand the number of high-intensity commodities available, the geographic spread of their availability, and the range of types of needs for which commoditized satisfactions exist.

Sustainability implies reduction of waste material and energy, less manipulation of the natural environment and more adaptation to our understanding of it, and arguably higher employment (Hueting 1996). Much of this prescriptive worldview is implicit in *Our Common Future*[1], which led to the United Nations Conference on Environment and Development and to Agenda 21, which emerged from it and has become part of the general discourse of sustainable development. But despite significant progress in improving efficiency in the use of materials and energy per unit of production, overall consumption of consumer goods and the environmental deterioration that necessarily accompanies it continue to rise at a dramatic pace that shows no sign of slowing down. What is to be done?

The first step is to get clearer about what the problem is and what it is not. There are many suggestions as to the root cause of unsustainability: human greed (Hardin 1968), ignorance (Orr 1992), spiritual detachment and/or malaise (Gore 1992), addictions (Catton 1980), or simply the inevitable consequence of human activity (Cross and Guyer 1980). The problem is not fundamentally about individual human greed but more about the *systems* of rewards in place that reinforce greed. It is not only about ignorance of ecology or the problems of environmental degradation, but more about *coevolutionary processes* that reward and reinforce environmentally destructive choices. It is not just about spiritual malaise or addictions to material goods, although both may result from *commoditization* pressures. Unsustainability is in the end the natural consequence of dynamics in the modern political economy, which systematically favor exactly those forms of goods and services that have the greatest environmental impact.

There are at least three sets of constraints that together act to select economic survivors: consumer choice, physical limits including resource availability, and the ability to attract research and development investment. These three constraints can be illustrated in the design of a car. Physical laws determine the range of design options and as a result most cars look fundamentally similar: height, width, wheel span, steering mechanisms, etc. Designs that veer too far from the physically optimal pay the price in higher fuel demands, safety risks, or other inefficiencies and are selected out. Consumer choice determines most of the variability within the range of what physical laws determine is practical. These choices are the result of the interplay of options and motivations, including disposable income, status seeking, comfort, and practical considerations such as size of family, the purposes to which the vehicle would be put to use, etc. The combined result of these factors leads to a range of available vehicles and features on the market that represent the optimal balance of possible customer satisfactions. Neither the physical limits nor consumer choices, however, account for the selection of automobile transport over other, lower commodity intensity forms of transportation such as adequate public transport, redesigned cityscapes that minimize transport needs, etc.

This phenomenon, the selection of high over low commodity intensity solutions to personal and social needs, can be observed in sector after sector (see Table 20.2). It is a self-reinforcing, positive-feedback mechanism. The key variable is investments in research and development. Since high commodity intensity solutions receive by far the greater amount of research and development (R&D), they invariably appear to be more advanced and competitive. It is then logically compelling to utilize these solutions and apparently irresponsible to suggest the adoption of lesser-developed alternatives. Communal solutions therefore always appear less capable of meeting human needs.

Unfair Comparisons

To understand how this works, consider as a hypothetical example two competing schools using contrasting approaches to teaching. Assume that both methods are based on sound pedagogy. For some reason school A, perhaps because its methods require considerably more inputs than school B, receives annual investments of $10,000 per student to develop its teaching methods. School B receives $1 per student to do the same. After several years, standardized tests are given to students in both schools. Unsurprisingly, students in school A score significantly higher. Parents making rational choices send their students to school A. The school receives even greater amounts of financial support for its methods. Other schools adopt the methods. Most conclude that school A's teaching methods are superior. Few people bother with school B's methods any longer. Occasionally supporters of the B methods try to make a case for why their approach should be used. Small pockets of B teachers form networks of enthusiasts around the country. Occasionally their methods have a resurgence of support. There are newsletters and conferences and many small successes. Their adherents strongly believe that if everyone were just taught the benefits of B, they would rationally choose B over A. But over and over, A receives the overwhelming amount of R&D, its teachers make more money, and on and on. B has a chance only if its proponents can find a way to counterbalance the overwhelming disadvantage they face in the competition for R&D investments.

It may well be that A is a superior pedagogy, but this can be determined only once the imbalance in R&D investment is corrected. Perhaps some synthesis of A and B may work best. But syntheses work best between methods that are at similar stages of development, or the more developed will likely reassert its dominance over time until its partner is virtually eliminated. The original competition between A and B was measured by a criterion, average test scores or points per pupil, that was independent of the investment variable. If instead, test scores were measured as points per dollar invested per pupil, the resulting evaluation would be far different.

This is precisely what happens in sector after sector in the competition between high and low commodity intensity goods. High commodity intensity satisfactions for human needs receive far more R&D investment than

TABLE 20.2

Some Characteristics of Commodities the Economy "Selects" over Those of Noncommodities, and Associated Environmental Effects

Attributes of Goods and Services with Low Commodity Potential	Attributes of Goods and Services with High Commodity Intensity	Negative Effects of Commoditization	Positive Effects of Commoditization
Openly accessible. Difficult to establish rights, widely available, difficult to accurately price	**Appropriable, Excludable, Enclosable, Assignable.** Simpler to establish right of ownership, easier to establish price	Privatization accelerates decline of sense of community and the common good and increases commercialization of all aspects of life	Releases individual and corporate entrepreneurial energy
Rooted. In local ecosystem and community	**Mobile.** Transferable, easy to package and transport	Propensity for mobility increases flows and export of energy and materials	Makes trade possible, increases choice
Particular, Customized, Decentralized and Diverse. Each culture potentially derives the best practices for its particular environmental context, leading to diverse customized goods and practices	**Universal, Standardized, Centralized and Uniform.** Adaptable to many contexts	Reduces cultural and geographic diversity, standardized methods may not be suited to particular ecosystems, as a result efficiency potential is reduced	Allows rationalization of production, economics of scale, and transfer of skills
Systems-Oriented. Development occurs in the context of a whole system; goal is system optimization; product is developed to serve the system	**Product-Oriented.** Development focuses on maximizing output of products; goal is profit maximization; system is developed to serve the product	Discourages systems thinking, keeps attention on parts rather than wholes, undermines capacity for ecosystem approaches to decision-making, overdevelops competitive skills and underdevelops collaborative skills	Produces cornucopia of products
Dispersed Energy. Energy is used and dissipated at the site of the activity or point of exchange or consumption	**Embedded Energy.** Production is energy intensive; packaging, transportation, and promotion add to energy embedded in the product	Concentration of energy causes ecological disruption at the point of its release; commoditization of fuel facilities causes dramatic increase in energy availability and use	Increased energy production is tied to wealth production
Disperse Knowledge and Skills, Convenience Is Not Goal. Use requires relevant knowledge and skills	**Embedded Knowledge or Skills, Convenient.** Use inherent in design and material	Impoverishes knowledge base particularly at the personal, local, and regional levels	Convenience frees human attention for other activities

Low Capital Intensity, High Energy Productivity, High Labor Intensity, Low Labor Productivity	**High Capital Intensity, Low Energy Productivity, Low Labor Intensity, High Labor Productivity**	Eliminates jobs, encourages replacement of workers with fossil fuel energy	Increased productivity frees capital to invest in new productive activities, creating new jobs
Consumption and Use Involve Cooperative Relationships	**Consumption by Individuals**	Promotion of individual consumption reduces the efficiency gains made possible by sharing, increases flow of energy and materials	Increased individual autonomy and freedom
More Variable, Unpredictable, Unreliable	**More Stable, Predictable, Reliable**	Predictability tends toward simplification, including loss of diversity and redundancy in ecosystems	Increased predictability and reliability benefits all human activities
Design Follows and Mimics Natural Flows and Cycles	**Design Resists and/or Alters Natural Flows and Cycles**	Failure to promote and use ecological designs leads to increased energy use and more waste	Overcoming ecological contraints opens more possibility
Concrete. Tied to physical and biological constraints	**Abstract.** Less direct ties to physical base of reality	Reduces knowledge and awareness of physical basis of human life and culture	Overcoming physical constraints opens more possibility
Coevolutionary and Traditional. Evolves in the context of specific ecosystem and culture, relationships often structured by custom	**Path-Breaking.** Break from bonds of place and tradition; relationships structured by contract	Loss of traditions and traditional knowledge	Overcoming cultural constraints opens more possibility
Complex. Involving multiple relationships, embedded in social and ecological web	**Simple.** Self-contained, extracted from relationships	Simplification leads to general loss of diversity, redundancy, and resilience	Narrowing focus to one or few variables makes production more manageable
Long term. Stable returns	**Short term.** Large return on investment	Increases speculation, reduces investments in sustainable opportunities	Increases wealth and its accompanying benefits
Sufficient. Optimal service for minimal expenditure of material and energy	**Efficient.** The most exchange value for the least investment	Reduces capacity to develop low-impact living, accelerates commoditization	Efficiency frees reserves for other wealth-producing activities
Contributes Little to GNP. The less commoditized a good or service, the less it contributes to GNP	**Contributes to GNP.** GNP growth measures commoditization	Public policy goals become tied to growth in size of economy rather than improvements in quality of life	GNP represents accurate measure of economic activity and is closely related to improved quality of life

low commodity intensity alternatives. Over time they become more "developed" and more attractive, just like school A.

Industrial Agriculture vs. Organic Agriculture

The evolution of agricultural practices, particularly in industrialized economies, is highly susceptible to distortion by commoditization. Alternative, indigenous, and organic methods of farming rely heavily on local natural resources, community networks of cooperation, and personal skills, each of which is difficult to buy and sell. Organic farmers' approach to controlling pests, weeds, and diseases is one of prevention rather than treatment. Consider the differences between products and processes in the agricultural industry:

Agricultural System Products (High Commodity Potential)

Proprietary hybrid and patented seeds
Insecticides, herbicides and fungicides
Commercial fertilizers
Farm machinery
Fuel
Farm management books and magazines

Agricultural System Processes and Skills (Low Commodity Potential)

Soil maintenance
Water conservation and management
Knowledge of soil, climate, local pests
Energy conservation and management
Nutrient cycling and enhancement
Crop rotation and placement
Rural networks of mutual aid
Pest control and management

Commoditization operates at the level of inputs and practices, preferentially developing the inputs that can be purchased, and tools and techniques that best utilize these inputs. Commoditization also operates on the outputs, favoring standardized crops marketed broadly and selecting out varieties with characteristics that are adapted to unique soil and farming circumstances. Instead, the characteristics of the land itself are homogenized to accommodate the homogenized crops grown on it so that the same crops can be grown in many places regardless of their original ecological characteristics. In this way the qualities associated with commodities are maximized: long shelf lives, portability, standardization of products, and industrial-scale production.

Alternative approaches to agriculture, sometimes lumped together under the heading of sustainable agriculture, suffer from the same fallacy of unfair comparisons as the hypothetical educational approaches described earlier. The highly developed commoditized agriculture sector brags of increasingly high productivity to which the underdeveloped alternatives are then negatively compared. This is even worse when industrialized agriculture is compared with indigenous agricultural practices. These comparisons are made even more difficult and unfair as a result of the kinds of land each approach has been practiced on, particularly in countries with large inequalities of income distribution where the most fertile land is owned or controlled by the elite. Small and subsistence farmers are relegated to the least fertile, most inaccessible, and steep uplands. These farmers are also the ones least likely to adopt modern farming methods and are more likely to continue the traditional practices they learned from the previous generation. So when comparisons are made between the productivity of traditional and modern agricultural sectors, what is compared is not only the results of productivity differences between farming practices but also the entire history of unequal access to land and resources. It is all the more remarkable that traditional farming practices have survived at all in the competition with highly commoditized industrial agriculture.

As a result of the economic distortions brought about by commoditization, the farmer is at a distinct disadvantage compared to other participants in the food economy. What farmers control—land, soil, knowledge, labor, skills, and ties to land and community—has intrinsically low commodity potential. Farmers themselves, no matter how much they adopt the industrialized model of farming, are always at an economic disadvantage in a totally commoditized economy. Farmers who opt out of the industrial agriculture model are at an even greater disadvantage. The economic benefits of agriculture accrue most to those who control the key agricultural commodities: the crop once it leaves the farm and the key agricultural inputs, especially fuel, fertilizers, pesticides, and farm machinery. The economic interests that control the most commoditizable sectors of the food economy also control the direction of agricultural research and development. With stronger ownership rights in intellectual property by the seed and agricultural input industry, these private interests have become much larger players in agricultural research, which was once dominated by publicly funded research (Fuglie et al. 1996).

Health Care Products and Services

There is a persistent belief in many parts of the world that access to health care should be a right, not a privilege reserved for those who can pay. As a consequence, there is always some effective resistance to its complete privatization and commoditization. Health care has been treated at least in part as a public good and a public service whose provision is the collective responsibility of society. This does not mean that health care is not distorted by the same sort of pressures that affect agriculture. In order to understand the effects of commoditization in health care, as in agriculture, a useful distinction can be made between products and processes. Health care *products* inherently have greater commodity potential than health care *processes*. Some examples of this distinction are:

Health Care Products (High Commodity Potential)
Pharmaceutical drugs
Hospital/health care supplies and equipment
Vaccines
Diagnostic equipment
Vitamins and herbs
Health books and magazines
Exercise equipment

Health Care System Processes and Skills (Low Commodity Potential)
Disease prevention
Health maintenance education
Hands-on therapy and care
Doctor/patient interaction
Exercise/outdoor play
Personal hygiene/sanitation
Counseling

Hands-on or labor-intensive prevention and treatment have inherently low commodity potential and as a result will get short shrift in the commoditized health care industry. Diagnostic equipment to support a physician's observational skills (*products*) are highly developed, while the observational skills themselves (*processes*) grow increasingly and comparatively underdeveloped. This is also true of healing arts which, like agricultural practices, coevolve within a set of local dynamics peculiar to a given culture. Traditional herbal medicines, which rely on the cultivation and collection of local plants, receive far less attention from investors than do pharmaceutical medicines, which can be patented. This has changed somewhat in recent years as a result of consumer demand for access to alternative health care products. Within the alternative medicine field, the standardization, packaging, and marketing of herbs has now become a commodity-intensive industry.

Environmental Pollution Control and the 4Rs
The same forces drive the economics of environmental health and human health. As in health care, prevention may be preferable to treatment, but treatment involves products and services that can be readily marketed, whereas prevention requires systems changes and the reform of production and consumption patterns, which are not readily packaged solutions.

Environmental Products (High Commodity Potential)
Remediation equipment
Energy-efficient appliances
Biological enzymes
Low-impact pesticides
Waste incinerators
Photovoltaic cells
Biomass fuels
Parks and zoos

Environmental Processes (Low Commodity Potential)
Energy and materials conservation programs
Ecological design
Watershed management
Voluntary simplicity
Community building and resource sharing
Environmental education
Waste reduction programs
Extended producer responsibility
Habitat protection and conservation

There is a widely accepted formula for waste minimization, the 4Rs: Reduce, Reuse, Recycle, and Recover. These four approaches are typically depicted in order of effectiveness and priority. The priority ranking for the 4Rs is the exact opposite of the order of commodity potential. Although the 4Rs approach and prioritization are regularly advocated by environmental agencies in the United States and elsewhere, the actual practice reflect another set of priorities.

Commoditization, Oppression, and Liberation

Laura Westra, in her chapter on environmental violence in this volume, lists 14 forms of ecoviolence; each of these is related to increased throughput caused by commoditization. This section presents a conceptual basis for understanding the link between oppression and commoditization. Commoditization is not simply an abstract and victimless process. It is at the center of what is meant by oppression, while the overcoming of its negative effects implies liberation from important features of that oppression. Understanding the politics of commoditization will also help to explain why liberation politics are potentially so closely linked with the movement for sustainable development. The systematic privileging of commodities and underprivileging of common goods means that those qualities and that "know-how" which are not commoditizable are systematically starved for material, energy, and attention. But these qualities and knowledge—local connectedness, conviviality, ecological attentiveness, cultural and individual distinctiveness, and long-term care and maintenance—are inherent human qualities, and their gradual emisseration by the free reign of commoditization and enclosure diminishes all human beings.

Human intelligence has the capacity to invent many solutions to the problems of providing for human welfare. Yet only solutions with high commodity potential can predictably depend on the support of the larger community in the form of investments of material and energy. This means that the vast potential of human intelligence is systematically stunted. This amounts to a form of oppression that damages all human beings. Of course the group most systematically excluded from the benefits of the liberal market economy has been people of African descent whose forbears were subject to the worst form of commoditization, human slavery, as well as the many colonized people of the world whose material and energy resources were exploited to fuel the Western development from the fifteenth to the mid-twentieth centuries.

Peoples whose energies focus on the particular, the local, or the community are expending energies on services that are not rewarded because by being local and particular, they are less suitable as commodities. Not surprisingly, the community-building tasks, which are inherently local and particular, are selected out as the people who devote themselves to those tasks find it increasingly difficult to sustain themselves. The geniuses of community organizing and caretaking easily fall victim to self-deprecation, as the primary vehicle for social valuation in a commoditized society, purchasing power, is systematically denied them. Thus the oppression is systematically internalized as a belief in the lesser value of the oppressed group, or it simmers as a deeply felt resentment against faceless and nameless oppressors. This difficulty with naming oppression is realistic: it results from the fact that the dynamics of oppression are simply the flip side of the dynamics of commoditization, which are embedded in the system and are not necessarily the result of individual decisions to oppress other human beings.

While the noncommodity ties of community suffer from lack of resources, in every oppressed group there exists a small but growing middle class that is blessed with or had forbears blessed with talents, ambitions, or economic luck that makes them "fit" for surviving or thriving in a commodity niche. Because of some improvements in the democratization of access to markets and capital in the past half-century, particularly in Western industrialized countries, there are always some opportunities for success among individuals in oppressed groups. Many succeed and their success is often presented as case arguments against the charge of racial or class bias. "Successful" individuals from oppressed groups experience at the same time the impoverishment of the common goods that are the lifeblood of their community. Their privileged position and/or wealth allow them to purchase the ever-increasing number of commodity replacements for common goods (security devices instead of community spirit, professional services instead of extended families, etc.).

This imbalance, personally and painfully felt, simply mirrors the fundamental imbalance created by commoditization pressures throughout society. It is felt most acutely by members of oppressed groups exactly because the system, which has been responsible for their oppression, appears to be the only practical alternative for promoting individual and social welfare. Since the system appears as perfectly neutral and open for everyone, those who have been left out experience it as their own fault. And as more and more spheres of human needs and wants become dominated by commodity satisfactions, participation or membership in social life itself depends on the ability to participate in the market. At the same time, certain aspects of oppressed people's culture are commoditized by the entertainment and sports industries so, for example, opportunities to experience the rhythms and power of African American culture can be purchased for the price of a CD or a ticket to a basketball or football game, while images of Native American culture are commoditized and marketed by Disney and Hollywood. This is an example of how commoditization pressures operate to simplify and stereotype by highlighting and marketing the most commoditizable aspects of complex social and cultural phenomena and ignoring or suppressing those aspects that resist commoditization.

The situation for indigenous people is particularly painful. The economic system that has evolved out of commoditization pressures selects out an important component of their very being, their connection with the ecosystem within which they have coevolved. In addition, inasmuch as the resources of their lands have been degraded by participation in the commodity economy, their previous way of life is often impossible to sustain as it once was. Since the commodity economy has expanded to the point where its allocation principles totally dominate the distribution of materials, energy, and human attention, it is almost impossible to opt out in favor of traditional ways. The end result is a form of cultural genocide. There is no doubt that tremendous potential exists for sustainable economic and cultural development in indigenous communities, but the realization of this potential will require substantial investments in research and development directed by indigenous peoples themselves. But these investments are systematically outcompeted by investments in commodities. It is no surprise that the economies of many indigenous communities in North America have become dominated by classic and destructive goods that are the almost pure commodities: gambling, gasoline, and nicotine.

The story of the oppression of women is not very different (Hynes 1993). The productive spheres in which women and women's innovations have predominated are also those that have been historically most resistant to commoditization. Expectations in many, if not most, cultures are that women attend to the least commoditized spheres of life: childrearing, caretaking, domestic maintenance, and interpersonal relationships. Again, as the economy becomes more commoditized, the distribution of material, energy, and human attention becomes more dominated by commoditization pressures, and the least commoditizable spheres of life become increasingly emisserated. In addition, saddled with the responsibilities for essential common goods, women tend to be less mobile and have less free time to invest in commodity production. At a time when the U.S. economy was less commoditized, income was expected to be distributed so that a worker could support both himself as a participant in commodity production and the noncommodity spheres of his household and community, the so-called family wage. As the noncommodity spheres have become increasingly marginalized, this is no longer viable. Hence the sphere of "women's work" has grown increasingly emisserated to the point that women and men can no longer afford to spend much of their time there. Again, only countervailing forces against commoditization pressures can effectively invigorate the non-commodity domestic and community spheres with material, energy, and the attention of women or men.

Commoditization brings more and more of civil society (all those previously independent noncommodity, or less commoditized, spheres) under the domination of the market. Hence success in achieving greater justice and equality in the spheres of civil society means access to an increasing share of a decreasing source of power. According to Michael Walzer in his influential book *Spheres of Justice* (1983), this is the very meaning of tyranny, when those who succeed in one sphere of social life (such as money and commodities) deliberately and unjustly wield the power and influence gained there to dominate in another sphere of social life (such as political influence).

Liberty, according to this formulation, requires active defense of the boundaries between the spheres. But commoditization, which also leads to domination by one sphere (money) over all others, is a "natural" outcome of system dynamics, and the methods of defending against it are not nearly so clear as those in the struggle against a tyrant who can be named and constrained or removed from power. Nonetheless, the movement for liberation from oppression involves much the same institutional framework that Walzer prescribes for the defense of liberty: "a strong welfare state run, in part at least, by local and amateur public officials; a constrained market; an open and demystified civil service; independent public schools; the sharing of hard work and free time; the protection of religious and familial life; a system of public honoring and dishonoring free from all considerations of rank or class; workers' control of companies and factories; a politics of parties, movements, meetings and public debate" (Walzer 1983, p. 318). Such an institutional framework would need to consider the way economies evolve through selection pressures and deliberately design public policy instruments that provide countervailing forces to the pressures of commoditization. In addition to reinvigorating presently impoverished spheres of communal life, this would reduce the amount of materials and energy needed per unit of social welfare (see Daly and Cobb 1989).

Recommendations and Conclusions

Western-style development has succeeded largely because societies invented legal and institutional mechanisms that favored commoditization and economic growth. If human welfare and ecological integrity are to be the goal of policy, then legal and political instruments designed to favor the noncommodity satisfaction of human wants must be invented to counterbalance the force of commoditization. Commercial law is now evolving into a global legal framework designed to unleash commercial energies worldwide by minimizing the capacity of states to restrict access to markets. As a result, commoditization pressures are expanding into all potential niches worldwide. Since the legal and political actors unleashing these forces operate at the global level, countervailing pressures must also operate globally. But since noncommodity solutions to human needs and wants are inherently local, the effects of these countervailing forces must be felt at the local level. New legal and political capacity to stimulate investment in community-based, less commoditized satisfactions for human needs and wants must devolve to the level nearest to the people with those needs and wants. There have been several efforts to describe the emergence of global civil society as a precursor to a governance capacity that can act with some effect and authority at both the global and local levels (Walzer 1983, Princen et al. 1994, Lipschutz 1996, Wapner 1996). At the same time, nation-states must invent new legal frameworks that allow localities to innovate economically and that protect them from the colonizing impulses of global forces and actors.

   Policy instruments to counterbalance commoditization pressures fall into
the following main categories:

- *Increased public investment in research and development* of non–commodity
  satisfactions to social and individual needs.

- *Taxes and fees* that increase the cost of energy and materials to better reflect the amount of environmental and social damage their mobilization
  causes. Examples include the 1990 U.S. tax on ozone–depleting chemicals, taxes and fees linked to discharges of carbon dioxide in Sweden
  and Norway.

- *Investing in "natural capital":* Various methods to encourage or require
  investments in protecting and restoring the natural environment to an
  equivalent degree to which profit–making activities deplete the natural
  environment.

- *Protecting ecological integrity:* Mandating limits to human disruption of
  key ecological regions and global ecosystemic processes, thereby
  forcing the development of alternative forms of human settlement and
  prosperity.

- *Investing in "social capital":* High levels of social development—evaluated in terms of such quality of life indicators as mortality rates and
  levels of life expectancy, education and literacy, and political participation—are consequences of public policies and strategies based not on
  economic growth considerations (through commoditization) but, instead, on *equity* considerations.

- *Tax reforms:* that decrease taxes on income from labor (the least commoditizable of production inputs), thereby decreasing the cost of labor
  in relation to energy and materials (Rees 1995a, 1995b).

- *Rationalizing subsidies:* to abolish environmentally harmful subsidies and
  subsidizing environmentally beneficial activities (Roodman 1996).

- *Protecting the rights of workers in the low–wage economy:* Low wages and
  poor working conditions subsidize massive commoditization and make
  noncommodity, highly labor–intensive local alternatives unable to
  compete (Daily and Ehrlich 1996).

- *Empowering local and indigenous communities:* (particularly those whose
  livelihoods depend on the long–term viability of local resources).

   The most important policy goal is increasing the amount of research and
development into non- or lower-commodity goods for the satisfaction of
human needs and wants: alternative agriculture, health maintenance and
disease prevention, lifelong learning, vital communities, low-impact trans-

portation. This investment, because it is directed toward development of goods and services with lower commodity potential, will require considerable involvement of governmental actors at all levels. What is clearly needed is democratically based authority that can act at the same international scale as the multinational corporations: an international labor movement, an international consumers' movement, an international people's movement with the capacity to initiate and sustain some forms of governance capacity that can counterbalance the global pressures of commoditization. At the same time, noncommodity alternatives to human need satisfaction are inherently local, and any governance reform for sustainable development must include increased civic capacity at both local and global levels, as has been nicely pointed out by Ronnie Lipschutz (1996) and others.

Although we are far from attaining parity between investment in high-intensity and low-intensity commodity development, there are hopeful signs that we are headed in the right direction. The movement for sustainable development, in all its myriad forms, poses a dramatic challenge to Western forms of production and consumption. So far material industrial society has avoided such questions in the production–consumption debate. The development of governing capacity at the appropriate levels to issue that challenge and invent and develop alternatives marks what can be seen as the deciding moment of politics in our era.

NOTES

1. Implicit it is, but also *deliberately not explicit.* The governments of modern nation-states act in effect as industrial development organizations. When they gather in international negotiations and receive the collected input of the global environmental movement, they tend to accept the consensus information about the causes of the environmental crises and their potential solutions without acknowledging the politically difficult implications for patterns of production and consumption that undergird the modern global economy. In fact, the authors of *Our Common Future* reached conclusions regarding the need for increased economic growth that were in direct contradiction to the logic of the arguments they presented in the report.

REFERENCES

Ausubel, J. H., "Can technology spare the Earth?" *American Scientist* 84: 166–178, 1996.

Catton, W. R., *Overshoot,* University of Illinois Press, Urbana, 1980.

Cross, J. G. and M. J. Guyer, *Social Traps,* University of Michigan Press, Ann Arbor, 1980.

Daily, G. C. and P. Ehrlich, "Socioeconomic equity, sustainability, and Earth's carrying capacity," *Ecological Applications* 6: 991–1001, 1996.

Daly, H. E. and J. B. Cobb Jr., *For the Common Good: Redirecting the Economy toward*

Community, the Environment and a Sustainable Future, Beacon Press, Boston, 1989.

Fuglie, K., N. Ballenger, K. Day, C. Klotz, M. Ollinger, J. Reilly, U. Vasavada, and J. Yee, *Agricultural Research and Development: Public and Private Investments under Alternative Markets and Institutions,* U.S. Department of Agriculture, Agricultural Economic Report Number 735, Washington, DC, May 1996.

Gore, A., *Earth in Balance: Ecology and the Human Spirit,* Houghton Mifflin, Boston, 1992.

Hardin, G., "The tragedy of the commons," *Science* 162: 1243–1248, 1968.

Hueting, R., "Three persistent myths in the environmental debate," *Ecological Economics* 18: 81–88, 1996.

Hynes, P. H., *Taking Population Out of the Equation: Reformulating I=PAT,* Institute on Women and Technology, North Amherst, 1993.

Lipschutz, R. D., *Global Civil Society and Global Environmental Governance: The Politics of Nature from Place to Planet,* State University of New York Press, Albany, 1996.

Miller, G. T. Jr., *Living in the Environment: Principles, Connections, and Solutions,* Wadsworth Publishing, Belmont, 1996.

Odum, H. T., *Environmental Accounting: Energy and Decision Making,* John Wiley, New York, 1996.

Orr, D. W., *Ecological Literacy: Education and the Transition to a Postmodern World State,* University of New York Press, Ithaca, 1992.

Princen, T. and M. Finger (w/contributions of J. P. Manno and M. L. Clark), *Environmental NGOs in World Politics: Linking the Local and the Global,* Routledge, London, 1994.

Rees, W. E., "More jobs, less damage: A framework for sustainability, growth, and employment," *Alternatives* 21, 24, 1995a.

Rees, W. E., "Taxing combustion and rehabilitating forest: Achieving sustainability, growth, and employment through energy policy," *Alternatives* 21, 31, 1995b.

Roodman, D. M. *Paying the Piper: Subsidies, Policies, and the Environment.* Worldwatch Paper 13, Worldwatch Institute, Washington, DC, 1996.

Schmidt-Bleek, F., "MIPS—a universal ecological measurement," *Fresenius Ecological Bulletin* 1: 306–311; also in *Fresenius Ecological Bulletin* 2: 8 (1993), a special edition on the Material Inputs per Unit of Service (MIPS) project of the Wuppertal Institut für Klima, Umwelt, und Energie (Wuppertal, Germany), 1993.

Wackernagel, M. and W. E. Rees, *Our Ecological Footprint: Reducing Human Impact on the Earth,* New Society, Gabriola Island, 1994.

Walzer, M., *Spheres of Justice: A Defense of Pluralism and Equality,* Basic Books, New York, 1983.

Wapner, P. K., *Environmental Activism and World Civic Politics,* State University of New York Press, Albany, 1996.

The State of the Planet at the Five-Year Review of Rio and the Prospects for Protecting Worldwide Ecological Integrity

Donald Brown

This book examines what needs to be done to assess and protect global ecological integrity. This chapter examines the prospects for protecting ecological integrity in light of recent environmental trends and failures in hoped-for international cooperation called for at the 1992 United Nations Conference on Environment and Development (UNCED) held in Rio de Janeiro.

The recently concluded United Nations five-year review of the Rio Earth Summit provided a rare opportunity to comprehensively and rigorously analyze how nations were doing in protecting the global environment and what nations are willing to do to reverse negative trends. Although this review showed that some progress has been made since Rio, it revealed many alarming global environmental trends as well as some disturbing social patterns. To many observers of the five-year review of Rio, the most troubling development was the continued absence of international cooperation between the rich and poor countries called for in Rio. In fact, to many observers, bitter suspicion and mistrust had grown between rich and poor nations.

This chapter first describes the deal struck between these countries in 1992 at Rio to solve the interrelated problems of environment and development. Next the chapter provides a detailed description of positive and negative environmental, economic, and social trends since Rio. This is followed by a description of what happened in negotiations among countries at the five-year review of Rio, and of the major barriers blocking progress in reversing trends that show continuing degradation of global, regional, and local ecosystems. The last section examines current prospects for protecting ecosystem integrity worldwide.

The Rio Deal

A report prepared for the United Nations by the World Commission on Environment and Development in 1987 pushed the concept of sustainable development to center stage in international affairs. This report, entitled *Our Common Future,* received extraordinary international attention because it concluded that rapid deterioration of the global environment was threatening life on Earth and that decisive political action was needed to ensure human survival. *Our Common Future* identified several environmental trends that threatened "to radically alter the planet, and many species upon it, including the human species" (WCED 1987). Environmental deterioration identified in the report included: (1) rapid loss of productive dryland that was being transformed into desert, (2) rapid loss of forests, (3) global warming caused by increases in greenhouse gases, (4) loss of the atmosphere's protective ozone shield due to industrial gases, and (5) the pollution of surface and groundwater (WCED 1987).

Until very recently, the problems of environmental degradation and poverty were viewed as unrelated, but *Our Common Future* also focused world attention on the futility of separating economic development problems from environmental issues. The report explained how some forms of development erode the environmental resources upon which they must be based, and how environmental degradation undermines economic development. For instance, development that can't afford to pay for treatment of sewage creates water pollution, and polluted water limits future development options. In addition, in many developing countries, in the absence of help from the developed world, rapid depletion of natural resources is the only hope of eradicating poverty. Thus, the report concluded, "poverty is a major cause and effect of global environmental problems." That is, there is no hope of solving the global environmental problems unless the international community works rapidly to resolve problems of human development throughout the world. Thus, for the first time in human history, *Our Common Future* forced the international community to see problems of poverty, population growth, industrial and social development, depletion of natural resources, and destruction of the environment as closely interrelated.

To solve the twin problems of environmental degradation and development, *Our Common Future* called for a world political transformation that supported "sustainable development" throughout the world. Sustainable development was defined as development that meets the needs of the present without compromising the ability of future generations to meet their needs. *Our Common Future,* because of its identification of the interrelationship between environmental destruction and poverty, put sustainable development on the front burner throughout the world.

In December 1989, the General Assembly of the United Nations, in reaction to the problems identified by *Our Common Future,* called for an unprecedented international meeting—a meeting of all the nations of the world. The United Nations Conference on Environment and Development, generally known as the Earth Summit, was held in Rio de Janeiro in June 1992 in response to *Our Common Future.* The Earth Summit was the largest and most ambitious international conference in history as measured by the number of issues under consideration and the size and number of international delegations. Assembled at the Earth Summit were 110 heads of state, more than any other previous international conference.

Five documents were signed in Rio. They were: (1) the Treaty on Climate Change; (2) the Treaty on Biodiversity; (3) the Convention on Forest Principles; (4) the Rio Declaration; and (5) Agenda 21.

Although it did not receive as much publicity in some parts of the world as the treaties on climate change and biodiversity, Agenda 21 was viewed by many as the most significant of all the Earth Summit agreements. This document was an 800-page blueprint for international action in the twenty-first century. It contains 40 chapters focused on solving the twin problems of environmental protection and sustainable development.

Agenda 21 was the international community's response to the issues raised by *Our Common Future.* It called for governments not only to adopt new environmental programs but to commit to significant economic, social, and international institutional reforms.

To follow up on the implementation of Agenda 21, the United Nations created the United Nations Commission on Sustainable Development (CSD). The CSD annually reviews progress made on specific Agenda 21 chapters.

To get the South to commit to the environmental protection objectives of Agenda 21, the North had to strike a deal with the South. The heart of this deal between North and South was contained in chapter 33 of Agenda 21, which covers financing of sustainable development. This chapter called for the developed countries to contribute 0.7 percent of GNP for direct assistance to the developing world. Section 33.13 of Agenda 21, which was never agreed to by the United States in Rio, states that:

> Developed counties reaffirm their commitments to reach the accepted United Nations target of 0.7% of GNP for Official Development Assistance (ODA) and to the extent they have not achieved this target, agree to augment their aid programs in order

to reach that target as soon as possible and to ensure prompt and effective implementation of Agenda 21.

Before Rio, the ODA—that is, foreign aid—from the North to the South was running above 0.3 percent of GNP worldwide.

In addition to this ODA target in chapter 33 of Agenda 21, other provisions of Agenda 21 that called for the North to help the South included the following chapters:

> *Chapter 3, "Combating Poverty."* This chapter states that all countries share responsibility for combating poverty, and that policies for increasing the sustainability of resource use must avoid increasing poverty. It also states that poverty within nations has both domestic and international causes that call for all countries to cooperate and share responsibility (United Nations 1992).

> *Chapter 4, "Reduction in Unsustainable Production and Consumption Patterns."* This chapter asserts that a major cause of global environmental deterioration is unsustainable production and consumption patterns in the developed countries. Reducing this phenomenon will require reorienting patterns of development in industrial countries that are being copied in much of the developing world. This chapter also calls on developed countries to take the lead in researching and moving toward sustainable resource use (United Nations 1992).

> *Chapter 34, "Capacity Building and Transfer of Technology."* This chapter calls for the developed world to assist the developing world in obtaining access to technology that will promote sustainable development. Transfer of technology includes exchanges of knowledge, goods, services, and organizational procedures (United Nations 1992).

These provisions of Agenda 21 were the heart of global international cooperation called for at Rio. This Rio deal between North and South was a core element in putting the planet on a sustainable development track. At the five-year review of Rio it was clear that the rich nations had not only failed to live up to this deal but had actually moved in the wrong direction.

The State of the Planet at the Five-Year Review

In Rio it was agreed that the nations of the world should review progress in implementing Agenda 21 in 1997. In preparation for the United Nations

General Assembly Special Session (UNGASS) on the five-year review of Rio, the United Nations prepared many detailed reports on the environmental, social, and economic health of the planet in 1997. These UN reports showed that the world had changed dramatically in the five years since the Earth Summit. The most momentous development since Rio was the rapid globalization of the economy entailed by astonishing increases in private foreign investment. The UN reports prepared for UNGASS concluded that large increases in private sector–led growth had become both the source of great hope of many of the world's poorest people and the cause of concern for others. On economic and a few social issues there were some positive trends that were mainly caused by increases in trade-related private sector–led growth. On the other hand, UN data indicated that most of the serious environmental problems of great concern at Rio not only had continued to deteriorate but had actually been exacerbated by the private sector–led growth.

Positive Economic, Social, and Environmental Trends
The following positive major economic, social, and environmental trends were noted in the UN reports prepared for UNGASS.

ECONOMIC

1. During the period 1992–96 growth of GDP in the developing world averaged 5.3 percent per year compared with 3.1 percent in the 1980s and 4.2 percent in 1991–92. The acceleration of GDP growth permitted the per capita growth rate to rise by more than 3 percent per year during 1992–96. The exception to these growth rates was sub-Saharan Africa and the least developed countries, where growth rates continued to fall (United Nations 1997a).

2. The developing world's export volume grew more rapidly than world trade, averaging about 12 percent per year from 1994 to 1996 (United Nations 1997a).

3. Net capital flows of private investment, portfolio investment, and commercial bank lending dramatically increased in the period 1992 to 1995 (United Nations 1997a).

4. The percentage of those living in poverty in developing nations declined slightly between 1990 and 1993, but most improvement was in East Asia and the Pacific (United Nations 1997a).

5. Despite significant sharp energy use rise worldwide, there is no short-term scarcity in energy, although there are significant problems in energy (United Nations 1997a).

SOCIAL

1. Life expectancy increased between 1990 and 1995 (United Nations 1997a).

2. Per capita dietary energy supply (kilocalories) increased in almost all regions of the world except eastern Europe and sub-Saharan Africa (United Nations 1997a).

3. A number of infectious diseases may be decreasing in the future, including polio, leprosy, guinea worm, and neonatal tetanus, but others, namely malaria and dengue, are increasing (United Nations 1997a).

4. Indicators of education such as enrollment ratios and adult literacy show improvement. Rates of illiteracy among adults appear to have declined steadily in developing regions, including South Asia and sub-Saharan Africa (United Nations 1997a).

5. Population growth rates slowed from 2 percent in 1970 to 1.6 percent per year in 1995. Yet middle-level population growth rates see world population above 9 billion by 2050, possibly reaching 11 billion by 2100 (United Nations 1997a).

ENVIRONMENTAL

1. Consumption of some materials is stabilizing in the developed world, although increases in demand have picked up so that use of materials continues to rise (United Nations 1997a).

2. Developed market economies have achieved a significant reduction in energy intensity due to improvements in generation and end-use efficiency. However, the increased volume of economic activity has offset these gains, and in particular, increases in carbon dioxide continue (United Nations 1997a).

3. Some developed countries and a number of middle-income developing countries have experienced significant reduction in energy-related emissions, notably sulfur dioxide (United Nations 1997a).

4. Lead exposure levels are down, due largely to a move toward nonleaded gasoline (United Nations 1997a).

Negative Economic, Social, and Environmental Trends
The following negative major economic, social, and environmental trends were noted in the UN reports prepared for UNGASS.

ECONOMIC

1. In sub-Saharan Africa and the least developed countries, GDP per capita continued to fall since Rio (United Nations 1997a).

2. In the period of high growth after Rio, 1.5 billion people did not share in growth due to unequal distribution (United Nations 1997a).

3. Net flows of Official Development Assistance as a percentage of GNP in the countries of the Organization for Cooperation and Development (OECD) declined from 0.34 percent in 1992 to 0.27 percent in 1995 (United Nations 1997a).

4. Globally, the number of people living in absolute poverty rose to 1.3 billion in 1993 (United Nations 1997a).

SOCIAL

1. Over 2 billion people do not have access to public and/or commercial energy (United Nations 1997a).

2. Growth in population fell faster, national fertility declines were broader and deeper, and migration flows larger, than previous estimates indicated. The latest medium fertility variant projection shows the world population will stabilize at 9.4 billion in 2050, almost half a billion lower than projected in 1994 (United Nations 1997a).

3. Eight hundred and forty million people in the world suffer from malnutrition (United Nations 1997a).

4. Excessive environmental pollution is affecting the health of urban agglomerations in developing counties (United Nations 1997a).

5. In spite of efforts since the start of the International Drinking Water Supply and Sanitation Decade in 1981, some 20 percent of the world's population lacks access to safe water and 50 percent lacks access to safe sanitation (United Nations 1997a).

6. The World Health Organization estimates that more than 5 million people each year die from diseases caused by unsafe drinking water and lack of sanitation (United Nations 1997a).

ENVIRONMENTAL

1. World energy consumption grew more than 40 percent between 1973 and 1993 (United Nations 1997a).

2. Consumption of energy in the developing world is rising rapidly (United Nations 1997a).

3. Global demand for water has increased dramatically over the past century, and it is estimated that 8 percent of the world's population now lives in countries that are highly water stressed and another 25 percent in countries that are experiencing moderate to high water stress. If current trends continue, two-thirds of the world's population could be living in countries experiencing moderate or high water stress by 2025 (United Nations 1997a).

4. Unless managed with a view to achieving much greater efficiency, for which there is considerable potential, water resources could become a serious factor limiting socioeconomic development in many developing countries (United Nations 1997a).

5. As much as 10 percent of the Earth's vegetated surface is now moderately degraded. Continued degradation of the agricultural land base will have serious implications for food supply at the local level (United Nations 1997a).

6. While the medium-term prospects for increasing food production are good, trends in soil quality and the management of irrigated land raise serious questions about longer-term sustainability (United Nations 1997a).

7. For the period 1980 to 1990, the annual estimated loss in natural forest area was 12.1 million hectares. The rates and causes of deforestation differ greatly between countries and regions; determining factors include population density and growth rates, levels and rates of development, and the structure of property rights and cultural systems. Rates of tropical deforestation increased in each of the past three decades in all tropical regions and currently are highest in Asia. The largest losses of forest area are taking place in the tropical moist deciduous forests, the zone best suited to human settlement and agriculture; recent estimates suggest that nearly two-thirds of tropical deforestation worldwide is due to farmers clearing land for agriculture (United Nations 1997a).

8. Coastal ecosystems, including wetlands, tidal flats, saltwater marshes, mangrove swamps, coastal nursery areas, and the flora and fauna that depend upon them, are particularly at risk from industrial pollution and urban land conversion (United Nations 1997a).

9. According to the FAO, 25 percent of the world's marine fisheries are being fished at maximum productivity and 35 percent are overfished (yields are declining) (United Nations 1997a).

10. Biodiversity is increasingly under threat from development, which destroys or degrades natural habitats, and pollution from a variety of

sources. One to 11 percent of the world's species per decade may be threatened by extinction. Major threats to species are related to threats to the ecosystems that support them from both development and pollution (United Nations 1997a).

11. Domestic and industrial waste production continues to increase in volume and per capita terms, worldwide. In the developed world, per capita waste generation has increased threefold over the past 20 years; in the developing world it is highly likely that waste generation will double in the next decade (United Nations 1997a).

12. Approximately 100,000 chemicals are now in commercial use. Persistent organic pollutants are now so widely distributed by air and ocean currents that they are found in the tissues of people and wildlife everywhere; they are of particular concern because of their high levels of toxicity and persistence in the environment. Pollution from heavy metals, especially from their use in industry and mining, is also creating serious health consequences in many parts of the world. Incidents and accidents involving uncontrolled radioactive sources continue to increase (United Nations 1997a).

13. Emissions and concentrations of greenhouse gases continue to rise even as scientific evidence assembled by the Intergovernmental Panel on Climate Change and other relevant bodies continues to diminish the uncertainties and points ever more strongly to the severe risk of global climate change (United Nations 1997b). Assuming the best estimate of climate sensitivity, the temperature increase worldwide will be on the order of 2°C by 2100, which would lead to global sea-level rise of 50 centimeters between the present and the year 2100 (United Nations 1997c). Global warming would also induce changes in continental temperate precipitation patterns, with impacts on soil moisture and potentially more-severe droughts and floods in some places and less severe ones in other places (United Nations 1997c).

14. The ozone layer continues to be degraded despite international success in getting over 149 countries to ratify the Montreal Protocol (United Nations 1997c). Nevertheless, it is believed that if the rapid phase-out of ozone-attacking chemicals called for by the Montreal Protocol is implemented by all nations, ozone concentrations may return to normal levels by 2045 (Parson 1996).

In summary, although some progress had been made since Rio, the globalization of the economy seemed to be accelerating environmental degradation of global, regional, and local ecosystems. Moreover, the Rio deal between the rich and poor countries had failed to materialize. These were the facts that confronted delegates at the United Nations five-year review of Rio.

Backwards from Rio

For six weeks in 1997, nations came to the United Nations to review progress since Rio in an attempt to reinvigorate the spirit of Rio. As the United Nations General Assembly Special Session on the five-year review of Rio came to a close in the early hours of Saturday, June 28, 1997, many weary delegates were wondering whether the spirit of Rio had been seriously wounded. At about 12:20 A.M., summing up the gloomy mood that had gained momentum during the last week of UNGASS, General Assembly president Razali Ismail reluctantly observed that this was not the time to paper over the cracks in the celebrated global partnership for sustainable development, but was instead a time for a sober assessment, an honest acknowledgment that progress to operationalize sustainable development remains insufficient, and that enormous difficulties of overcoming short-term and vested interests were blocking implementation of Agenda 21.

At the close of UNGASS sometime after 1:00 A.M., many disheartened delegates were troubled because not only had the UNGASS text failed to make progress on many important issues, but on some it may actually have weakened Agenda 21 provisions.

Although significant progress in implementation of Agenda 21 had been achieved on few issues since Rio, an acrimonious North-South debate over the content of a political statement in the last few days of UNGASS was viewed by many as another important but failed opportunity to make progress toward a sustainable future. That is, despite some notable successes since Rio in the creation of over one hundred national sustainable development bodies, the initiation of 1,800 local Agenda 21s worldwide, and the entry into force of several treaties, disputes between the developed and developing world over such issues as finance, technology transfer, law, and capacity building continued to block meaningful international agreement on further implementation of Agenda 21.

Attendees at yearly United Nations meetings on Rio could see that a handful of nations had taken Agenda 21 quite seriously, others had made promising starts, some had never moved far out of the starting blocks, and a number of the poorer nations had openly proclaimed that sustained economic growth rather than sustainable development was the national goal they intended to pursue.

Many negotiators had hoped to reinvigorate the spirit of Rio at UNGASS but feared that the CSD had become the hospice for the goal of international cooperation called for by Agenda 21, the UNCED blueprint for solving the interrelated environmental and development problem. Although the CSD had been created to review the implementation of Agenda 21, it too often had become the battleground for renegotiating carefully structured Rio compromises between the North and the South.

Because many poor people around the world had seen real increases in their standard of living due to foreign private investment, these large increases in worldwide trade since Rio were seen by many as the basis for great hope to alleviate the suffering of the more than one billion people still living in absolute poverty. Yet others were concerned about these trends because public foreign aid had actually decreased since Rio, and some of the world's poorest people were not benefiting from private sector–led growth. Moreover, huge increases in private sector foreign investment worried many because evidence has been mounting that private sector–led growth may be exacerbating the global environmental degradation of forests, biodiversity, climate, oceans, and fisheries.

Therefore, the gridlock blocking forward movement on the international sustainable development path that was so apparent at UNGASS was seen by many as a truly tragic development because this standoff was in neither the North's nor the South's interest. This is the case because evidence is accumulating that future generations in rich and poor countries alike will suffer from a degraded environment unless Rio's call for new international cooperation on sustainable development is taken seriously.

Extraordinarily wide income disparities and pollution loadings currently exist between rich and poor countries and between rich and poor within countries.

For instance, the median per capita income of the United States is $35,000 per person (Hammond 1998). This means that the average citizen in the United States earns in a year what the citizen of Africa or India earns in a lifetime (Hammond 1998). In Brazil, the top fifth of income is 32 times the bottom fifth (Hammond 1998).

Moreover, future projections show the gap increasing. By 2025, if current trends continue, the top fifth of the world will exceed the bottom fifth by a factor of 100 (Hammond 1998). The United States is the most unequal of global industrial societies, with the bottom fifth below the poverty line (Hammond 1998).

In pollution loading, the rich countries are contributing far more than their share of pollution on most issues of concern. For instance, the United States emits 20.5 thousand tonnes of CO_2 per capita versus 9.3 for the United Kingdom, 6.7 for Bulgaria, 2.7 for China, 1.0 for India, and 0.8 for Nigeria (Hammond 1998). The United States, Canada, and

Europe account for about 67 percent of the cars on the road. The United States has about one car for every 2 people, while Canada has one car for every 2.1 people. In Bangladesh there is one car for every 2,250 people. In 1994, in China there were 6 cars per 1,000 people (Hammond 1998).

As long as these disparities exist, the developing nations are not likely to take steps to protect global ecology. This was the position that the South consistently articulated during the five-year review of Rio.

Barriers to Protecting Global, Regional, and Local Ecology

The conflict between rich and poor nations on how to move forward is the central barrier to international cooperation to protect global ecology. The poor nations strenuously argue that if the richer countries want to advance the goals of sustainable development adopted at Rio in 1992, they must help the poor countries financially. That is, the South argues that the rich countries must live up to the Rio deal. The poor countries also argue that because the rich countries caused much of the global pollution problems threatening the world, the rich countries have greater responsibilities to cut back on unsustainable consumption patterns.

These two concerns raised by the poor nations, i.e., the call for more development assistance and the differentiated responsibilities of the richer countries to reduce pollution, have become the major unresolved issues that have most frequently prevented progress since Rio. These issues must be faced if the world is to reverse environmental degradation trends.

The key to reversing the dangerous threats to global ecosystems lies in resolving North–South conflicts over international equity. Within the concept of international equity there are several problem areas. These include international finance for sustainable development, unsustainable production and consumption patterns in the developed world, and technology transfer.

The South has been quite understandably nervous about relinquishing any claim to the 0.7 percent GNP for official development assistance contained in Agenda 21, for they fear the North will establish a set of constraints on development that will freeze the South in place developmentally. Yet without diminishing its position on the importance of ODA, the South should support a more focused and expanded analysis of the potential of the private sector to finance sustainable development, because such analysis is likely to more clearly identify the continuing and legitimate needs for ODA.

Reduction of unsustainable production and consumption patterns is also a great source of rich-versus-poor-nation conflict. Because the North emits much higher levels of pollution than the South on a per capita basis, the

North must agree to curb its emissions at a level that takes international equity into account. The North must take the lead on reducing pollution levels.

At the five-year review of Rio, the European Union came closest to initiating a meaningful debate about production and consumption patterns. They called for all industrial nations to reduce materials and energy use by a factor of 4 in the short term and a factor of 10 by 2030. The United States objected to this proposal because it did not target energy and materials practices that cause environmental problems. The rich nations must develop more specific reduction targets if this issue is to be taken seriously.

Agenda 21's call for reduction of unsustainable production and consumption patterns is obviously a very important sustainable development goal, but this subject must be grounded in better factual analysis if it is to be taken seriously. Analytical tools are starting to emerge that will help make better sense of this issue. For instance, the World Resources Institute has produced an analysis of worldwide energy and materials flows that has the potential to foster better understanding of consumption and production issues. However, future discussions on consumption and production must be put on a factual basis following the strategic approach if progress is to be made.

Prospects for Protecting Global, Regional, and Local Ecosystems

At the international level, conflicts between rich and poor countries have become the transcendent issues blocking progress and the largest barrier to protecting global ecosystems. Unless the richer nations agree to curb pollution loadings to a level that takes into account the relevant contribution of nations, and unless the North helps the South fight poverty and finance sustainable development, the trends showing worsening environmental destruction identified at the five-year review of Rio will continue. At the same time, the developing nations must commit to protecting ecosystems to the maximum extent possible.

Other parts of this book examine the concept of ecosystem integrity and make recommendations about what needs to be done to protect ecosystem integrity. Specific recommendations are made about how to measure integrity in a number of different types of ecosystems and how to establish indicators that will monitor changes in ecosystem integrity and warn of degradation. The ability to analyze ecosystem integrity is a necessary but insufficient basis for protecting ecosystem integrity. That is, even if the world established reliable indicators of ecosystem integrity, unless conflicts between the rich and poor nations are greatly reduced, worldwide ecosystem integrity is likely to continue to rapidly decline. Therefore, a first-order problem in protecting ecosystem integrity worldwide that must be faced is the lack of vigorous support of the North for protecting ecosystems in the South. An honest analysis of the failure to make progress at the five-year review of Rio must lead to pessimistic conclusions about current prospects of protecting global ecosystems. Political support in the rich countries for much-expanded financial assistance for the poorer countries' sustainable development activities does not exist at this time. Without such support, the rapid decline in ecosystem integrity will likely continue.

REFERENCES

Hammond, A. 1998. *Which World?: Scenarios for the 21st Century*, Island Press, Washington, DC.

Parson, E.A. 1996. International Protection of the Ozone Layer, in *Green Globe Yearbook*, Oxford University Press, United Nations, New York.

United Nations. 1992. *Agenda 21*, New York.

United Nations. 1997a. *Overall Progress Achieved since the United Nations Conference on Environment and Development*, United Nations, New York.

United Nations. 1997b. *Program of Further Implementation of Agenda 21*, United Nations Special Session of the General Assembly, United Nations, New York.

United Nations. 1997c. *Assessment of Activities That Pose a Major Threat to the Environment*, United Nations, New York.

WCED (World Commission on Environment and Development). 1987. *Our Common Future*, Oxford University Press, New York.

PART VI

Synthesis

CHAPTER 22

Implementing Global Ecological Integrity: A Synthesis

Donald Brown, Jack Manno, Laura Westra, David Pimentel, and Philippe Crabbé

The Global Integrity Project has brought together ecologists, epidemiologists, philosophers, lawyers, economists, and other social scientists to consider the practical meaning of the concept "ecological integrity." Although the U.S. Clean Water Act and the U.S.–Canada Great Lakes Water Quality Agreement include references to ecological integrity in their statements of purpose, other than Karr's index of biological integrity (see Karr, ch. 12 this volume), the concept has never been fully defined and applied in day-to-day environmental decisionmaking. Instead decisionmakers have mostly relied upon isolated measures of chemical and physical parameters, such as dissolved oxygen, bacteria, and turbidity in water; metals in sediments; and productivity in forests when measuring or anticipating the environmental impacts of human actions. By focusing on individual physical and chemical attributes to measure the condition of ecosystems, the whole picture, the integrity of the system, is lost. Such a limited focus has proven to be too narrow to prevent widespread ecosystem degradation throughout the world.

The Integrity Project first set out to evaluate a common understanding of the most important elements constituting ecological integrity and proceeded to look at what happens when integrity is lost or compromised. Next we looked at how integrity can be measured over time so that trends might be determined and ecological systems more effectively protected throughout the world.

In examining ecological integrity we have also looked at related concepts such as wilderness, the wild, and ecological health. We have studied the relationship between ecological integrity and human health as well as ethical and policy arguments for protecting ecosystem integrity. We also considered the question of which policies logically followed if human activities are to be ethically constrained to protect ecosystem integrity.

This chapter summarizes the conclusions of the Integrity Project and identifies additional steps and principles that should be followed to protect and restore ecological integrity. Information is presented in the following sections:

FINDINGS

>   Our Most Urgent Conclusion

>   Concept of Ecological Integrity

>   State of Ecological Integrity Worldwide

>   Measures of Ecological Integrity

>   Relationship between Human Health and
>   Ecological Integrity

>   Causes of Ecosystem Degradation and Barriers to
>   Protecting Ecosystems

>   Ecological Integrity and Human Values

GENERAL PRINCIPLES FOR PROTECTING ECOLOGICAL INTEGRITY

ADDITIONAL STEPS FOR INTERNATIONAL INSTITUTIONS AND GOVERNMENTS TO PROTECT ECOLOGICAL INTEGRITY

Findings

The following are the major findings of the Integrity Project.

Our Most Urgent Conclusion

The Integrity Project believes that one of its conclusions needs to be stressed above all others: that there is an urgent need for rapid and fundamental change in the ecologically destructive patterns of collective human behavior. We must quickly reverse worldwide ecological degradation now taking place at all ecological scales. Because the developing world appears to be committed to following the destructive development path of the developed world and because the developed world's production and consumption patterns are already exceeding the ability of ecosystems to respond, human development is moving on an increasingly dangerous trajectory.

The course corrections needed to avoid disaster are not minor ones; they entail hard-to-imagine U-turns and transformations of policy. For instance, to prevent serious degradation from human-induced climate change, the developed world will have to reduce fossil fuels use by 80 to 90 percent below current usage during a time when business-as-usual growth in fossil fuels consumption is expected to climb to between four and six times current usage. Pressure on forests, fish stocks, remaining arable land, and freshwater supplies creates similar daunting needs for dramatic consumption reversals. To turn around current degradation trends, humans need to rapidly reinvent the completely ecologically dysfunctional political and economic systems of our times. In the words of William Rees, humans need to turn from managing the environment to managing themselves.

The Concept of Ecological Integrity

The Integrity Project has brought together scientists and philosophers who are interested in clarifying the concept of ecological integrity. Included in this group have been some who were somewhat skeptical of the basic intelligibility of some elements of the concept in light of the random and contingent natural forces that initially shape and continue to change ecosystems over time (e.g., see Sagoff, ch. 4). Others in the Integrity Project have responded to the skeptics' concerns while accepting a number of the skeptics' points (e.g., Partridge, ch. 5; Westra et al., ch. 2; Holland, ch. 3; and Ulanowicz, ch. 6). This interchange among participants in the Integrity Project has been stimulating and fruitful in clarifying the concept of ecological integrity.

In addition to this examination of the fundamental meaning of "ecological integrity," the Integrity Project sought to distinguish the concept of ecological integrity from such terms as the "ecosystem approach" and "biodiversity." The major conclusions of the Integrity Project's inquiry in regard to these conceptual issues are:

- Ecological integrity should be defined as an ecosystem's undiminished ability to continue its natural path of evolution, its normal transition over time, and its successional recovery from perturbations. (Westra et al., ch. 2)

- The concept of ecological integrity denotes the quality of the ecosystem and its biota that is the product of evolutionary and biogeographical processes with minimal influence from human society. (Karr, ch. 12)

- In protecting ecological integrity, we are seeking to protect or reestablish not a specific structural configuration (at least for the areas defined as wild) but an optimum structural capacity that reflects the system's evolutionary history. (Westra et al., ch. 2)

- Ecosystems comprise thousands of species interacting in dynamic relationships, the properties of which cannot be predicted from knowledge of the individual species in isolation. Species invade or disappear, evolve or become extinct, and many system variables are in constant flux. Yet ecosystems have structure, pattern, and predictability despite the radically contingent forces that may have created them. The structure, pattern, and function of ecosystems provide "goods and services" upon which all life depends. (See Westra et al., ch. 2; Partridge, ch. 5)

- Below global scale, demarcation of ecosystems into subsystems is often made for practical reasons, and therefore any identified ecosystem should be understood to have epistemological rather than ontological significance (see Miller and Ehnes, ch. 9). That is, there is some flexibility in making demarcations of ecosystems where decisions of scale are often made on the basis of the problems one is trying to address.

- The concept of ecological integrity should be understood to be a species of an "ecosystem approach" to understanding human–environment interactions with an added normative element. That is, the concept of ecological integrity entails protection of ecosystems at a level that would preserve the integrity of the ecosystem. By contrast, an "ecosystem approach" is understood to require analysis of human-induced impacts on entire ecosystems but does not specify what level of protection should be achieved through policy implementation. Governments could, for instance, adopt an ecosystem approach to assure that water quality meets drinking water standards. Yet managing a watershed to meet drinking water standards would not necessarily prevent channelization of a river, a dramatic modification to the ecosystem that could severely degrade benthic biota. By contrast, the concept of ecological integrity should be understood to entail an ecosystem approach that targets protecting or restoring the integrity of an ecosystem as its goal.

- The concept of ecological integrity is distinguishable from the idea of sustainable development. The concept of sustainable development can also be understood to be an idea that entails normative elements. That is, development is sustainable if it does not degrade the environment. In addition, the idea of sustainable development is also understood to include the normative prescription that governments should integrate environmental, economic, and social goals in developing policy, a necessary approach to achieving global ecological integrity. The concept of sustainable development, however, does not contain any specific policy endpoint that establishes the environmental protection goal to be reached by development projects, nor does the concept of sustainable development specify how conflicts should be resolved between competing environmental and development goals. Under the concept of sustainable development, for instance, one could also decide to manage a watershed to provide drinking water as the highest use of the water, a goal that does not prohibit channelization and concomitant degradation of benthic biota. Such degradation would be incompatible with the concept of ecological integrity.

- Protection of ecological integrity is a broader goal than protecting either biodiversity or endangered species because ecosystem integrity can be threatened before loss of biodiversity or species is experienced. In protecting ecosystem integrity, it is not individual species, the quantities of stocks and productivity, or resource use by humans that is of paramount importance, but the ecological system they all depend on that is the focus of concern.

State of Ecological Integrity Worldwide

Many members of the Integrity Project reviewed the condition of ecological systems worldwide in preparing their work for the Integrity Project and in making contributions to this book (see Miller and Rees, ch. 1; Westra et al., ch. 2; Goodland and Pimentel, ch. 7; Rees, ch. 8; Loucks, ch. 10; Pauly, ch. 13; Westra ch. 16; McMichael, ch. 14; Brown, ch. 21). The Integrity Project's conclusions about the state of ecological systems worldwide are as follows:

- Ecological integrity is greatly threatened worldwide and for all types of ecosystems (terrestrial, aquatic, polar, ocean, and coastal) at all scales (global, regional, and local). (Passim)

- Almost all ecosystems on the planet, including those that have been preserved by governments in protected areas and those in the remotest of unprotected wild areas, have been affected by human activity through the long-range transport of toxic substances and human-induced climate change (Goodland and Pimentel, ch. 7; Rees, ch. 8; Westra, ch. 16; McMichael, ch. 14; Brown, ch. 21).

- Current human-induced stresses on ecosystems are threatening to degrade ecosystems beyond threshold points, that is, the points at which additional degradation will trigger irreversible collapse of ecosystems. It

is not currently known, however, at what levels of degradation ecosystem threshold levels will be triggered. It is now possible, however, to
measure the biological state of affairs of ecosystems that appear to have
relatively high levels of ecological integrity and compare these unaffected ecosystems to threatened ecosystems of similar types. As stated
more fully above, the Integrity Project recommends two general
methods of measuring ecological integrity.

- Efforts to protect endangered species of plants and animals or to protect
  biodiversity through habit protection in protected areas are grossly inadequate because they are not extensive enough to protect worldwide
  threatened species habitat, nor do they deal with ecological impacts in
  protected areas caused by human activities outside the protected areas.
  In other words, ongoing efforts to protect endangered species or biodiversity have not designated a sufficient amount nor appropriate placement of wild lands nor begun to deal with the buffer effects of human
  activities where buffer effects are understood to be those impacts on
  wild lands caused by human actions outside the wild lands. (See Noss,
  ch. 11)

- Appropriate goals for conservation of landscapes are: (1) representing all
  kinds of ecosystems, across their natural range of variation, in protected
  areas; (2) maintaining viable populations of all native species in natural
  patterns of abundance and distribution; (3) sustaining ecological and
  evolutionary processes within their natural range of variability; and (4)
  building a conservation network that is adaptable to environmental
  change. (Noss, ch. 11)

- Most existing protected areas are too small to remain viable over the
  long run unless they are buffered and connected. The answer to how
  much additional protected area is needed to conserve landscape ecosystems must be developed empirically, case by case. Nevertheless, most
  estimates of the area needed in reserves in order to attain well-accepted
  conservation goals range from 25 to 75 percent of the ecoregion. (Noss,
  ch. 11; Westra et al., ch. 2)

- Stresses to the biosphere are causing tensions between human communities that can create conflict and its attendant damage to public health.
  Of particular concern from the standpoint of international tensions is
  the growing scarcity of fresh water because almost 40 percent of the
  human population is facing water scarcity. (McMichael, ch. 14)

- Some types of ecological degradation are of particular concern, including worldwide degradation of fresh water, rapid destruction of
  forests and coastal ecosystems, loss of biodiversity and species, and

degradation of fisheries stocks and soil quality needed to feed growing world populations. (Rees, ch. 8; Goodland and Pimentel, ch. 7; McMichael, ch. 14; Pauly, ch. 13; Brown, ch. 21)

- Human-induced climate change presents an immense threat to ecological integrity and human welfare because of its great potential to create rapid stresses on species and ecosystems that far exceed their ability to adapt and because of its great human health consequences to many of the poorest people around the world. (Schrecker, ch. 17; Rees, ch. 8; Goodland and Pimentel, ch. 7; Westra, ch. 16; McMichael, ch. 14; Pauly, ch. 13; Brown, ch. 21)

- The degradation of fish stocks in coastal waters is approaching or has already exceeded threshold levels around the world. As fish species high on the food chain have disappeared, humans are fishing further down the food chain to meet human consumption needs, a development that further threatens to trigger disastrous threshold responses. (Pauly, ch. 13)

- There is growing evidence that forests around the world may be approaching threshold points due to air pollution–induced degradation of soils and biota. (Miller and Ehnes, ch. 9; Loucks, ch. 10)

- Various well-known environmental trends—zone depletion, fisheries collapse, human-induced climate change, falling water tables—are not first-order problems, but rather are symptoms of fundamental human ecological dysfunction of current economic and government systems. (Rees, ch. 8)

- Recent plateauing of the productivity of our main terrestrial and marine food-producing ecosystems raises serious questions about our ability to feed growing human populations. (Goodland and Pimentel, ch. 7)

- There is no possibility of global ecological integrity or health or even sustainability on the current global development track, which assumes 9 billion people and a five- to eightfold expansion of world economic product by 2050, particularly assuming known technologies. (Rees, ch. 8)

- Sustainable development requires a 90 percent reduction in energy consumption in industrial countries. (Rees, ch. 8)

- Despite significant increases in world GNP initiated by private sector–led growth in an increasing globalized economy, the gap between the richest and poorest countries is widening and the pace of environmental degradation has been increasing. (Brown, ch. 21)

Measures of Ecological Integrity

To make the idea of ecological integrity practically useful, the Integrity Project has examined a variety of approaches to measuring ecological integrity. Many parameters of ecosystems are currently frequently measured, such as air and water quality, landscape type and distribution, biomass productivity, and biological diversity. Although these measurements are often of value and need to be continued, they fail to give a holistic understanding of ecological integrity and thereby may fail to indicate important negative trends in the ecological state of affairs or an appropriate level of restoration. To correct these limitations, the Integrity Project recommends certain measurements of ecological integrity be initiated by policy makers. In addition, because there is growing evidence that demonstrates a relationship between degradation of both ecological systems and human health, the Integrity Project recommends greater use of epidemiological tools that can more precisely determine ecology–health relationships. The conclusions of the Integrity Project in regard to measuring ecological integrity are as follows:

- There are two basic approaches to measuring ecological integrity that are recommended. The first is a direct measurement of biological conditions of an ecosystem compared to baseline conditions of wild nature using multimetric biological indices. Karr (ch. 12) pioneered this first method with the development of the index of biological integrity (IBI). IBI was initially developed for river ecosystems and is being used around the world. There are also a number of ongoing attempts to extend IBI to terrestrial ecosystems.

- In developing multimetric biological indices for IBI, five tasks are critical (Karr, ch. 12). They are: (1) classification to define homogeneous sets; (2) selection of appropriate metrics; (3) development of sampling protocols; (4) analysis of data to reveal biological patterns; and (5) communication of biological conditions. (Karr, ch. 12)

- Loucks (ch. 10) adopted Karr's basic approach to measure pollution impacts on forest ecosystems, yet, rather than measuring biota, Loucks's approach focuses primarily on forest productivity. This approach is entitled mean functional integrity (MFI).

- Miller and Ehnes (ch. 9) also use Karr's IBI as a point of departure for developing indicators for the midboreal forests of Canada. This work examines several issues that need to be considered in extending IBI to forests.

- The second general approach to measuring ecological integrity is the method proposed by Ulanowicz (ch. 6), which measures characteristics of ecosystems' organization, structural flows, vigor, and resilience.

- Because integrity is not a unitary attribute of an ecosystem but a product of various attributes, multiple measures of ecosystem integrity are recommended.

- To extend IBI beyond watershed approaches and beyond that which has been recommended by Loucks, additional theoretical and empirical research may be necessary. (See Miller and Ehnes, ch. 9, for a description of issues that must be considered.)

- The recommended scale of concern for measurement of the integrity of landscapes is the ecoregion. (Miller and Ehnes, ch. 9)

- William Rees's "ecological footprint" analysis should be widely used for a variety of purposes, including informing people around the world about the impacts of their actions on ecosystems at a distance from their own communities, and to encourage all to limit their footprint to an equitable share of the Earth's carrying capacity while protecting global ecological integrity. (See Rees, ch. 8; also Wackernagel and Rees 1996)

- Epidemiological tools should be used more widely to understand cause-and-effect relationships between ecological degradation and human health. (Soskolne et al., ch. 15)

Relationship between Human Health and Ecological Integrity

Because of growing but sometimes inconclusive evidence that links ecological degradation to human health, the Integrity Project has been interested in examining this relationship between human health and degradation of ecological integrity. Although human health indicators have improved on average throughout the world in the last several decades, there is increasing evidence that links ecological degradation to human disease. Some ecological trends pose enormous long-term threats that could terminate or reverse the recent positive trends in human health.

The major conclusions of the Integrity Project in regard to the relationship between ecological integrity and human health are:

- Epidemiological tools should be used more widely to understand cause-and-effect relationships between ecological degradation and human health. (Soskolne et al., ch. 15)

- Environmentally related risks to human health arise from:

  - Increased exposure to UVA/UVB radiation due to loss of strato-spheric ozone

  - Physical and disease impacts of climate change

  - Exposure to toxic wastes

  - Exposure to the hazardous by-products of industrial pollution

  - Exposure to chemical food additives and chemical residues

  - Long-term, disseminated exposure to persistent organic chemicals

  - The loss of nature's "goods and services" through loss of biodiversity fragmentation of natural landscapes, deforestation, and increased presence of particulate and other air pollutants

  - Decline in safe water supplies

  - Direct contact with pathogens through encroachment with the wild

  - Potential hazards from bioengineered food and transgenics

  - Exposure to antibiotic-resistant strains of pathogens

  - Increases in communicative disease risk caused by increased human migration (Westra, ch. 16; McMichael, ch. 14)

- The poorest people in the world are most likely to have their health harmed by environmental degradation, the very people who have the least medical resources on which to rely in case of disease or sickness caused by increased human migration. (Schrecker, ch. 17; McMichael, ch. 14; Westra, ch. 16; Brown, ch. 21)

- Human-induced climate change will change rates of mortality and morbidity due to heat waves and thermal stresses in general, the respi-ratory consequences of change in exposure to aeroallergens, and the di-rect, often physical, hazards of any increases in extreme weather events—including storms, floods, and droughts. The indirect health ef-fects of climate change include alteration in the range and activity of vector-borne infectious diseases (such as malaria, leishmaniasis, and dengue); changes in the transmission of person-to-person diseases (in-cluding food poisoning and waterborne pathogens); nutritional and health consequences of local and regional changes in agricultural pro-ductivity; and the various consequences of rising sea levels. There would also be more diffuse public health consequences due to popula-tion displacement, migration (both "economic" and "distress" migra-tion), and enforced loss of employment due to disruptive effects of climate change on various economic sectors and vulnerable locations. (McMichael, ch. 14)

- The rapidly expanding human population and the environmental degradation it causes are contributing to various health problems. (McMichael, ch. 14)

- Increasing environmental degradation is increasing the risks of malnutrition, ultraviolet radiation exposure, the spread of pathogenic microbes, and releases in chemical and biological pollution to food, air, water, and soil. Chemical pollutants include use of pesticides, water pollution due to the absence of sewage treatment, and air pollution, which includes biomass cooking and tobacco smoke. All of these pollution problems will be compounded further as the world population increases from 6 billion to as many as 10 billion in the next 50 years. (Passim)

- Global change processes that pose risks to human health are of two broad types. At one extreme are changes that transcend their point of origin and entail change in truly global "commons." This category includes "greenhouse"-mediated climate change and stratospheric ozone depletion. A different type of global change comprises the mosaics of multiple local changes, which tend to aggregate and span most of the world. This category includes deforestation, land degradation, the spread of irrigation, the depletion of fresh water (especially aquifers), loss of biodiversity, and depletion or displacement of ocean fisheries. Both types of degradation create adverse consequences for human health. (McMichael, ch. 14)

- There is growing evidence that human health is already being adversely affected by climate change. This includes evidence of increased vector-borne disease, malaria, dengue, and meningitis. (McMichael, ch. 14)

- The health impacts of stratospheric ozone loss include increased sunburn, skin cancer, various eye disorders, and perhaps immune suppression. (McMichael, ch. 14)

- Some of the poorest countries in the world are likely to suffer most from climate change. These countries include Bangladesh, Egypt, Pakistan, Indonesia, and Thailand, where populations are threatened by rising sea level, loss of fishing mangroves, tropical cyclones, and droughts. (McMichael, ch. 14)

- There are serious health impacts caused by growing land degradation stemming from erosion, desertification, nutrient exhaustion, waterlogging, and salinization. The poorest countries are also at most risk from land degradation, including sub-Saharan Africa, the foothills of the Himalayas and the Andes, Haiti and Honduras, and Central and South America. Poor people in the growing cities throughout the world also experience increased obesity, hypertension, cigarette smoking, sedentism, and traffic-related diseases. (McMichael, ch. 14)

Causes of Ecosystem Degradation and Barriers to Protecting Ecosystems

To make recommendations on how to reverse recent adverse trends, the Integrity Project explored causes of worldwide ecological degradation and barriers to protecting ecosystems. Although the Integrity Project has not attempted to describe all causes of ecological degradation and barriers to greater ecological protection, it believes that certain causes and barriers need to be stressed based upon our investigations. The major conclusions of the Integrity Project relating to causes of degradation and barriers to protection include the following:

- Vast increases in human population coupled with the enhanced technical ability and power to cause adverse ecological impacts have enabled humans to create, for the first time in history, truly global ecological impacts while creating unprecedented destruction of regional and local ecosystems. (Passim)

- Often the global ecological consequences of individual human actions are not visible at the place where the action is initiated because consequences are felt long distances from where the damaging activity takes place. That is, without an attempt of governments or individuals to understand their global ecological footprints, individuals are unable to tie their actions to global consequences. (Rees, ch. 8; Wackernagel and Rees 1996)

- Most protected areas are too small to remain viable over the long run unless they are buffered and connected. The answer to how much additional protected area is needed must be developed empirically, case by case. Nevertheless, most estimates of the area needed in reserves in order to attain well-accepted conservation goals range from 25 to 75 percent of each ecoregion. (Noss, ch. 11)

- The richer nations have utterly failed to live up to their obligations to the developing world to assist with financial resources, poverty alleviation, and technology transfer, and to refrain from unsustainable patterns of production and consumption. (Brown, ch. 21)

- Recent large increases in private sector–led growth worldwide have been characterized by accelerating global environmental degradation. In many parts of the world, large increases in economic activity are taking place in nations that have neither adequate environmental laws and regulation nor the financial resources to implement a modern environmental law regime. (Brown, ch. 21)

- The developed world has neither reduced unsustainable levels of production and consumption nor assisted the developing world with financing sustainable development despite promises to do so at the Earth Summit in Rio de Janeiro in 1992. (Brown, ch. 21)

- Most agricultural practices around the world are seriously unsustainable because, among other reasons, fuel prices and water use and irrigation pumping costs don't reflect external environmental damage. (Goodland and Pimentel, ch. 7)

- Economic systems worldwide fail to internalize environmental costs, value natural capital, or deal with questions of distributive justice. (Goodland and Pimentel, ch. 7; Brown, ch. 21)

- Most economists have not yet acknowledged that the economy is an open, growing, wholly dependent subsystem of a materially closed, nongrowing, finite ecosphere. (Rees, ch. 8)

- Ecosystem integrity is threatened by direct human impacts, such as point source discharges into streams, and indirect impacts, such as deposition of air pollutants that travel long distances in the atmosphere. (Noss, ch. 11; Westra, ch. 16; Brown, ch. 21)

- Our survival depends on many of nature's "goods and services" that are invisible to markets and the economy. (Rees, ch. 8)

- Government boundaries do not match ecosystem boundaries, and governments sharing ecosystems with others have failed to create government decisionmaking institutions that match ecosystem management needs. (Miller and Ehnes, ch. 9; Brown, ch. 21)

- Current market-based methods of determining value fail to value important functions of ecosystems that produce and support life on Earth. (Manno, ch. 20; Brown, ch. 21)

- The economy rewards innovations that promote commoditization with investments and research and development and does not reward those innovations that are less commoditized. Thus the economy drives the evolution of human activity toward increasing commoditization and a corresponding increase in the mobilization of the Earth's material and energy resources, a trend in the exact opposite direction from what is typically recommended as the path toward sustainable development. (Manno, ch. 20)

- A bitter North versus South fight over who will pay for sustainable development has been responsible for increasing global ecological degradation. (Brown, ch. 21)

- The rich countries continue to contribute larger shares of pollution loading at a time when differences in income between rich and poor countries are increasing, and many of the burdens of ecological degradation will fall most heavily on the poorest nations. (Schrecker, ch. 17; Brown, ch. 21)

- Existing laws do not create sufficient civil or criminal sanctions for those who engage in activities that are jeopardizing human health through environmental degradation. (Westra, ch. 16)

- Despite international recognition of the precautionary principle as the appropriate standard for dealing with scientific uncertainty about the consequences of human actions when the environment is being seriously threatened, the precautionary principle has not been widely adopted by governments in domestic decisionmaking. (Partridge, ch. 5; Westra, ch. 16; Brown, ch. 21)

Ecological Integrity and Human Values

The Integrity Project started with th e assumption that environmental problems are fundamentally interdisciplinary in nature and that implementation of policies to solve these problems must attempt to integrate environmental science, economics, law, and ethics in problem analysis, synthesis, and solution. Although most members of the Integrity Project have been scientists, the work of the Integrity Project was initiated by the work of a philosopher, Laura Westra. In addition to Dr. Westra, other philosophers who have made major contributions to the work of the Integrity Project have included Ernest Partridge, Mark Sagoff, Peter Miller, James Sterba, Alan Holland, and Ted Schrecker. Believing that values and ethical assumptions of society are important considerations for determining whether a concept is implementable, the Integrity Project examined the ethical basis for protecting ecological integrity. Contributions about the ethical basis for our conclusions came not only from the philosophers but also through active participation by most members of the Integrity Project in discussions about the ethical underpinnings of proposed policy. Although Westra and Sterba are acknowledged biocentrists, other philosophers examined the ethical basis for protecting ecological integrity from other ethical points of view. The major conclusions of the Integrity Project relating to the ethical basis for protection of ecological integrity are as follows:

- Natural ecosystems are valuable to and in themselves, for their continuing support of life on Earth, for their aesthetic features, and for the "goods and services" they provide for humankind. (Westra et al., ch. 2; Sterba, ch. 19)

- The focus of human value and ethical systems must be expanded to include consideration of human impacts on ecological integrity because all life depends upon protection of ecological integrity. (Sterba, ch. 19)

- Although biocentric ethical arguments made by Westra, Sterba, and others strongly support protection of ecological integrity as having value in itself, because environmentally destructive human activities are degrading and seriously threatening human health, anthropocentric ethical positions also support taking a tougher stand on outlawing ecological degradation than is now accepted by governments. (Westra, ch. 16; McMichael, ch. 14; Sterba, ch. 19)

- The human race needs to develop an ecological ethic that gives more weight to international and intergenerational distributive justice. (Schrecker, ch. 17; Brown, ch. 21)

- Ecosystem integrity—retention of a full complement of species, the capacity for continued self-production, and retention of full developmental potential—is of value in its own right. (Westra et al., ch. 2)

- Most ethical systems require humans to consider the consequences of actions before taking action. For this reason, humans must learn to see the ecological consequences of actions that are experienced far from where an initiating action takes place now that it is clear that local human actions have global consequences. For this reason, communication about the ecological footprint of one's own community is ethically compelled. (Rees, ch. 8)

- Society has chronically undervalued the biological components of ecosystems, a fact that is antithetical to many ethical norms. (Goodland and Pimentel, ch. 7; Sterba, ch. 19; Westra, ch. 16)

- Because the poorest people in the world will suffer most from degradation of ecological integrity, the rich nations have ethical obligations to both: (1) refrain from unsustainable patterns of production and consumption, and (2) assist the poorest countries to move to a sustainable future. In addition, the richest nations may have ethical responsibilities to pay damages for harm to ecological systems caused by the developed world in the developing world. (Schrecker, ch. 17; Westra, ch. 16; McMichael, ch. 14; Brown, ch. 21)

- A biocentric ethic strongly supports protection of ecological integrity because ecosystems promote the good of humans and plants and animals, the center of value in a biocentric ethic. (Sterba, ch. 19)

- Although the developed nations have failed to fulfill their responsibilities to the poorer nations on a variety of issues, the richer nations have a particularly important ethical responsibility to the poorer nations to alleviate the suffering caused by human-induced climate change that is taking place and will take place with greater force in the developing world. (Schrecker, ch. 17; Westra, ch. 16; McMichael, ch. 14; Brown, ch. 21)

- Because the diets of the developed world include large quantities of meat from cattle that feed on grains that are needed to feed the starving and undernourished in the developing world, those in the developed world should eat less meat. (Goodland and Pimentel, ch. 7)

General Principles for Protecting Ecological Integrity

The Integrity Project has examined general principles that should be followed by all to protect ecological integrity. The following principles are norms that the Integrity Project believes should be binding on all:

- Because we should not engage in activities that are potentially harmful to natural systems and life in general, humans should protect ecological integrity. (Westra 1998)

- We should accept an "ecological worldview" and thus reject an "expansionist worldview" that entails an unlimited ability to expand energy and materials use. (Westra 1998)

- We need to be aware of our ecological footprint and reduce it to levels that are protective of global ecological integrity based upon principles of international and intergenerational equity. (Rees, ch. 8; Wackernagel and Rees 1996)

- In order to protect and defend ecological integrity, we must start by designing policies that are capable of dealing with complexity. In this regard, human activities should be limited by the requirements of the precautionary principle. (Westra 1998; Partridge, ch. 5; Brown, ch. 21)

- When human-induced stresses begin threatening ecosystem thresholds, we will have reached the point at which irreversible ecosystem collapse will take place, yet there is some scientific uncertainty about when thresholds will be exceeded. Therefore decisionmakers and governments must apply the precautionary principle to decisions that may affect ecosystems. (Partridge, ch. 5; Brown, ch. 21; Westra, ch. 16)

- Environmental, social, and economic sustainability are interrelated concepts. There can be no economic or social sustainability without environmental sustainability. (Goodland and Pimentel, ch. 7)

- To be sustainable, use of renewable resources must be kept within the regenerative capacities of the natural systems that generate them. (Goodland and Pimentel, ch. 7)

- Depletion rates of nonrenewable resources should be set below the rate at which renewable substitutes are developed by human invention and investments. (Rees, ch.8)

- To assure sustainability, waste emissions from a project or action should be kept within the assimilative capacity of the local environment or risk degradation of ecological integrity. (Rees, ch. 8)

- Economic subsidies that encourage unsustainable use of resources should be removed. (Goodland and Pimentel, ch. 7)

- Humans must understand that everyone lives in a buffer zone for protected areas because human activities are already affecting protected areas and the remotest of wilderness areas. (Noss, ch. 8; Westra 1998)

- Agricultural practices must be transformed so that they are sustainable and in particular assure that soil quality is maintained, water quality is not degraded, and water quantity is conserved. (Goodland and Pimentel, ch. 7)

- Humans must expand the definition of human welfare to include impacts on ecosystem integrity. (Rees, ch. 8)

- Humans must understand the global ecosphere, human society, and the global economy as complex systems, with the latter a subsystem of the former. (Rees, ch. 8)

- Waste emissions must be kept within the assimilative capacity of ecological systems. (Rees, ch. 8)

- The criteria for selecting protected areas are: (1) protection of special elements, (2) representation of all habitats, and (3) meeting the needs of focal species. Protected areas must be protected by buffers and connected by corridors. (Noss, ch. 11)

- The principles of protected area design must be reexamined upon their application. Nevertheless, the starting principles of protected area design are: (1) species well distributed across their native range are less susceptible to extinction than species confined to small portions of their range; (2) large blocks of habitat, containing large populations, are better than small blocks with small populations; (3) blocks of habitat, containing large populations, are better than blocks far apart; (4) habitat in contiguous blocks is better than fragmented habitat; (5) interconnected blocks of habitat are better than isolated blocks; and (6) blocks of habitat that are roadless or otherwise inaccessible to humans are better than roaded and accessible habitat blocks. (Noss, ch. 11)

- An ecosystem approach to a city requires that cities must be clean (i.e., not impair the uses of ecosystems), green (i.e., protect natural ecosystem functions), usable by people according to diversified tastes, open (i.e., physically accessible and aesthetically inviting), accessible to all, continuous so as not to break the ecosystem artificially, affordable, and attractive while valorizing nature. (Crabbé, ch. 18)

Additional Steps for International Institutions and Governments to Protect Ecological Integrity

In addition to the general principles that should be followed by all, the following are steps that should be taken by international institutions and governments to better protect ecological integrity:

- International institutions and governments at all levels need to immediately communicate the urgency of our findings. In particular, people should be informed about the tenuous state of affairs of global, regional, and local ecosystems and that threshold points are likely being approached for many ecosystems worldwide.

- International institutions and governments need immediately to begin to measure ecological integrity in accordance with the recommendations in this book and develop additional indicators of ecological integrity and relationships between ecological integrity and human health, while examining the social and economic causes of degradation of ecological integrity. These measurements need to be developed at all geographical scales, and measurement at various scales should be coordinated so that measurements at lower scales can be used at higher scales. Measures of integrity should be initiated on a strategic planning basis with the most important and vulnerable ecosystems being measured first. International institutions such as the United Nations Environment Programme, the United Nations Development Programme, and the World Health Organization, supported by the Bretton Woods institutions, should coordinate global monitoring of ecological integrity.

- International institutions and governments around the world need to determine which human activities outside protected areas may have impacts on ecological integrity inside protected areas and outlaw activities that may cause any degradation within the protected areas. In this regard, it is imperative that governments proceed as quickly as possible to reverse human-induced climate change and the long-range transport of toxic substances.

- International institutions and governments around the world need to take steps to greatly increase the quantity of areas protected from human activities while assuring that those ecosystems of significant ecological importance are included in such protected areas. Protected areas must be buffered and connected by corridors. (Noss, ch. 11)

- International institutions and governments need to assure that economic incentives and disincentives are structured to protect global ecological integrity.

- Because it is sometimes difficult for citizens to understand the consequences of their actions on places far from where the initiating action takes place, international institutions and governments need to use, develop, and frequently publicize the ecological footprints of the relevant societies' activities on global ecosystems. (Rees, ch. 8)

- The developed nations must immediately live up to their obligations to the poorer nations to assist in financing sustainable development, to give much greater assistance to alleviate poverty, and to transfer technology on concessional terms. The developed nations also have special obligations to adjust unsustainable production and consumption patterns because the developed world is producing pollution and consuming resources at a greatly disproportionate rate. (Schrecker, ch. 17; Brown, ch. 21)

- International institutions should calculate the amount of assistance that the developing world needs to protect global ecological integrity. Nations in the developed world need to dedicate themselves to providing financial and technical assistance to the developing world. To do this, all developed nations should begin to fulfill their promises made at the 1992 Earth Summit to provide 0.7 percent of GDP for financing sustainable development in the developing world. (Brown, ch. 21)

- International institutions and nations must increase their efforts to stabilize population while reducing consumption. (Goodland and Pimentel, ch. 7)

- Governments must create institutions or cooperate with other governments so that government actions relating to any individual ecosystem are coordinated by assuring that ecosystem boundaries match government jurisdictions.

- International institutions must create protected areas for all native ecosystem types and serial stages across their natural range of variation. (Noss, ch. 11)

- International institutions and governments must protect viable populations of native species in natural patterns of abundance and distribution through the creation of protected areas. (Noss, ch. 11)

- To protect ecosystems, governments must maintain evolutionary processes, such as disturbance regimes, nutrient cycles, and biotic interactions. (Noss, ch. 11)

- Governments must manage landscapes and communities to be responsive to short- and long-term environmental change and to maintain the evolutionary potential of biota.

- Governments need to set aside appropriate areas for wild reserves while designing for reserve networks and provide for standard buffers and corridors. (Noss, ch. 11)

- To determine the "ideal" size for reserves, governments must target the primary biota for protection and restoration. (Noss, ch. 11)

- To retain integrity of marine ecosystems, governments must abolish subsidies for fishing, support transition to small-scale fishing wherever possible, establish large marine protected areas, enforce limits, and rapidly implement market-based, community-based, and ecology-based mitigation measures. (Pauly, ch. 13)

- Governments should consider the expansion of criminal law to include human activities that threaten human health through degradation of ecological integrity. (Westra, ch. 16)

- Governments should support greater use of epidemiological tools to understand cause-and-effect relationships between loss of ecological integrity and human health. (Soskolne et al., ch. 15)

- International institutions and governments should assure that public health statistics are augmented by indices of sustainable public health so that the potential damage to public health that may be entailed by adverse environmental trends will be counted for a more realistic picture. (McMichael, ch. 14)

- Richer nations need to compensate poorer nations for protecting global ecological integrity. (Schrecker, ch. 17)

- To reduce urban sprawl, governments need to reduce transportation subsidies and invest in public transportation. (Crabbé, ch. 18)

- To protect ecological integrity threatened by cities, city governments should use tools available to cities, including official plans, zoning, protection of essential functions of ecosystems, building codes, investment in transit systems and pollution prevention, taxes and subsidies, and education. (Crabbé, ch. 18)

- Governments must intervene in markets to effectively counterbalance commoditization pressures and adopt policy instruments that would result in (a) increased public investment in research and development for noncommodity products; (b) taxes and fees for energy and materials that internalize environmental and social costs; (c) laws that protect ecological integrity; (d) more investment in social and natural capital; (e) tax reforms on labor; (f) abolishing harmful subsidies; (g) protecting workers' rights; and (h) empowering local and indigenous communities. (Manno, ch. 20)

REFERENCES

Wackernagel, M. and W. Rees, 1996, *Our Ecological Footprint*, New Society Publishers, Philadelphia.

Westra, L., 1998, *Living in Integrity*, Rowman & Littlefield, Lanham, Maryland.

About the Contributors

DONALD A. BROWN is senior counsel for sustainable development for the Commonwealth of Pennsylvania, Department of Environmental Protection, where he counsels Pennsylvania on the creation of sustainable development programs. Before holding this position, Brown was project manager for United Nations organizations and the U.S. Environmental Protection Agency, Office of International Environmental Policy. From 1995 until 1998, Brown represented the USEPA on eight U.S. delegations to United Nations meetings to negotiate agreements relating to the world's freshwater problems, biodiversity and forest loss, climate change, ocean degradation, and international hazardous and nuclear waste problems. Brown has also served in a number of senior positions with Pennsylvania and New Jersey environmental programs, worked as an engineer, and taught philosophy, environmental law, and sustainable development at various universities. He received a B.S. in commerce and engineering sciences from Drexel University, a Juris Doctor from Seton Hall University School of Law, and an M.A. in liberal studies, majoring in philosophy and art, from the New School for Social Research. Brown has written and lectured extensively on the interface between environmental ethics, science, law, and economics. The author of many publications, he most recently coedited *Sustainable Development, Science, Ethics, and Public Policy* (Kluwer Academic Press, 1995).

PHILIPPE CRABBÉ is the principal investigator of a $0.6 million Community-University Research Association grant devoted to adaptation to climate change impacts on water resources in eastern Ontario. Previously, he was the principal investigator of the $2.25 million ecoresearch project Ecosystem Recovery on the St. Lawrence, one of the 10 such projects funded by Environment Canada under the Green Plan. He was born in Belgium, where he obtained a Doctorate of Law and a master's degree in economics. He also obtained a degree in quantitative economics in Paris. Crabbé spent five years at Harvard working on quantitative economics and on the valuation of human lives in economic decisions. He worked for the National Energy Board on the econometrics of the demand for energy and the exploration for oil and gas, and in 1969 joined the University of Ottawa Department of Economics, where he became professor of economics of natural resources and of the environment and later served as chair of the department. He is a past president of the Société Canadienne de Sciences Économiques, and was the first director of the Institute for Research on Environment and Economy (IREE) at the University of Ottawa, an interdisciplinary sustainable development research institute that involves professors and students from most faculties on campus.

Crabbé was the coeditor of one of the first books on the economics of natural resources and the environment in Canada and is widely published in forestry, fishery, mining, and environmental economics.

JAMES W. EHNES is president of ECOSTEM Ltd. and a research scholar in the Department of Biology, University of Winnipeg, Manitoba. He holds a B.A. Honours in economics from the University of Manitoba, an M.Phil. in economics from the University of Cambridge, England, and a Ph.D. in botany from the University of Manitoba. During the seven years between his M.Phil. and Ph.D., he worked as a commercial and residential real estate developer, overseeing new projects from Ontario to British Columbia. His main interest is to ensure that our forests are used sustainably. Ehnes devotes most of his time to scientific research in boreal forest ecosystems. He also works with government and industry translating scientific information into operational tools, guidelines, and procedures. He currently leads a project that is designing, implementing, and monitoring timber harvest practices, with the overall goal of maintaining forest ecosystem health. Some of his past research activities include the comparison of the effects of wildfire and harvesting on vegetation recovery and the design of a forest bird monitoring program. Ehnes has also served as a volunteer for numerous organizations promoting the sustainable use of our forests.

ROBERT GOODLAND is a tropical ecologist who worked in Brazil, Malaysia, Indonesia, and elsewhere as an environmental consultant to the private sector for more than a decade. He is currently the Environmental Adviser to the World Bank, where he received Presidential Excellence Awards in 1998 and 1999. He was elected metropolitan chair of the Ecological Society of America in 1989, president of the International Environmental Assessment Association in 1993, and independent commissioner of Canada's Great Whale Hydro in 1994. The International Society of Ecological Economics awarded their first Kenneth Boulding Prize jointly to Goodland and Herman Daly in 1994.

ALAN HOLLAND is professor of applied philosophy at Lancaster University, United Kingdom; editor of the international, interdisciplinary journal *Environmental Values;* and member of the U.K. Home Office Ministry's Animal Procedures Committee. He has recently coedited collections of articles on global sustainable development and animal biotechnology, and is a partner in several European research projects, including Environmental Valuation in Europe (funded by the European Commission), Deliberative and Inclusionary Processes (funded by the U.K.'s Economic and Social Science Research Council), and Social Psychology and Economics in Environmental Research (funded by the European Science Foundation). Holland has written widely on issues in environmental and applied philosophy and contributed the entries on "sustainability" for the *Blackwell Companion to Environmental Ethics* and on "ecological balance" for the *Encyclopedia of Applied Ethics.*

JAMES R. KARR is a professor of fisheries and zoology and an adjunct professor of civil engineering, environmental health, and public affairs at the University of Washington, Seattle. He holds a B.S. in fish and wildlife biology from Iowa State University, and an M.S. and Ph.D. in zoology from the University of Illinois, Urbana–Champaign. He served on the faculties of Purdue University, University of Illinois, and Virginia Tech University; he was also deputy director and acting director of the Smithsonian Tropical Research Institute in Panama. Karr has taught and done research in tropical forest ecology, ornithology, stream ecology, watershed management, landscape ecology, conservation biology, ecological health, and science and environmental policy. He is a fellow in the American Association for the Advancement of Science and the American Ornithologists' Union. He developed the index of biological integrity (IBI) to directly evaluate the effects of human actions on the health of living systems. Karr's earlier Island Press books include *Entering the Watershed* with B. Doppelt, M. Scurlock, and C. Frissell, and *Restoring Life in Running Waters* with E. W. Chu.

ORIE L. LOUCKS is Ohio Eminent Scholar of Applied Ecosystems Studies and professor of zoology at Miami University, after teaching for many years at the University of Wisconsin at Madison. He received his undergraduate and master's degrees in forestry from the University of Toronto and a Ph.D. in botany from the University of Wisconsin at Madison. Although trained as a forester and biologist, Loucks has collaborated with scholars in many other fields, particularly engineering, economics, the law, political science, and certain humanities. His research has focused on the dynamics of lakes and forests, but has also included policy-related work on pollution effects, biodiversity conservation, the integrity of forest landscapes, and the sustainability of cities. He has served on boards for UNESCO, the U.S. National Research Council, The Nature Conservancy, and numerous professional associations.

JACK P. MANNO is a cross-disciplinary scholar and writer, the executive director of the New York Great Lakes Research Consortium, and an adjunct associate professor of environmental studies at the State University of New York College of Environmental Science and Forestry in Syracuse, New York. He is also president of Great Lakes United, a coalition of 170 organizations in Canada and the United States including environmental activists, First Nations and Native American organizations, conservationists, hunting and fishing clubs, and others working for the protection and restoration of the Great Lakes–St. Lawrence Ecosystem of North America. For the past three years, Manno has been affiliated with the Global Integrity Project, a multidisciplinary team of ecologists, philosophers, legal scholars, and economists working to improve understanding of the practical implications of the concept of ecological integrity in a range of ecosystems around the world. Manno has written extensively on the dynamics of social and political systems, including the militarization of the U.S. space program and the role of nongovernmental organizations in world environmental politics. His new book, *Privileged Goods: Commoditization and Its Impact on Environment and Society,* is available through CRC Press at www.crcpress.com.

A. J. MCMICHAEL is professor of epidemiology at the London School of Hygiene and Tropical Medicine, London, United Kingdom. After graduating in medicine from the University of Adelaide, he gained a doctorate in epidemiology at Monash University. He has subsequently worked in a variety of research positions and fields: occupational disease research, studies of diet and disease, environmental epidemiologic studies of lead exposure and early childhood intellectual development, studies of air pollution and health, and, more recently, in studies relating to global environmental changes and their potential health impacts. During 1990–92, he chaired the Scientific Council of the International Agency for Research on Cancer (WHO). McMichael has been a frequent adviser to WHO, the World Meteorological Organization, and the World Bank. During 1994–96 he chaired the health impacts assessment task group for the UN's Intergovernmental Panel on Climate Change (Second Assessment Report)—and is currently doing likewise for the IPCC's Third Assessment Report. He has written widely on aspects of global environmental change and health, including climate change, stratospheric ozone depletion, and biodiversity loss. His book *Planetary Overload: Global Environmental Change and the Health of the Human Species* (Cambridge University Press/Canto, 1995) explored these and other issues.

PETER MILLER is a senior scholar in the Department of Philosophy and a member of the Centre for Forest Interdisciplinary Research (C-FIR) at the University of Winnipeg in Manitoba, Canada. He is also an adjunct professor at both the Natural Resources Institute and the Department of Philosophy, University of Manitoba; and an associate of that university's Centre for Professional and Applied Ethics. He earned his Ph.D. at Yale University. His research focus in recent years has been in value theory, environmental ethics, and ecological integrity and sustainability, with applications to recycling and forest policy. Miller also serves on the Manitoba Environmental Council (which is advisory to Manitoba's Conservation Minister) and participates in forest issues as vice president of TREE (Time to Respect Earth's Ecosystems—a coalition of Manitoba environmental groups) and chair of the Social Issues Working Group of the Manitoba Model Forest. In the recent past he has served as chair of the Department of Philosophy and in various other capacities, including president of the Canadian Society for the Study of Practical Ethics.

REED NOSS is chief scientist for Conservation Science, Inc., an international consultant and lecturer, president of the Society for Conservation Biology (1999–2001), and science editor for *Wild Earth* magazine. He has adjunct appointments in forest science and fisheries and wildlife at Oregon State University. Noss is the author of more than 170 scientific articles and three previous Island Press books: *Saving Nature's Legacy* (1994), coauthored by Allen Cooperrider; *The Science of Conservation Planning* (1997), coauthored by Michael O'Connell and Dennis Murphy; and *The Redwood Forest* (1999), which he edited. His present research involves the application of natural science to conservation planning at regional to continental scales. He lives with his family in the foothills of the Oregon Coast Range outside Corvallis.

ERNEST PARTRIDGE is a research associate in philosophy at the University of California, Riverside, and a lecturer-consultant in applied ethics and environmental ethics. His doctoral dissertation from the University of Utah was titled *Rawls and the Duty to Posterity*. Partridge has published numerous papers dealing with moral philosophy, moral psychology, policy analysis, and environmental ethics, and he has presented many papers before the American Philosophical Association and other scholarly societies in the United States, Canada, Japan, Italy, and Russia. He has served on the board of editors of *Environmental Ethics* and the *Journal of Environmental Education*. Under a grant from the Rockefeller Foundation, Partridge conducted original research relating to the moral question of the duty to posterity. One product of that research, an anthology titled *Responsibilities to Future Generations* (Prometheus Books), was published in 1981. His current research, also supported by the National Science Foundation, concerns the ethical and policy implications of "disequilibrium ecology." In Russia, Partridge has participated in scholarly and environmental conferences and has established productive and ongoing communication and cooperation with international scholars and scientists involved in global environmental issues. Partridge maintains a Web site, The Online Gadfly (www.igc.org/gadfly), which contains his recent publications as well as news and opinions regarding environmental ethics and policy.

DANIEL PAULY is a professor at the Fisheries Centre, University of British Columbia, Vancouver, Canada, where he has taught since 1994. He is a French citizen who grew up in the French-speaking part of Switzerland, but completed high school and university studies in the Federal Republic of Germany, where he acquired a master's degree in 1974 and a doctorate in fisheries biology in 1979 at the University of Kiel. In 1979, he joined the International Center for Living Aquatic Resources Management (ICLARM) in Manila, Philippines, as a postdoctoral fellow, and gradually took responsibilities as associate, senior scientist, then program and division director. In 1985 he obtained the "Habilitation," again at Kiel University. His scientific output, reflecting broad international experience in Africa, Asia, and Latin America and covering fish biology, fisheries management, and ecosystem modeling, comprises over 350 items, including journal articles, reports, books, and software used throughout the world. His present interests include further development of a large online database on fish (see www.fishbase.org), creation of a similar database on tools for ecosystem modeling (www.ecopath.org), and following up on the implications of "fishing down marine food webs," a global process he first documented in *Science,* February 6, 1998.

DAVID PIMENTEL is a professor of ecology and agricultural science at Cornell University, Ithaca, New York. His Ph.D. is from Cornell University. His research spans the fields of basic population ecology, ecological and economic aspects of pest control, biological control, biotechnology, sustainable agriculture, land and water conservation, natural resource management, and environmental policy. Pimentel has published more than 500 scientific papers and 20 books and has served on many national and government organizations, including the National Academy of Sciences; President's Science Advisory Council; U.S. Department of Agriculture; U.S. Department of Energy; U.S. Department of Health, Education and Welfare; Office of Technology Assessment of the U.S. Congress; and U.S. State Department.

WILLIAM E. REES received his Ph.D. in bioecology from the University of Toronto and has taught at the University of British Columbia in Vancouver since 1969. He served as director of the university's School of Community and Regional Planning from 1994 to 1999, and is currently a professor there. Rees's teaching and research focus on the public policy and planning implications of global environmental trends and the necessary ecological conditions for sustainable socioeconomic development. Much of this work is in the realm of human ecology and ecological economics, where he is best known for his "ecological footprint" concept.

MARK SAGOFF is senior research scholar at the Institute for Philosophy and Public Policy in the School of Public Affairs at the University of Maryland, College Park. He has an A.B. from Harvard and a Ph.D. in philosophy from the University of Rochester. He is the author of *The Economy of the Earth* (Cambridge University Press, 1988) and has published widely in journals of law, philosophy, and the environment. Sagoff was named a Pew Scholar in Conservation and the Environment in 1991; served from 1994 to 1997 as president of the International Society for Environmental Ethics; and, for the academic year 1998–99, was awarded a fellowship at the Woodrow Wilson International Center for Scholars. He taught at Princeton, the University of Pennsylvania, the University of Wisconsin at Madison, and Cornell before coming to the University of Maryland, College Park.

TED SCHRECKER is an adjunct assistant professor in the Faculty of Environmental Studies, University of Waterloo, and lecturer in the Department of Political Science, Huron College, University of Western Ontario. As a consultant, he has specialized in studying the value dimensions of public policy in science-based fields; his current academic research interests involve the economic determinants of human health and the social impacts of transnational economic integration and technological change. He is the editor of *Surviving Globalization: The Social and Environmental Challenges* (Macmillan, 1997), as well as numerous articles and book chapters.

H. MORGAN SCOTT is a graduate veterinarian (Saskatchewan, 1988) and holds a Ph.D. in veterinary epidemiology from the University of Guelph, Ontario, Canada. He has most recently been engaged as a postdoctoral fellow in the Department of Public Health Sciences at the University of Alberta, Edmonton, Canada. His professional experiences range from a rural veterinary practice, through conducting clinical field trials and animal health studies on dairy farms, to environmental and veterinary epidemiologic studies of the impacts of oil and gas processing activity on the health and productivity of livestock in western Canada. Scott's current research interests include the impacts of environmental degradation on the health of all species.

LEE E. SIESWERDA works for Novartis. He completed his bachelor of education degree in 1996 and, after some teaching and research experience, came under the tutelage of Colin Soskolne at the University of Alberta, Edmonton, Canada. Sieswerda completed his M.S. degree in epidemiology in 1999 with a thesis entitled *Towards Measuring the Impact of Ecological Disintegrity on Human Health*. He has developed case studies in public health ethics and has coauthored chapters and papers for the World Health Organization, Ecosystem Health, and EpiSource. He has also presented his work to the International Society for Environmental Epidemiology, for whom he is also the founding webmaster.

COLIN L. SOSKOLNE is professor of epidemiology in the Department of Public Health Sciences, University of Alberta, Canada. His career began as a statistician in the human sciences domain in South Africa before moving into biostatistics and occupational epidemiology. He was awarded the Society for Epidemiologic Research annual student prize for his doctoral dissertation, completed at the University of Pennsylvania in 1982. He was among the first in Canada involved in HIV-AIDS research, education, and policy formulation. Shortly after receiving his Ph.D., he became a prime mover in focusing epidemiology on professional ethics. In 1999, he completed a sabbatical year as a visiting scientist with the European Centre for Environment and Health, World Health Organization, Rome Division. There, concerns about the human health consequences of environmental degradation resulted in a Soskolne first-authored Discussion Document entitled *Global Ecological Integrity and "Sustainable Development": Cornerstones of Public Health,* accessible on the Web at www.who.it/Emissues/Globaleco/ globaleco/htm. In 1999, he was elected to the board of the International Society for Environmental Epidemiology. Soskolne is associated with more than 120 publications.

JAMES P. STERBA is professor of philosophy at the University of Notre Dame, where he teaches moral and political philosophy. His Ph.D. is from the University of Pittsburgh. He has written more than 150 articles and published 18 books, including *How to Make People Just; Contemporary Ethics; Feminist Philosophies,* 2nd ed; *Earth Ethics,* 2nd ed; and *Morality in Practice,* 5th ed. His latest book, *Justice for Here and Now,* published by Cambridge University Press, was given the 1998 Book of the Year Award by the North American Society for Social Philosophy. He is past president of the International Society for Social and Legal Philosophy, the American Section, past president of Concerned Philosophers for Peace, and past president of the North American Society for Social Philosophy, and has lectured widely in the United States and Europe, the Far East, and Africa.

ROBERT E. ULANOWICZ has pursued research in theoretical ecology at the University of Maryland's Chesapeake Biological Laboratory in Solomons, Maryland, since 1970. He is a native of Baltimore, where he graduated in 1961 from the Baltimore Polytechnic Institute. He received a Ph.D. in chemical engineering from the Johns Hopkins University in 1968 and taught chemical engineering at the Catholic University of America. Ulanowicz's major areas of interest are the quantitative analysis of ecosystem trophic exchange networks, ecological thermodynamics, information theory in ecology, and the nature of causality in living systems.

LAURA WESTRA presently holds the Barbara B. and Bertram J. Cohn Professorship in Environmental Studies at Sarah Lawrence College. She received her Ph.D. from the University of Toronto in philosophy (1983). She has nine published books: *Freedom in Plotinus* (Edwin Mellon, 1990); *An Environmental Proposal for Ethics: The Principle of Integrity* (Rowman & Littlefield, 1994); *Faces of Environmental Racism—Confronting Issues of Global Justice* (Rowman & Littlefield, 1995); *Ethical and Scientific Perspectives on Integrity* (Kluwer Academic, 1995); *The Greeks and the Environment* (Rowman & Littlefield, 1997); *Technology and Values* (Rowman & Littlefield, 1997); *Ecological Sustainability and Integrity: Concepts and Approaches* (Kluwer Academic, 1998); *Living in Integrity* (Rowman & Littlefield, 1998); and *The Business of Consumption* (Rowman & Littlefield, 1998). Westra also has roughly 60 published papers and chapters in books, most on environmental ethics, 150 presented papers at meetings, and 50 invited papers. She has been funded by Canadian sources such as the Social Sciences and Humanities Research Council of Canada and by NATO (Advanced Research Workshop, June 1999, Budapest); she has arranged meetings and conferences at both philosophical and scientific venues on related topics. She is the founder of the International Society for Environmental Ethics (ISEE), and has held the position of secretary since 1990. Westra has also worked as a consultant for professional associations, including the World Health Organization.

Index

Absolutism, 304, 308
Africa, 128, 250–251, 281. *See also specific countries*
Agenda 21, 299, 353, 371–373, 381
  North-South agreements and, 16, 371–372, 378–379
Agglomeration economies, cities as, 327
Aggression, defense against, 343, 349n.24
Agriculture, 14, 116–136, 397, 401
  aquaculture and, 130–131
  biotechnology and, 73–74, 132
  chemicals/pesticides for, 131–132, 282–283, 395
  climate change and, 124, 242
  commoditization of, 358–359
  energy resources for, 125–126
  export *vs.* self-sufficient, 125
  extensified *vs.* intensified, 124
  food consumption and, 132–136
  land resources for, 126–128
  pollution and, 131–132
  productivity in, 242, 248, 249, 376
  regeneration in, 121, 122
  Serafian rule and, 121–123
  trade-offs in, 123–124
  water resources for, 128–130, 213
Agroecosystem Health Project, 273
Air pollution, 286
Altruism, 336–339, 347nn.4–10, 348n.21
Amazon, 310
Analysis of Variance (NOVA), 170
Anthropocentrism, 340–342
Anthropogenic systems, 51, 54. *See also* Human interference
Aquaculture, 130–131
Aquatic systems, assessment of, 218. *See also* Rivers
Ascendency theory, 44, 107–109, 110–111
Assessment, biological, 217–222
Australia, 283
Autocatalysis, 104, 144

Automobiles, 354, 380
Autopoietic capacity, 20
Average mutual information (AMI), 33, 105–107

Balance, in ecosystems, 83–84
Baltic Sea, 109–110
  urban areas of, 147, 217, 253
Basic needs, 343–344, 348n.21
  equity and, 305–307, 312
Bayes' Theorem, 105
Bears, grizzly (*Ursus arctos*), 39, 40, 201
Beef/meat consumption, 134, 400
Behavior:
  counterintuitive, 8
  human, 116, 153
  predictability of, 320
Bell, E. A., 286
Benchmark condition, 28, 214–215
Benign utopia scenario, 234
Bethell, T., 47
Biocentric ethics, 15, 298, 399. *See also* Ethics
Biodiversity, 200
  assessment of, 218
  conservation of, 13, 151, 163, 301–302
  conservation planning for, 191, 194
  economic benefits of, 216
  global strategy for, 38, 390
  hotspots of, 194, 199
  loss of, 250, 376–377
  safe minimum standards for, 305
  species level of, 192
Biological assessment, 217–222
  multimetric indices for, 219–222
Biological integrity, 25, 27, 29
  human activity and, 145–146, 212–213
  see also Ecological integrity
Biology and Philosophy (journal), 48
Biomass, in forests, 179, 180–181
Biophysical integrity, 4

Biosocial regional integrity, 162, 172
Biosphere, 2, 88
Biotechnology, 73–74, 132, 287
Bishop, Richard, 305
Boltzmann, L., 104
Bormann, F. E., 180
Botkin, Daniel, 80, 82–83, 90, 95n.8, 96n.15
Bottom-up approach, to conservation, 206
Boundary Waters (Minnesota–Ontario), 83
Brazil, 310, 379
Brent Spar oil platform (North Sea), 53
Brown, Donald A., 16, 299–300, 407
Brown, James H., 62
Brundtland Commission, 36, 163, 303, 306
Buffer maxim, 26–27, 41
Bulletin of the Ecological Society of America, 73
Business Council on Sustainable Development, 152

California, 198
Callicott, Baird, 51
Canada, 14, 149, 229, 318. *See also* Forest management, sustainable
Canada Forest Accord (1992), 116–117, 157, 162, 171
Cancer, 249, 266, 270, 281, 282
Capacity, of systems, 19–21, 27
Carnivores/predators, 37–38, 86–88, 145, 201–202
  grizzly bears, 39, 40, 201
  lynx-hare cycle, 87–88, 90–91
  wolverines, 201, 202
  wolves, 86, 201–202
Cartesian dualism, 7, 140
Case-control study, in epidemiology, 265
Catastrophic, *vs.* gradual effects, 273. *See also* Disaster
Catastrophic intervention, 91
Causation, in epidemiological studies, 262
Channelization, 213
Chaos theory, 8, 50, 88, 90
Chemical products, 284, 290–291
  agricultural, 131–132, 282–283, 395
Chesapeake Bay ecosystem, 102–103, 109–110
Chilean desert, 19–21
China, 126, 127, 128, 134
  water consumption in, 129, 130

Cholera, 255–256, 286
Cigarette smoking, 266, 270
Cities. *See* Urban areas
Civilization, environmental burden of, 3–4
Civil society, commoditization of, 364–365
Clean Water Act (US), 29, 214
Clearcutting, 178–179, 180, 181, 195–196. *See also* Timber harvest
Climate change:
  agriculture and, 124, 242
  global warming, 227, 228, 261–262, 306, 307, 377
  health effects of, 242, 247–248, 281, 285, 390–391, 394
Climax stage, 84, 86
Clinton, William, 203
Club goods, 326
Coastal ecosystems, 376
Codfish, demise of, 229
Cohort epidemiological study, 263–265
Colborn, Theo, 284, 289, 291
Colorado, 213
Commoditization, 16, 351–367, 405
  of agriculture, 358–359
  economy and, 299, 356–357
  environmental health and, 360–361
  globalization and, 365
  of health care, 359–360
  hypothetical example of, 355
  oppression and liberation and, 361–365
  policy to counter, 365–367
  range of potential, 351–353
  sustainability and, 353–354, 397
Community, 362, 366
Compensation regime, 296–297, 308–312
Complementary effects, 328
Complexity, trend toward, 54
Complex systems, urban areas as, 319–323
Compromise, morality as, 339, 341–342, 344
Confounding, in epidemiological studies, 270
Congress, US, 214
Conrad, Michael, 63
Conservation planning, 191–206
  development of, 196–198
  ecoregional assessments for, 192–196
  ecosystem approach to, 192, 204–205, 390

focal species in, 200–202
habitat corridors in, 201, 202
protected areas in, 197, 200, 203
special elements and, 198–200
top-down *vs.* bottom-up approach to,
    205–206
see also Environmental conservation
Conservation policy, 150–153, 302, 303,
    308–310
Constant change, 80, 82–84
Constraint, on ecosystems, 104–106
Consumerism, 140, 150, 153
Consumption levels, 28–29, 256, 372
Cooking efficiency, 123
Cooperation, 322
Cooperrider, A. Y., 36, 38
Coral reef formation, 49
Coronary heart disease, 266
Corporate interests, 280
Costanza, R., 32, 101, 216
Crabbé, Philippe, 297–298, 407–408
Creationist theory, 85
Critique for Ecology (Peters), 99
Cross-sectional studies, 265–268, 270–272
Culture, commoditization and, 363

Daly, Herman, 304, 306
Darwin, Charles, 44, 64–65, 89
Darwinian paradigm, integrity and, 45–58,
    64–66
    human impact and, 50–54
    quantification of, 54–56
    radical contingency and, 47–50
    see also Evolution
Data aggregation. *See* Cross-sectional
    studies
Death/mortality, from disease, 254, 266,
    269
Deforestation, 376. *See also* Clearcutting;
    Timber harvest
Degradation, 9–10
    ecological, 17, 300, 389, 390, 393–395
    ecosystem, 119–120, 243–244, 395–398
    human activity and, 160, 161
    measurement of, 29
    soil, 149
    see also Land degradation
Demand management, food, 133
Democratization, 362–363
Demographic entrapment, 250–251

Descartes, René, 7
Desert areas, capacity of, 19–21
Determinism, stochasticity and, 100
Developing nations, 126, 130, 289,
    380–381, 403
    economic aspirations of, 256
    water needs of, 287
    see also North–South disparity; Poorer
    countries
Development, 104, 312, 386–387
    economic, 116, 296–297, 370
    see also Growth; Sustainable
    development
Diet:
    food chain and, 133–136, 146
    vegetarian, 28, 127, 133
Directionality, 100
Disasters, 281–282. *See also* Catastrophic
Disease, 131, 210, 286–287, 375
    cholera, 255–256, 286
    climate change and, 242, 247
    infectious, 251–252, 255–256, 285, 374,
    394
    mortality from, 254, 266, 269
    see also Epidemiological methods
Disproportionality principle, 344–345,
    346, 349n.23
Distinctiveness, bioregional, 194
Distinctive traits, species, 340
Distributive justice, 313–314, 391. *See also*
    Equity/equality
Diversity, 31, 171, 198. *See also*
    Biodiversity
Dominance, economic, 324
Dynamic externalities, in urban areas, 329

Earth Summit (Rio, 1992), 16, 396. *See
    also* United Nations Conference on
    Environment and Development
Ebola virus, 287
Ecological degradation, 17, 300, 389, 390,
    393–395
Ecological destruction, 23
Ecological footprint, 146–150, 153n.7,
    275, 286, 403
    analysis, 34, 35, 216–217, 393
    global, 149–150, 396
    integrity and, 400
    of urban areas, 35, 147–149, 217,
    252–253, 298

Ecological health, 30, 32, 118–119, 160, 210–212
Ecological integrity, 11–12, 29, 261, 366, 387
  defined, 99
  global overview of, 389–391, 402–405
  health and, 290, 393–395
  human needs and, 24, 399
  themes of, 20–21
  see also Biological integrity; Global Integrity Project
Ecological restoration, 196
Ecological stability, 6, 96n.15
Ecologic bias, 270
Ecologic study. *See* Cross-sectional study
Ecologists, 44, 62, 74
Ecology, 6–11
  and economics, 6, 7, 8–9, 215–216
  global, 380
  holistic view of, 9, 10
  scientific approach and, 7–9
  see also Theoretical ecology
Economic development, 116, 296–297, 370
Economic growth, 6, 210, 378
Economic policy, conservation and, 302, 303, 308–310
Economics:
  and complex systems compared, 320–322
  dominance of, 324
  ecology and, 6, 7, 8–9, 215–216
  ethos of, 256–257
  human ecology and, 141
  machine of, 14–16
  natural law and, 142
  system of, 56, 397
  trends, since Rio summit, 373, 375
  of urban areas, 323–329
  see also Commoditization; Globalized economy
Ecoregions, 118, 193
Ecosystem design, context for, 61–75, 89–90
  Darwinian paradigm and, 64–66
  ecological theory and, 70–73
  and ecosystem defined, 68–70
  Mill on nature and, 66–68
  reductionist challenge to, 73–74
  theories for, 62–63

Ecosystem performance, measurement of, 101–108
  average mutual information, 105–107
  exchanges/flows in, 101–106
Ecosystems, 22, 93, 151, 298, 404
  approach, 192, 388
  assessment of, 193–194
  coastal, 376
  conservation planning for, 192, 204–205
  constraint on, 104–106
  degradation, 119–120, 243–244, 395–398
  equilibrium, 83–84, 87, 96n.15, 141
  health of, 56, 317
  inscrutability of, 94–95
  integrity of, 24, 26, 381–382, 399
  management of, 118, 397
  marine, 227–228, 232, 234, 236–237, 404
  natural selection and, 80–81, 88–92
  organization of, 32, 80, 101, 104, 107
  as oxymoron, 80, 87
  resilience, 22, 33–34, 101, 108–109
  trophic flows in, 32–34
  value of, 21
  variables in, 388
  vigor of, 32, 101, 102, 106–107
Ecosystems, urban areas as. *See* Urban areas, as ecosystems
Ecoviolence, institutionalized, 15, 279–292
  climate change effects, 281, 285
  corporate interests and, 280
  disease and, 285, 286–287
  endocrine disruptors and, 284–285
  ethical dimensions of, 288–291
  sexual liberation and, 285–286
  toxic substances and, 279, 282–284, 286
Edge-of-Appalachia Preserve (Ohio), 183–184, 185
Education, 374
Egoism principle, 336–339
Ehnes, James W., 116–117, 392, 408
  on forest ecosystems, 12, 14, 170, 171
Ehrenfeld, D., 205
Ehrlich, Paul, 61, 88
El Serafy, S., 121–123
Empiricism *vs.* theory, 70–71
Endangered Spaces program (Canada), 163
Endangered Species Act (US, 1973), 192, 218

Endocrine disruptors, 284–285
End of Nature, The (McKibben), 67
Energy use, 125–126, 373, 375, 381, 387
English Environment Agency, 55
Entropy, 31–32, 141
Environment, civilization and, 3–4
Environmental change, health and. *See* Health, global environmental change and
Environmental conservation, 301–314
  absolutism and, 304, 308
  basic needs and, 305–307
  compensation regime for, 308–312
  ethics and public policy, 304–305
  hypothetical case for, 302–303
  of landscape, 118
  policies for, 307–310
  prospects for, 313–314
  sustainability and, 12–14, 301
  see also Conservation planning
Environmental deterioration, 370, 394
Environmental impact statements, 218
Environmental integrity, human interference and, 344–346. *See also* Ecological integrity
Environmentalism, 140–142
Environmental policy, 212–213, 296–297
Environmental regulations, 214. *See also* *specific regulation*
Environmental sustainability, 56, 121, 401
Environmental trends, 374, 375–377
Environmental Values (perodical), 51
Epidemiological methods, health assessment, 243–244, 261–276, 392, 393, 404
  bias in, 269, 270
  case-control study, 265
  causation and, 262
  cohort study, 263–265
  and confounding, 269
  cross-sectional studies, 265–268, 270–272
  gradual *vs.* catastrophic effects, 273
  need for ecological model for, 273–274
  overview of findings in, 274–276
  randomized controlled trial, 262
Equilibrium, ecosystem, 83–84, 87, 96n.15, 141
Equity/equality:
  basic needs and, 305–307, 312

distributive justice, 313–314, 391
income, 139–140, 307–308, 311, 313, 398
international, 380, 400
Erosion, soil, 127–128
"Essay on Man" (Pope), 61
Estimated Ecological Daily Intake, 284
Ethics:
  biocentric, 15, 298, 399
  of economics, 256–257
  of ecoviolence, 288–291
  and income, 311
  of integrity, 26, 28, 39, 40–41, 398–400
  of preservation, 81
  and public policy, 304–305
  wilderness preservation and, 304
  see also Morality
Europe:
  Baltic Sea area of, 109–110, 147, 217, 253. *See also* Rich countries
European Union, 134, 381
Evaluation, of ecosystems, 92–93. *See also* Assessment
Evolution, 44, 45, 54, 65–66, 82
  ecosystems and, 80–81, 88–92
  radically contingent, 47–50
  randomness in, 322–323
  see also Darwinian paradigm
Exchanges/flows, in ecosystems, 101–106
Export crop production, 125
Exposure assessment, for disease, 265
Extensification, agricultural, 124
Externalities, urban economic, 326–327, 329
Extinction, 36, 37, 81, 250, 377
  human-induced, 150
  prehistoric, 143, 144

Falsifiability, 84–85
Farmers, 75, 359. *See also* Agriculture
Fatalism, 16
Fertility, soil, 121
Fertilizers, 129–130
Finis mundi scenario, 232. *See also* Catastrophic effects; Disasters
Fire:
  in forest management, 160–161, 165, 166, 171, 178–179
  suppression, 194–195, 196
First World, 150. *See also* Rich countries

Fisheries, 119–120, 227–237, 376, 404
    decline in, 130–131
    demise of cod, 229
    economic factors and, 231–232
    ecosystem degradation and, 119–120
    global warming and, 227, 228
    human demand and, 229–231, 391
    market-based approaches and, 234, 236
    protected areas for, 234, 236–237
    scenarios for, 232, 234–235
Florida, 213
Flows, in ecosystems, 101–106
Focal species analysis, 200–202
Folke, C., 147, 253
Food consumption, 132–136
    chain, 133–136, 146
    vegetarian diet, 28, 127, 133
Food production, 123, 144, 250, 391
    land degradation and, 249, 376
    see also Agriculture
Forcella, Frank, 73
Foreign aid, 371–372, 375, 380
Foreign investment, 373, 379
Forest integrity, measurement of, 177–189
    biomass decomposition, 179, 180–181
    hydrolic flux, 179, 180
    mean functional integrity, 12, 117,
        181–182, 184–188, 392
    net primary production of, 164–170,
        178–179, 180
    nutrient cycling, 164, 167, 179, 181,
        185
    pollutant deposition studies in, 182–186
    secondary production of, 179
    species loss and, 179, 187–188
Forest management, sustainable, 14,
        157–173
    approaches to integrity, 158–162
    conservation planning for, 194–195
    ecosystem-based, 163–164
    human impact and, 164–165, 169
    implementing, 162–164
    measurement of integrity and, 116–118
    natural state envelope, 165–166, 172
    old-growth, 56
    outcome maintenance envelope,
        166–168
    regional scale, 169–170, 173
    timber harvest, 164, 168
Forman, David, 39

Fossil depositions, 84–85
Fossil fuels, 126, 387
Foster, D. R., 56
Fowler, C. M. R., 53
Free-market philosophy, 257
Frost, Robert, 75
Frost Center Forest (Ontario), 183, 185
Function, ecosystem, 24, 101. See also
        Vigor
Functional integrity, measure of, 28, 35.
        See also Mean functional integrity
Fundamentals of Ecology (Odum), 193
Future realization, 21

Gause, G. F., 90
Geertz, Clifford, 65
Gilbert, F., 63
Ginzburg, Lev, 72
Global ecology, 380
Global Integrity Project, 9–10, 36, 39, 99
Global Integrity Project, findings of,
        385–405
    conclusion, 386–387
    ecosystem degradation and, 395–398
    human health, 393–395
    human values and, 398–400
    institutions and government role,
        402–405
    integrity concept and, 387–389
    measurement, 391–393
    principles for protecting integrity,
        400–402
    and worldwide integrity, 389–391
Globalized economy, 252, 300, 373, 377
    commoditization and, 365
    distributive justice and, 313–314, 391
Global warming, 227, 228, 261, 306, 307,
        377
God, 61, 66, 68
Goodland, Robert, 13, 14, 116, 304, 306,
        408
Gould, Stephen J., 49, 65
Government:
    boundaries of, and ecosystems, 397
    compensation regime and, 311–312
    health and, 257
    protection of integrity by, 402–405
Gradual vs. catastrophic effects, 273
Grain import/export, 125, 127
Grant, Peter and Rosemary, 71

Geographic information system (GIS), 268
Gray wolf (*Canis lupus*), 201–202
"Great Chain of Being" cosmology, 61,
    68, 75
Great Lakes Water Quality Agreement, 24
Green History of the World, A (Ponting), 3
Greenhouse gases, 227, 232, 245, 377,
    395. *See also* Global warming
Green revolution, 132, 249
Grimm, Volker, 69, 77n.27
Grizzly bear (*Ursus arctos*), 39, 40, 201
Growth:
    economic, 6, 210, 378
    private sector-led, 373, 379, 380, 396
    see also Development
Growth pole theory, 323–324

Habitat:
    corridors for, 201, 202
    fragmentation of, 36–37
    gradients, 200
    large blocks of, 118, 402
Haldane, J. B. S., 88
Happiness, wealth and, 14–15
Hardin, Garrett, 58, 87
Hazards, 15. *See also* Toxic wastes
Health, 15, 209–210, 243, 279
    commoditization of, 359–360
    ecological degradation and, 393–395
    ecosystem, 56, 317
    of forests, 166–169
    integrity and, 11, 24–25, 393–395
    see also Epidemiological studies, health
        assessment
Health, global environmental change and,
    245–257
    climate change and, 242, 247–248
    demographic entrapment, 250–251
    North *vs.* South, 251–252
    ozone depletion, 248–249
    policy setting for, 257
    population growth and, 245–246
    risk assessment, 246–247
    sustainability and, 253–256
    urban footprint, 252–253
Health sciences, 11–12
Heath ecosystem, 64–65
Henderson, D. A., 261–262
Herbicides, 132. *See also* Agricultural
    chemicals

Hierarchy, 21, 142, 153n.4
    in urban systems, 319–320, 322
Hirschman, A. O., 71
Historical process, evolution as, 45
History, natural, 55, 62, 69–70, 72
Holland, Alan, 11, 44, 408
Hoosier National Forest (Indiana), 184
Hotspots, of biodiversity, 194, 199
Hubbard Brook Experimental Forest
    (New Hampshire), 180, 181, 183,
    185
Hubris, technological, 4–5
Human:
    behavior, 116, 153
    choices, 39–40
    demand, 28–29
    distinctiveness, 340
    and landscape disturbance, 19
    and natural integrity, 66–68
    nature and, 36–37
    needs, 204–205, 296, 351
    preservation of, 343–345, 348n.20
    systems complexity of, 320–321
    welfare, 5–6, 16
    wildlands and, 38
Human activities, 160, 161, 212–213, 244
    ethical principles for, 41
    forest management and, 166–167
    in wild areas, 26–27, 401
    see also Ecological footprint
Human defense principle, 342–345,
    349n24
Human ecology, 7, 139–154
    biological integrity and, 145–146
    conservation policy and, 150–153
    ecological footprint and, 146–150
    environmentalism and, 140–142
    hunting–gathering, 142–144
    income disparity and, 139–140
    patch disturbance and, 142–146
Human health. *See* Health
Human impact/influence, 27, 90, 397
    environmental integrity and, 344–346
    integrity and, 22–23, 24, 50–54, 119,
        335
    on living systems, 209, 390
    in measuring integrity, 29–30
    patch disturbance, 142–146
    sustainable forestry and, 164–165
Human rights, 305, 313

Human use, regional integrity and, 162
Human value, 398–400
Humboldt, Baron Alexander von, 211
Hunter-gatherers, 142–144
Hydrolic flux (HF), 180

Income disparity, 139–140, 307–308, 311, 313–314, 398. *See also* Equity/equality
Indeterminacy, measurement of, 33–34
Index of biological integrity (IBI), 12, 23, 29–31, 110, 392–393
    forest management and, 117, 159–160, 177
    and other methods compared, 34–35, 219, 221–222
    skeptics and, 100–101
    see also Measurement, of integrity
India, 130
Indiana, 184
Indigenous people, 363
Individual Transferable Quotas, 234, 236
Industrialization, 236, 275, 310
Industrial revolution, 210
Industrial society, 4
Inequality, in income, 139–140, 307–308, 311, 313, 398. *See also* Equity/equality
Infectious disease, 251–252, 254, 285, 374, 394
    cholera, 255–256, 286
Information theory, 33, 104, 105–107
Infrastructure:
    of rich countries, 310–311
    urban, 328–329
Inscrutability, ecosystem, 94–95
Integrity. *See* Biological integrity; Ecological integrity; Environmental integrity; Global Integrity Project
Intensification, agricultural, 124
Intensive management, in forestry, 169
International community, conservation and, 308–310
International institutions, integrity and, 402–404
Irrigation, 129, 213
Ismail, Razali, 378

Jacobs, J., 329
Japanese Journal of Hygiene, 284

Jorgensen, Sven, 63
Journal of Health Services, 283

Karr, James R., 12, 28, 50, 179, 408–409
    definition of *integrity,* 166
    on ecological health, 118–119
    on integrity, 23–24, 335
    on succession, 22
    see also Index of biological integrity
Katz, Eric, 304
Kenya, 251
Kiester, A. R., 268
King, M., 250
Kissimmee River (Florida), 213
Klamath-Siskiyou ecoregion, 198–200, 201
Kumate, J., 285
Kyoto (Japan), 280

Land degradation, 127–128, 243, 248, 395
    food production and, 249, 376
Landor, Walter Savage, 61, 75
Landscape, 19, 118, 214–215
Land use:
    for agriculture, 126–128
    conservation planning for, 191, 390
    restrictions, 310
Law of limiting factors (Liebig), 85
Law of the Minimum (Liebig), 111
Law of the Sea, 229
Leopold, Aldo, 79, 94, 192, 205
Levels, of integrity, 54–56
Levin, Simon, 69, 70, 71–72
Liberation, and commoditization, 361–365
Liebig, Justus von, 85, 111
Life expectancy, 253–254, 255, 261
Likens, G. E., 180
Lipschutz, Ronnie, 367
Literacy, 374
Livestock production, 131, 134, 136
Living systems design. *See* Ecosystems design
Local ecosystems, 4
Localization economies, 327
Logging, 195–196. *See also* Clearcutting; Timber harvest
London (UK), 148
Longleaf pine (*Pinus palustris*), 195–196
Loucks, Orie L., 13, 24, 26, 28, 40, 409
    MFI concept of, 12, 35, 117–118, 392

"Lucretius versus the Lake Poets" (Frost), 75
Lynx-hare cycle, 87–88, 90–91

Madagascar, 309
Manitoba (Canada), 170, 172
Manno, Jack P., 16, 298–299, 409
Marine ecosystems, 227–228, 232, 234, 236–237, 404. *See also* Fisheries
Marketing of nature. *See* Commoditization
Mayr, E., 100
McCoy, E. D., 99
McGinn, Colin, 54
McIntosh, Robert, 345, 346
McKibben, Bill, 67, 74
McLachlan, J. S., 56
McMichael, A. J., 242–243, 409–410
Mean functional integrity (MFI), 12, 35, 117–118, 181–182, 184–188, 392
Measurement, of integrity, 31–35, 44, 99–111, 391–393, 402
   ascendency theory and, 32–34, 107–109, 110–111
   ecosystem performance and, 101–108
   entropy production and, 31–32
   functional, 28, 35
   human impact and, 54
   methods compared, 34–35
   multimetric indices for, 12, 29, 119, 392
   resilience potential, 108–109
   see also Index of biological integrity
Measurement of integrity, in Forests. *See* Forest integrity, measurement of
Meat consumption, 134, 400
Mexico, 307
MFI. *See* Mean functional integrity
Migration, 5, 242, 247, 297, 319
Mill, John Stuart, 66–68, 73, 74
Miller, Peter, 11, 12, 14, 116–117, 392, 410
Models, for integrity, 215
Monetary value, of nature capital, 216
Montreal Protocol (1996), 377
Moral authority, 311
Moral duty, 6, 11, 298
Morality:
   as compromise, 339, 341–342, 344
   and ecosystem inscrutability, 94–95
   and self-interest, 337, 339
   see also Ethics

Moral reasons, 57, 335–339, 347nn.4, 8–10
Morgenstern, H., 267
Mortality, from disease, 254, 266, 269
Mount St. Helens, 83–84
Mozambique, 125
Muddling through scenario, 234
Multimetric indices, for assessment, 12, 29, 119, 392. *See also* Index of biological integrity
Multiple group comparison, 268

Naess, Arne, 39
National Environmental Policy Act (US, 1969), 217–218
Natural capital, 216, 366
Natural history:
   ecologists and, 44, 62
   ecology and, 69–70, 72
Natural selection, 11, 45, 47–48, 65–66
   ecosystems and, 80–81, 88–92
   see also Darwinian paradigm
Natural state, constant change in, 82–84
Natural state envelope, 165–167, 172
Natural systems, 11, 53–54, 398. *See also* Ecosystems
Nature:
   counterintuitive behavior of, 8
   human relations to, 142, 345–346
   legacy of, 20, 36–40
   Mill on, 66–68, 73, 74
   reductionist approach to, 73–74
   scientific culture and, 140
   services of, 286, 290
Nature Conservancy, The, 198
Nature (periodical), 53
Netherlands, 253
Net primary productivity (NPP) of forests, 164–170, 178–179, 180
   natural state and, 165–166, 172
   outcome maintenance and, 166–168
Network effects, 326–327
Newfoundland (Canada), 229
Newtonian mechanics, 7, 74
Nicolis, G., 321
Nigeria, 20
Niño, El, 19, 27, 248, 251
Nisbet, E. G., 53
Nonrenewables, depletion of, 121–123
Northern cod (*Gadus morhua*), 229

North–South antagonism, 251–252, 300,
      380–382
   Agenda 21 and, 16, 371–372, 379
   disparity and, 288–289, 299, 380–381
Northwest Forest Plan, 203
Noss, Reed, 24, 26, 39, 40, 118, 410
   on nature's legacy, 36–38
Nuclear industry, 282
Nutrient cycling, in forests, 164, 167, 179,
      181, 185

Odum, Eugene P., 53, 62–63, 108, 147,
      193
Oechsli, Lauren, 304
Official direct assistance (ODA), 371, 375,
      380
Ogallala aquifer (US), 129
Ogoniland (Nigeria), 20
Ohio, 183–184, 185
Oil production. See Fossil fuels
Olson, J. S., 180
Oppression, and commoditization,
      361–365
Optimum capacity, of ecosystems, 109
Oregon, 198
Organisms, 69, 89
Organization, ecosystem, 32, 101, 104,
      107
Origin of Species (Darwin), 64
Orr, David, 211
Orwig, D. A., 56
Our Common Future (report), 353, 367n.1,
      370–371
Overpopulation, 133–134. See also
      Population growth
Owen, J., 63
Ozone depletion, 243, 248–249, 377,
      395

Pacific fisher (Martes pennanti pacifica), 201
Partridge, Ernest, 11, 44, 410–411
Patch disturbers, humans as, 142–146
Pauly, Daniel, 13, 119–120, 411
Pearce, David, 151, 310
Peppered moth (Biston betularia), 47
Periphery dependence, urban areas, 324
Perroux, F., 324
Pesticides, 131–132, 282–283, 395
Peters, R. H., 72, 99
Physics, ecology and, 7

Picket, Steward, 63
Pierce, Charles Saunders, 100
Pimentel, David, 13, 14, 116, 216, 411
Plotinus, 62
Policy:
   against commoditization, 365–367
   for conservation, 150–153, 302, 303,
      307–310
   for development, 386–387
   environmental, 212–213, 296–297,
      304–305
   for health, 257
   income inequality and, 313–314
   for sustainability, 299, 305, 388
   for urban economy, 325
Pollution, 377, 379, 380–381, 394–395,
      398
   and agricultural sustainability, 131–132
   air, 286
   controls for, 360–361
   deposition, in forests, 182–186
Ponting, Clive, 3, 4
Poorer countries, 250–251, 301
   Agenda 21 promise and, 299–300, 378,
      380–381
   assistance to, 16, 399, 403
   climate change and, 242–243, 395, 400
   ecosystem integrity and, 381–382
   health of, 244, 251–252
   income parity and, 307, 398
   see also Developing nations;
         Poverty/Poor; and specific countries
Pope, Alexander, 61
Popper, Karl, 100
Population growth, 132, 133–134, 152,
      254, 396
   current trends in, 139, 374, 375
   fisheries and, 229
   food production and, 124, 144
   human health and, 131, 245–246
   urban, 5
Poverty/Poor, 5, 296, 372, 373, 379
   in developing world, 289
   diet of, 133
   environment and, 370
   health of, 252, 394
   industrial activity and, 139–140
   see also Poorer countries
Precautionary principle, 398, 400
Predators. See Carnivores/predators

Preservation ethic, 81. *See also*
    Conservation planning
Prigogine, I., 321
Primer of Ecological Theory (Roughgarden),
    71
Principle of Integrity, The (Westra), 335
Private sector-led growth, 373, 379, 380,
    396
Production, sustainability in, 372, 381
Productivity:
    agricultural, 242, 248, 249, 376
    of aquaculture, 131
Propensity concept, 100
Protected areas, 31, 36–38, 163, 200, 396
    conservation of, 13, 197, 203, 390
    design of, 202–203, 401–402
    human activities in, 26–27, 403
    marine, 234, 236–237
    selection of, 118
    see also Wild areas; *and specific areas*
Public goods, 326

Quantifying integrity, 109–110. *See also*
    Measurement of integrity
Quasi-sustainability, 122. *See also* Serafian
    rule

Racism, 282, 283
Radical contingency, Darwinian, 47–50
Radon gas, 270
Randomized controlled trial (RCT), 263
Randomness/stochasticity, 100, 321,
    322–323
Reduce, Reuse, Recycle, and Recover
    (4Rs), 361
Reductionism, and theoretical ecology,
    73–74
Redundancy, 50
Rees, William E., 12, 22, 28, 116, 159,
    411–412
    ecofootprint analysis of, 34, 35, 150,
    393
Regeneration, in agriculture, 121, 122
Regeneration (report), 318
Regional integrity, biosocial, 162, 172
Regional policy, for urban areas, 325
Representation approach, to conservation,
    200
Research & Development (R&D) invest-
    ment, 355

Reserve design, 202–203. *See also*
    Protected areas
Resilience, 22, 33–34, 101, 108–109
Resources, for urban areas, 252–253
Restoration, 81, 151, 196
Rich nations, 149–150, 261, 296
    Agenda 21 promise and, 299–300,
    379–380, 396
    ethical obligations of, 399, 400, 403
    income disparity and, 307, 398
    see also Wealth
Ridley, M., 47
Rio Convention on Biological Diversity
    (1992), 163
Rio Summit (1992), 299. *See also* United
    Nations Conference on Environment
    and Development
River systems, 23, 119, 213, 219–222, 246
RIVPACS, 219, 221–222
Roadless areas, 203
Robinson, W. S., 267
Rolston, Holmes, 56
Roughgarden, Jonathan, 71
Royal Dutch/Shell Oil, 20
Rural–urban relationship, 148–149
Rwanda, 250

Safe minimum standards (SMSs), 305
Sagoff, Mark, 48, 57, 95n.6, 349n.27, 412
    critique of theoretical ecology by,
    79–81, 84, 85–86, 88, 91–92
    on human interference, 345, 346
    on integrity, 44, 46
    on science, 99
Saving Nature's Legacy (Noss and
    Cooperrider), 36
Schrecker, Ted, 15, 296–297, 412
Science:
    culture of, and nature, 140
    specialization of, 211
    vs. ecological approach, 7–9
Science (magazine), 261
Scott, H. Morgan, 243, 412
Second order principles (SOPs), 26, 39,
    40–41
Self-interest, 7, 336–339, 347nn.4, 8–10
Self-sufficiency, in agriculture, 125
Serafian rule, 121–123
Sewage treatment, 130
Sexual liberation, 285–286

SFM. *See* Forest management, sustainable
Shannon, C. E., 33, 104
Shrader-Fréchette, Kristin S., 99, 305
Shue, Harry, 306
Sieswerda, Lee E., 243, 412
Simon, Julian, 4–5, 85
Skin cancer, 249
Smith, F. E., 47
Social capital, 366
Social goals, place for nature and, 57
Social life, commoditization of, 364–365
Social policy, for health, 257
Social trends, 374, 375
Societal values, 212–213
Society, living systems and, 215
Soil, 121, 127–128, 149
Soskolne, Colin L., 243, 412–413
Soulé, Michael, 79
South, North and. *See* North–South
    antagonism
Specialization, urban, 323–324
Species:
    biology of, 202
    concept of, 48
    distinctive traits of, 340
    endangered, 192, 196, 390
    extinction of, 143, 144, 377
    focal, 200–202
    imperilment of, 198, 218
    loss, 28, 179, 187–188
    nonmarket, 6
    value of, 81
Spectrum argument, 86
Spheres of Justice (Walzer), 364
Stability, ecosystem, 6, 96n.15. *See also*
    Equilibrium
Sterba, James, 11, 298, 305, 413
Sterner, Robert, 63
Stochasticity, 100, 321, 322–323
Stress, 33
Structure, 101. *See also* Organization
Subsidies, 366
Succession, 22
Survival strategies, 91
Susser, M., 272
Sustainability:
    absolutism and, 304
    commoditization and, 353–354, 397
    conservation and, 12–14, 301
    economic efficiency and, 307

environmental, 56, 121, 401
    as function, 27
    health and, 253–256
    integrity and, 22
    policy for, 299, 305, 388
    in production, 372, 381
    rural–urban relationships and, 149
Sustainable development, 299, 367, 378,
    380–381
    and commoditization, 362, 397
    defined, 370–371
    ecological integrity and, 388–389
    North–South fight over, 300, 379
Svirezhev, Y. M. and A. Svirejeva-
    Hopkins, 31
Systemic integrity, 159

Tallachini, M., 22
Taubes, Gary, 261–262
Taxes, 366
    food chain and, 134–135, 136
Technology, 4–5, 146, 372. *See also*
    Biotechnology
Teleology, 100. *See also* Ecosystem design
Thames Water Company (UK), 55
Theoretical ecology, 62–63, 69–74, 79–94,
    345, 346
    authentic knowledge of, 94
    constant change and, 80, 82–84
    and ecosystem evaluation, 92–93
    vs. empiricism, 70–71
    natural history and, 69–70
    natural selection and, 88–92
    reductionist challenge to, 73–74
    Sagoff's reconstruction of, 79–81, 84,
        85–86, 88, 91–92
    and system in ecosystems, 87–88
Thermodynamic law, 8, 31–32, 110, 116,
    141
Third World, 251–252. *See also*
    Developing nations; Poorer
    countries
Thünen, J. H. von, 317, 320
Three Essays on Religion (Mill), 66
Timber harvest, 125, 158, 170–171, 172.
    See also Clear-cutting
Top-down approach, to conservation,
    205–206
Touch-of-Nature Preserve (Illinois), 184
"Toxic Chemical Profile" (Colborn), 291

Toxic chemicals, 290–291. *See also* Chemical products
Toxic wastes, health effects of, 15, 279, 282–284, 286. *See also* Waste; and *specific substances*

Ulanowicz, Robert E., 11, 12, 35, 109, 392, 413
  ascendency theory of, 32–34, 44, 63, 69
  on integrity, 159
Ultraviolet radiation (UVR), 248–249, 266, 281
Understanding, of integrity, 10–11
United Kingdom, 53, 55
United Nations:
  Commission on Sustainable Development (CSD), 371, 379
  Conference on Environment and Development/Rio Earth Summit (1992), 16, 299, 353, 369, 371, 396
  Development Program Human Development Index, 307
  Food and Agricultural Organization (FAO), 250
  Intergovernmental Panel on Climate Change, 247
United Nations General Assembly Special Session (UNGASS), 373–379
  economic trends and, 373, 375
  environmental trends, 374, 375–377
  social trends, 374, 375
United States, 134, 198, 216, 318, 379
  Forest Service, 204
  models of integrity in, 215
  optimal population of, 152
  sustainable agriculture in, 125, 126, 127
  water use in, 128–129, 214
Unsustainability, 354. *See also* Sustainability
Urban areas:
  ecofootprint of, 35, 147–149, 217, 252–253, 298
  population growth of, 5
  sprawl of, 329, 405
Urban areas, as ecosystems, 297–298, 317–330, 402
  complex systems thinking, 319–323
  economic character of, 323–329
  health of, 317
  and integrity, 330
  migration to, 319

randomness/stochasticity in, 321, 322–323
  social benefits of, 319, 330
Useful variation, evolution and, 47

Value:
  human, 398–400
  of integrity, 11, 21, 212–213
  level of health and, 119
  in species, 81
Vegetarian diet, 28, 127, 133
Vigor, ecosystem, 32, 101, 102, 106–107
Violence, environmental, 15, 244. *See also* Ecoviolence, institutionalized
Vitousek, P. M., 216

Wackernagel, M., 150
Waide, Jack B., 72, 78n.39
Walzer, Michael, 364–365
Warfare, health effects of, 247
Waste:
  emissions, 122, 401
  from livestock production, 136
  minimization of, 361
  production, 377
  toxic, 15, 279, 282–284, 286
  water treatment, 130
Water resources, 286–287
  for agriculture, 128–130, 132
  for aquaculture, 130–131
  assessment of, 219–222
  disease and, 286, 375
  shortage of, 246, 376, 390
Wealth, 14–15, 133, 308. *See also* Rich countries
Well-being, 4, 210. *See also* Health
Westra, Laura, 11, 13, 27, 35, 413–414
  on ecoviolence, 15, 244, 361
  on humanmade environment, 38–39
  on integrity, 335
  second order principles of, 26, 39, 40–41
West Virginia Forest Inventory, 184, 186, 187
Wild areas, 13, 26–27, 30–31, 81, 304
  integrity of, 20
  proposals for, 39–40, 404
  see also Protected areas
Wildfire, forest management and, 160–161, 165, 166. *See also* Fire

Wildlands Project, 36
Wilson, E. O., 71, 91
Wolverine (*Gulo gulo*), 201, 202
Wolves, 86, 201–202
Women, commoditization and, 364
Wonderful Life (Gould), 49
Woods, Mark, 95–96
Workers' rights, 366
World Commission on Environment and
    Development, 370

World Health Organization (WHO), 248,
    267, 375
World Health Statistics Quarterly, 281
World Resources Institute, 381
World Wildlife Fund (WWF), 15,
    193–194, 198
Worster, Donald, 47, 51
Wulff, F., 109

Yodzis, Peter, 63

DATE DUE

APR 1 3 2003			
GAYLORD			PRINTED IN U.S.A.